PHARMACEUTICAL
DOSAGE FORMS

PHARMACEUTICAL DOSAGE FORMS

Tablets

SECOND EDITION, REVISED AND EXPANDED

In Three Volumes
VOLUME 3

EDITED BY

Herbert A. Lieberman

H. H. Lieberman Associates, Inc.
Consultant Services
Livingston, New Jersey

Leon Lachman

Lachman Consultant Services
Westbury, New York

Joseph B. Schwartz

Philadelphia College of Pharmacy and Science
Philadelphia, Pennsylvania

MARCEL DEKKER, INC. **New York and Basel**

ISBN: 0-8247-8300-X

This book is printed on acid-free paper.

MARCEL DEKKER, INC.
270 Madison Avenue, New York, New York 10016

Current printing (last digit):
10 9 8 7 6 5 4 3 2 1

PRINTED IN THE UNITED STATES OF AMERICA

Preface

Tablets are the most commonly prescribed dosage form. The reason for this popularity is that tablets offer a convenient form of drug administration, provide dosage uniformity from tablet to tablet, are stable over extended and diverse storage conditions, and can be produced on high-speed compression, labeling, and packaging equipment. As a result, tablet production technology is constantly undergoing improvements that enhance their ability to deliver, with precision, a desired drug in a dosage form intended for immediate or extended therapeutic effect. In addition, the growth of the generic industry as well as increased competition from both foreign and domestic markets require that a tablet manufacturer have greater concern regarding the economics of tablet production by introducing less labor-intensive, higher-productivity manufacturing methods for making the increasing number of tablet products available today. The changes in the science and technology of tablet formulation, production, and quality assurance to accomplish the above are reflected in the second edition of the three-volume series *Pharmaceutical Dosage Forms: Tablets*.

The first volume in this series describes the many types of tablet products, giving specific updated examples of typical formulations and methods of manufacture. These include single- and multilayered tablets, buccal and sublingual tablets, effervescent tablets, and diverse methods for manufacturing them by wet and dry granulations and by direct compression. In addition, medicated candy products are a form of drug delivery that has appeared in the marketplace; no complete chapter on this technology has been printed in any pharmacy text other than both editions of this series on tablets.

To manufacture tablets a number of unit processes are required, such as mixing, drying, size reduction, and compression. The economics of tablet production today require an update of the technologies for each of these pharmaceutical operations. The granulations and tablets produced have particular characteristics that must be analyzed and understood in order to produce superior tablets, particularly when new and sometimes faster methods of manufacture are introduced. No drug dosage form would be meaningful to the patient without the drug being bioavailable. The chapter on bioavailability in tablet technology is updated in the second edition of Volume 2. Finally, many advances in the specifications and care of tablet tooling and problem solving caused by faulty compression tools are expertly covered in the second volume.

Volume 3 in the series on tablets updates the special characteristics that should be considered for optimizing tablet production. Particular emphasis is given to design methods that should be considered when formulating a tablet product. Discussions of specialized granule and tablet-coating equipment are presented, discussing improvements or presenting new equipment developed since the publication of the first edition. Aqueous film coating is now firmly established in pharmaceutical coating processes, and thus, a shift in emphasis on coating procedures has been made in the revised chapter on coating. New coating pans and automation of aqueous film- and sugar-coating methods are covered. Fluid-bed processes and particle-coating methods, including theoretical considerations, are updated to reflect current practices.

No text on tablet technology could be considered complete without a full theoretical and practical updated description of current methods for formulating, manufacturing, and controlling the release of drug from sustained-release tablet and particle dosage forms. A chapter on sustained drug release through coating provides an updated and authoritative discussion of this popular form of drug delivery. There is an enhanced emphasis on the various polymers and their combinations used to attain sustained drug activity. Pilot operations must reflect production methods in order to minimize difficulties in transferring a product from preproduction to production. Granules prepared by precompression, wet and dry granulation, fluidized-bed granulation, and spray drying are compared. A new method for preparing a granulation, namely the moisture-activated dry granulation (MADG), is also suggested for more widespread pilot evaluation.

With the increasing emphasis on product uniformity from one tablet to another, or from one batch to another, whether the product is made sequentially or with long lag periods between batches, or whether the raw material source is from several different manufacturers, the concept of process validation is essential. An extensive chapter describing the essential considerations that should be evaluated in process validation has been added to the revised edition of this volume. Although the chapter presents a complete detailed description of many validation methods, it also shows how less detailed approaches, some of which are commonly used in the industry, are useful. Current tablet production methods are described with sample control charts to help the readers improve their tablet production methods. The importance of the several different functions of production departments, their particular skills, and the need for coordinated and cooperative work relationships are stressed in the chapter "Tablet Production" so that the combined, partnership efforts of all production personnel can lead to superior tablet production. Automation of tablet compression and coating is also part of the chapter concerned with the production of tablets.

In the discussion of stability, updated stability protocols to comply with recent FDA guidelines are presented. A new covariance analysis and statistical method for expiration date prediction are described. The chapter "Quality Assurance" upgrades tablet testing for uniformity, dissolution, assay limit, test methods, and compendial requirements for tablets to comply with current USP/NF requirements. Included are instructive figures for new schematic sampling plans, an update of the restrictions on the use of colors, and a recommended sampling method for raw materials. Thus, with this third volume on tablets, all the parameters currently concerned with the production of superior tablets are made current and discussed extensively.

An updated and full coverage of the many topics concerned with tablets requires highly knowledgeable authors for each of the many areas that must be covered. To compile and update the pertinent information needed for the various chapters in this book required a multiauthored text of technologists with specific expertise and experience in their chosen subject matter. Each of the authors was charged with teaching their subject in such a fashion that the novice as well as the experienced reader will profit. They were to offer basic scientific facts and practical information so that *all* readers can learn theory and apply it toward the knowledge that each needs to formulate, produce, and control tablet operations in a scientific rather than an empirical manner.

With this third volume, the editors have finished their task of updating the second edition on tablets. The editors are grateful to the authors for their fine contributions and, particularly, their patient response to the editors' suggestions for changes. The choice of the chapter topics, the authors, and the format are the responsibilities of the editors. It is hoped that these choices will prove fruitful to our readers by helping them solve their tablet technology problems and thereby advance industrial pharmacy's contribution toward improving both quality and efficiency in the manufacture of tablets.

Herbert A. Lieberman
Leon Lachman
Joseph B. Schwartz

Contents

Chapter 6   Tablet Production   369

*Robert J. Connolly, Frank A. Berstler,
and David Coffin-Beach*

Chapter 7.   The Essentials of Process Validation   417

Robert A. Nash

Contributors

Neil R. Anderson   Department Head, Pharmacy Research Department, Merrell Dow Pharmaceuticals, Inc., Indianapolis, Indiana

Gilbert S. Banker   Dean, College of Pharmacy, University of Minnesota Health Sciences Center, Minneapolis, Minnesota

Frank A. Berstler   Manager, Technical Service, Superpharm Corporation, Central Islip, New York

Charles H. Bruno   Director, Pharmaceutical Technical Services, Colorcon, West Point, Pennsylvania

Rong-Kun Chang   Principle Scientist, Formulation Development, Schering Research, Miami, Florida

David Coffin-Beach   Manager, Process Development, Schering-Plough, Inc., Kenilworth, New Jersey

Robert J. Connolly   Vice President, Manufacturing, Superpharm Corporation, Central Islip, New York

Samir A. Hanna   Vice President, Quality Assurance, Industrial Division, Bristol-Myers Squibb Company, Syracuse, New York

Charles I. Jarowski   Professor, Department of Pharmacy, St. John's University, Jamaica, New York

Robert A. Nash   Associate Professor, College of Pharmacy and Allied Health Professions, St. John's University, Jamaica, New York

Garnet E. Peck   Professor, Department of Industrial and Physical
Pharmacy, Purdue University, West Lafayette, Indiana

Stuart C. Porter   Vice President, Scientific Services, Colorcon, West
Point, Pennsylvania

Joseph R. Robinson   Professor of Pharmacy, Madison Center for Health
Sciences, University of Wisconsin–Madison, Madison, Wisconsin

Dale E. Wurster   Professor and Dean Emeritus, College of Pharmacy,
University of Iowa, Iowa City, Iowa

Contents of Pharmaceutical Dosage Forms: Tablets, Second Edition, Revised and Expanded, Volumes 1 and 2

edited by Herbert A. Lieberman, Leon Lachman, and Joseph B. Schwartz

VOLUME 1

VOLUME 2

Contents of Pharmaceutical Dosage Forms: Parenteral Medications, Volumes 1 and 2

edited by Kenneth E. Avis, Leon Lachman,
and Herbert A. Lieberman

Contents of Pharmaceutical Dosage Forms: Disperse Systems, Volumes 1 and 2

edited by Herbert A. Lieberman, Martin M. Rieger, and Gilbert S. Banker

VOLUME 2

1
Principles of Improved Tablet Production System Design

Garnet E. Peck

Purdue University, West Lafayette, Indiana

Neil R. Anderson

Merrell Dow Pharmaceuticals, Inc., Indianapolis, Indiana

Gilbert S. Banker

University of Minnesota Health Sciences Center, Minneapolis, Minnesota

I. INTRODUCTION

The old saying that all progress is change but not all change is progress is considered a truism by product manufacturers. Changes that are made in the production process of an established product are thoroughly evaluated from every point of view before implementation is allowed. The very existence of the company depends on its ability to produce products for sale. Therefore, any suggested change in the manufacture of an existing product must be viewed with suspicion until it can be shown that the change will indeed be advantageous to the company and not simply represent change for the sake of change. A company's prestige, profitability, and compliance with legal requirements are at stake when production changes are considered. Therefore, changes in the pharmaceutical industry must clearly be warranted before they are implemented. The object of this chapter is to introduce to the pharmaceutical scientist how changes can be accomplished in a pharmaceutical tablet production facility that will constitute progress for the company.

A. Unit Operations and Pharmaceutical Processing

A unit operation can be defined as a process designed to achieve one or more changes in the physical and/or chemical properties of the raw material(s) being processed.

Two or more unit operations that are designed to convert the basic raw materials into the final product or at least to have significantly improved the quality or value of the original raw material(s) describes a manufacturing system. In a tablet-manufacturing system, some of the unit operations may include (1) particle size reduction, (2) sieving or classification, (3) mixing, (4) particle size enlargement, (5) drying, (6) compression, (7) sorting, and (8) packaging.

The literature is well documented with various unit operations involved in the manufacture of tableted products which may impact on a number of final dosage-form quality features. The features include, but are not limited to, such items as content uniformity, hardness, friability drug dissolution properties, and bioavailability. The traditional responsibility of the development pharmacist has been to identify and control such impacts. This includes the establishment of specific operating limits for each unit operation to ensure that the production system is under sufficient control for the production of safe, effective, and reliable tablets. The scope and purpose of this chapter is to examine system design considerations, and as a result, the individual unit operations and their potential impact on product quality will not be covered. The authors assume that each unit operation has been thoroughly investigated and is under sufficient control to do what it is purported to do. Specific effects of processing variables on product quality are dealt with in the pertinent chapters in this book series.

B. Batch Versus Continuous Processing

Most pharmaceutical production operations are batch operations, whereby a series of manufacturing steps are used to prepare a single batch or lot of a particular product. The same quantity or batch of material, if processed en mass through the various production steps to produce the final product, will then typically be treated by the manufacturer and the U.S. Food and Drug Administration (FDA) as one lot. A relatively few pharmaceutical products are prepared by true continuous-processing procedures whereby raw materials are continuously fed into and through the production sequence, and the finished product is continuously discharged from the final processing step(s). In continuous processing, one day's production, the production from one work shift, the quantity of a critical raw material from a given lot, or a combination thereof may define a single lot of manufactured product. Development of continuous-processing procedures requires specially designed and interfaced equipment, special plant layouts, and dedicated plant space, which reduces plant flexibility. The equipment, special plant design requirements, and dedicated space are all factors leading to the high costs of setting up and maintaining a continuous-manufacturing operation for a product. Unless the volume of product being produced is very high, the cost of setting up a product-dedicated, continuous-production operation will not usually be justified. Since pharmaceutical products, even within a dosage-form class such as compressed tablets, differ materially in many important aspects, such as drug dosage, excipients used, critical factors, affecting product quality, manufacturing problems, and the like, it is usually not feasible or possible to set up a continuous-processing operation for one product and then apply it to several others. Thus true continuous-processing operations are largely limited in the drug industry to large-volume products, which often also have large doses (or high weights per tablet), such as Tums, Gelusil, Aldomet, or Alka Seltzer, for which tons of material must be processed each day, on an ongoing basis.

II. BENEFITS OF IMPROVED TABLET
PRODUCTION SYSTEMS

In either the batch or the continuous mode of operation, the objective of
the production function is to produce pharmaceutical tablets for sale.
Consequently, a production process should always be viewed as a candidate for progressive change in an effort to maintain the company's products in the marketplace. When looking at a process for possible changes,
one must be aware of the potential benefits for the company. The major
benefits that can be obtained, and which constitute the major valid reasons for changing or redesigning a pharmaceutical tablet manufacturing
process, are the following [1-5]:

> Regulatory compliance
> > Current good manufacturing practices (CGMPs)
> > Occupational Safety and Health Administration (OSHA)
> > Environmental Protection Agency (EPA)
> Increased production capacity and flexibility
> Decreased product throughput time
> Reduced labor costs
> Increased energy savings
> Broadened process control or automation for control, operator inter-
> > face, and reporting
> Enhanced product quality
> Enhanced process reliability

The benefits that can be derived from the redesign of a process are
dependent to a large extent on how "good" or "bad" the old process is.
With perhaps the exception of some CGMP, OSHA, or even EPA requirements, the expected benefits to be derived from proposed process design
changes are generally reduced to a dollar figure in order to compare the
cost of implementing the change with the expected savings to be generated
by the change. Proposed changes on a good facility may not be cost-
justifiable, whereas the same proposal on a bad facility can easily be cost-
justified. What can be justified and what cannot is a function of what can
be referred to as the corporate policy or corporate personality at the time
the proposal is made. A pharmaceutical company, like any company, is a
part of the community in which it resides and as such has responsibilities
to many other societal groups. These include governments, stockholders,
employees, the community, the competition, and customers. The interaction of all these groups with the company results in a corporate personality. Therefore, companies have different standards for evaluating different financial situations, different production philosophies, varying time
constraints for design and implementation, and varying technical support
available for design changes. All of these items will be given consideration and will influence the decision-making process when a redesign proposal is made.

III. PRODUCTION PROCESS DESIGN CONSIDERATIONS

A fact that should be well understood is that the production unit is not an
independent organization within the company. Any changes made in the

production unit impact on many other units that come in contact with the production unit. However, with the rising costs of materials, labor, inflation, and regulations being constantly added to the manufacture of pharmaceuticals, the pharmaceutical industry cannot afford to neglect change or the modification of existing processes simply because there are established standards that may be difficult to change. Increased productivity matched with a reduction in direct labor cost will probably be the way of the future. This can only be accomplished by a conscious effort on the part of those in process development. The development pharmacist should therefore be familiar with ways in which the manufacture of pharmaceutical products can be increased and labor reduced. Even though the development pharmacist will not be thoroughly knowledgeable in all areas of process design considerations, he or she should at least be aware that those considerations exist and be able to interact with experts in those fields to accomplish cost savings.

Major advances in efficiency have been made in tablet production over the last 20–30 years. These advances have come about by the development of methods; pieces of equipment, and instrumentation with which tablet production systems have been able to (1) improve materials handling, (2) improve specific unit operations, (3) eliminate or combine processing steps, and (4) incorporate automated process control of unit operations and processes.

A. Materials Handling

Materials-Handling Risks

Possibly the single largest contribution to the effectiveness of a manufacturing facility is made by the facility's materials-handling capabilities. In addition to a lack of efficiency, there are certain risks involved with improper or inefficient materials handling. These risks include increased product costs, customer dissatisfaction, and employee safety liabilities. Materials that are not handled efficiently can increase the cost of raw materials. For example, penalty charges are assessed (demurrage) when railroad cars are not loaded or unloaded according to schedule. If raw materials are not moved as required by production schedules, delays are incurred which can lead to situations in which machine time is wasted, personnel time is wasted, in-process inventories are increased, and the entire manufacturing process is slowed down. In addition, the improper handling and storage of materials can lead to damaged, outdated, and lost materials. Improper materials handling can place employees in physical danger. An increase in employee frustration generated by constant production delays due to poor materials handling can result in reduced morale.

Materials-Handling Objectives

A well-designed and efficiently operated materials-handling system should impart to the manufacturing facility reduced handling costs, increased manufacturing capacity, improved working conditions, and improved raw material distribution to the appropriate manufacturing areas. To achieve an efficient materials-handling system, as many of the basic general principles of efficient materials handling need to be implemented as practical.

Basic Principles of Materials Handling

SHORT DISTANCES. Raw materials used in the production process should only be moved over the shortest possible distances. Moving materials over excessive distances increases production time, wastes energy, creates inefficiency, increases the possibilities of delays, and adds to the labor costs if the material is moved by hand.

SHORT TERMINAL TIMES. When material is being transported, the means of transportation should not have to spend time waiting on the material to be picked up. Material should always be ready when the transportation is available.

TWO-WAY PAYLOADS. The transportation mechanism for raw materials should never be moved empty. For example, if tablet-packaging materials are being transported from a warehouse to a packaging line by means of a fork-lift truck, the return trip could be used, for example, for the removal of accumulated scrap material or finished product from the production line.

AVOID PARTIAL LOADS. The movement of quantities of raw materials that require only a partial use of the total capacity of the transportation system is a waste of time and energy. If the movement of such materials cannot be avoided, then the partial loads should be doubled up to make efficient use of the transportation system.

AVOID MANUAL HANDLING. The manual handling of raw materials is the most expensive way of moving them. A great deal of direct costs can be eliminated by mechanically moving material rather than having it moved by the production personnel.

MOVE SCRAP CHEAPLY. The movement of scrap material is a nonproductive function and scrap material should not be a primary work objective for a transportation system. Therefore, scrap material should be moved as inexpensively as possible. One way of achieving this is to handle the removal of scrap on return loads after delivering needed materials.

GRAVITY IS THE CHEAPEST POWER. The movement of material from top to bottom through multileveled facilities, if available, is the most efficient way of moving material.

MOVE IN STRAIGHT LINES. A basic theorem of geometry states that the shortest distance between two points is a straight line. Therefore, the most efficient movement of material is along the straightest and most direct path to its destination.

UNIT LOADS. Raw materials should be delivered to their ultimate destination in loads that will be completely consumed by the manufacturing process. This will eliminate the need for the excess raw materials to be handled at the point of use and to be returned to the storage place.

LABEL THOROUGHLY. Thoroughly labeled raw materials will eliminate or help to eliminate having the improper raw material delivered to a production site. Much time and effort is wasted in correcting raw materials errors.

Factors Affecting Materials-Handling Decisions

Of course, not all of the basic materials-handling principles can be applied or applied to the same extent in every situation. How a company designs its materials-handling facility and its production process is based on several different considerations. The type of process that is being designed, batch or continuous, will have a great influence on the type of materials-handling system used. The materials-handling system in a batch-oriented, multiproduct facility is significantly different from a single-product, continuous-process, materials-handling system. The type and quantity of product as well as the physical characteristics of the raw materials involved will also affect the materials-handling system. For example, fluids for granulating will have to be pumped, whereas solids will have to be handled in another manner, such as with vacuum devices of conveyors. The type of building that is available for the manufacturing process may exert the single greatest influence on the materials-handling system. The lack of a multistoried building will preclude the use of gravity for material flow. Like all company decisions, the costs of purchase, installation, operation, and maintenance as well as the useful life and the scrap value of the materials-handling system must be weighed against its advantages.

Greene [6] quotes an old cliché which best summarizes materials handling:

> The best solution to a materials-handling problem is not to move the material. If this is possible, then move it by gravity. And if this is not possible, usually the next best way is to move it by power. If people must move the material, it should be moved by the cheapest labor possible.

Examples of Materials-Handling Improvement

Improvements in the use of materials-handling techniques have been incorporated into the new product facilities of Merck Sharp & Dohme (MSD) and Eli Lilly and Company (Lilly). Figure 1 shows a schematic of the granulation and tableting area at MSD's new facility for the production of Aldomet. There is virtually no human handling of materials during or between processing steps. The movement of materials (solids and liquids) through the system is accomplished by a sophisticated materials-handling system. The system is built in a three-story building which allows the entire process to operate in three operational "columns." The system incorporates vertical drops to utilize gravity whenever possible and uses pumps, vacuum, and bucket conveyors to move material upward whenever necessary.

In the first processing column bulk raw materials are loaded into the system on the third floor and flow by vertical drop through holding and feeding hoppers into mixing equipment and then into continuous-granulating and drying equipment on the first floor. The dried granulation is then transported by vacuum back up to the third floor to start the second processing column for milling and sizing. By vertical drop the sized granulation flows down through the lubrication hoppers and mixer and then to the tablet compression machines on the first floor. The compressed tablets are then transferred by bucket conveyor back up to the third floor and the start of the third column. Here, the tablets are collected, batched, and transferred to feed the air suspension film-coating equipment located on the second floor. Once coated, the tablets are stored on the second

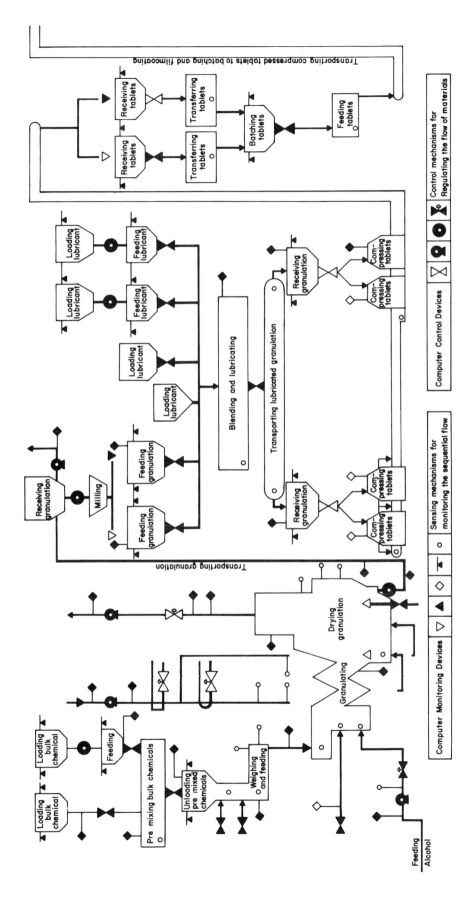

Figure 1 Granulation and tableting sections of the computer-controlled tablet-manufacturing process, Merck Sharp & Dohme Pharmaceutical Laboratories. (From *Innovation in Pharmaceutical Manufacturing: Compounding a Prescription Medicine by Computer Control* brochure, 1977, by permission of Merck & Co., Inc., proprietor.)

7

floor until required for packaging. During packaging operations the tablets flow by vertical drop from the second floor to the packaging lines on the first floor.

The Aldomet facility was built to meet the need for increased manufacturing capacity of Aldomet. The new Aldomet facility requires fewer production people, thus keeping direct-labor costs low. Since the facility is continuously monitored by computer throughout each phase of the process, Aldomet has a high degree of uniformity and reproducibility. The continuous monitoring also bring about a conservation of energy. As a result of the numerous and rigid in-process controls in the Aldomet process, quality control and the quality assurance costs have been reduced. Through the creation of a new building, MSD's compliance with the Good Manufacturing Practices regulations was greatly facilitated [7].

A study of Figure 2, schematically representing Warner-Chilcott's redesigned Gelusil manufacturing system, shows that the dedicated single-process system makes use of gravity, belts, and pneumatic devices to efficiently move material through the process. The old manufacturing operation was a semiautomated batch operation with a capacity limit of three shifts employing 14 persons. The capacity of the redesigned system for manufacturing Gelusil tablets is three times greater than that of the old process, and the unit throughput time for Gelusil manufacture was reduced to a third of the old process time. The output of the new extrusion process, in one shift with two persons, equals the total daily output from the old process. Obviously, another one of the benefits of the new process was a reduction in required manpower, which reduced the direct-labor costs involved in producing Gelusil [5,8].

While the previous examples involved very large volumes of product produced on a continuous basis, batch-oriented production systems have also been made more efficient by materials-handling improvements. Figure 3 shows a schematic of E. R. Squibb & Sons Inc.'s (Squibb) production process for Theragran M tablets. The vacuum transfer of the granulation to the tablet compression machines has been accomplished by a vertical drop from storage devices on a mezzanine above the tablet machines.

Lilly's new dry products manufacturing facility (Fig. 4) has increased their materials-handling efficiency by the use of (1) a driverless train which transports bulk raw materials from the receiving dock to the staging area, (2) vacuum powder transfer mechanisms, (3) direct transfer of in-process materials, and (4) the liberal use of vertical drops in the two-story operation [9].

B. Processing Step Combination or Elimination

The design of a new production facility should attempt to improve the old process by eliminating or combining certain processing unit operations. This could take the form of simply eliminating tasks that are no longer necessary or by the utilization of new pieces of equipment that can perform more than one of the unit operations required under the old processing system.

Direct Compression

Many processing steps have been eliminated in the manufacture of some pharmaceutical tablets as a result of the development of directly

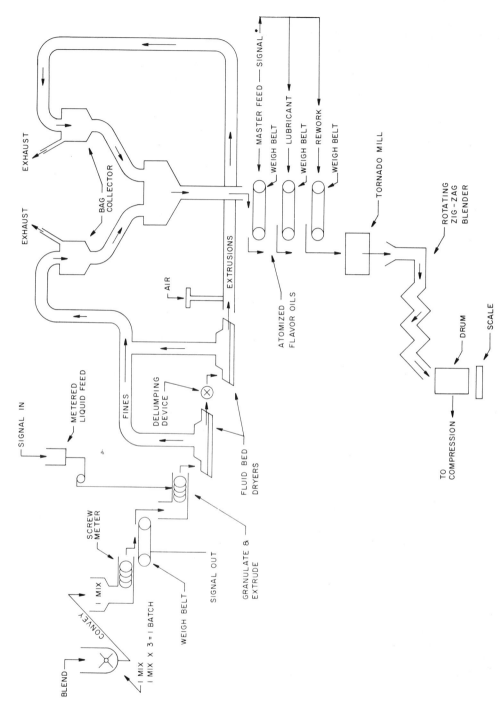

Figure 2 A schematic of the Warner–Chilcott Gelusil extrusion process. (Reprinted courtesy of Warner–Lambert Company.)

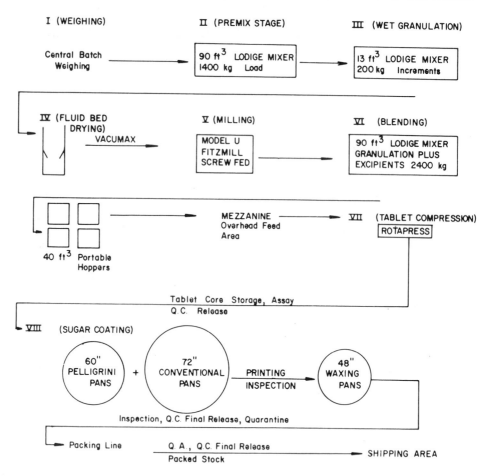

Figure 3   A schematic of the Squibb Theragram M tablet production process.   (Courtesy of E. R. Squibb, New Brunswick, New Jersey.)

compressible excipients, wherein powdered drug can be directly mixed with the excipient and then immediately compressed into a finished tablet. Direct compression is the method of choice in tablet manufacture, when the process may be employed to produce a high-quality finished product. Direct compression offers the most expeditious method of manufacturing tablets because it utilizes the least handling of materials, involves no drying step, and is thus the most energy-efficient method, and is also the fastest, most economical method of tablet production.

The reformulation of a product from a wet-granulated process to a direct-compression process to eliminate several process steps is illustrated in Table 1 by the comparison of Lederle Laboratories' (Leaderle) old and new tablet-manufacturing processes.   If reformulation to direct compression cannot be accomplished, purchasing the critical raw material in granular form could have the same effect from a processing standpoint.   While the cost of directly compressible raw material may be higher, the labor, time, and energy cost savings realized by eliminating the granulation, drying,

Table 1 Unit Processing of Solid Dosage Forms, Lederle Laboratories

Old tablet-manufacturing process (wet granulation)	New tablet-manufacturing process (direct compression)
1. Raw materials	1. Raw materials
2. Weighing and measuring	2. Weighing and measuring (automatic weigher and recording system)[a]
3. Screening	
4. Manual feeding	3. Gravity feeding
5. Blending (slow-speed planetary mixer)	4. Blending (Littleford blender)
6. Wetting (hand addition)	5. Gravity feeding from the storage tank[a]
7. Subdivision (comminutor)	6. Compression (high-speed rotary press)[a]
8. Drying (fluid bed dryer)	
9. Subdivision (comminutor)	7. Aqueous coating (Hi-Coater)
10. Premixing (barrel roller)	
11. Batching and lubrication (ribbon blender)	
12. Manual feeding	
13. Compression (Stokes rotary press)	
14. Solvent film coating (Wurster Column)	
15. Tablet inspection (manual)	

[a]In planning phase. To be installed later.
Source: Courtesy of Lederle Laboratories, Pearl River, New York.

and sizing of the raw material may more than justify the increased material cost.

Unfortunately, there are many situations in which direct compression does not lend itself to tablet production, for example, with low-dose drugs or where segregation and content uniformity are a problem, or with high-dose drugs which are not directly compressible or which have poor flow properties, or in the preparation of certain tablets or in many special tablet-manufacturing operations. When direct compression is not a feasible method of tablet manufacture, wet granulation is usually the method of choice.

Equipment for the Elimination/Combination of Processing Steps

Until relatively recently, wet granulation was a highly labor-intensive and time-consuming process. Figure 5 illustrates the various steps involved in batch wet-granulation processes in the 1960s and before. Typically, two

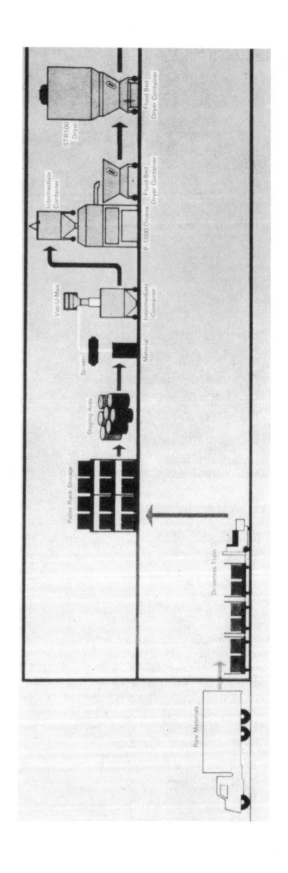

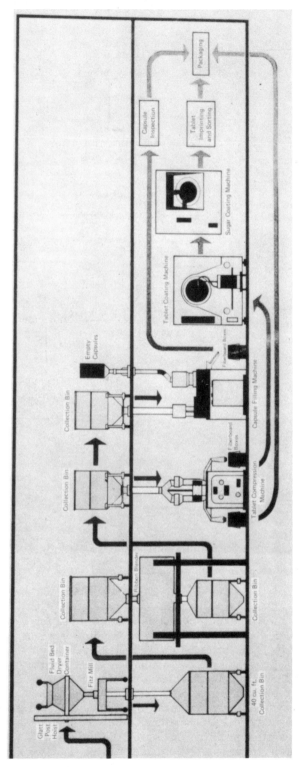

Figure 4 A pictorial representation of the Lilly dry products manufacturing facility. (Courtesy of Eli Lilly and Company, Indianapolis, Indiana.)

13

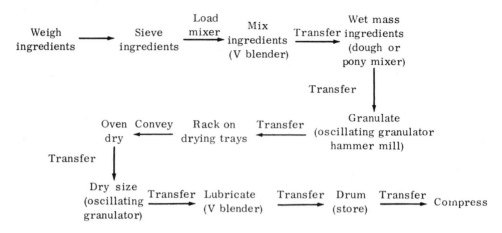

A. Standard processing steps in the 1960s and before

B. Standard Processing steps in the 1980s

C. Standard processing steps in the 1990s and beyond

Figure 5   Standard steps in batch wet granulation in the 1960s and 1980s.

separate mixing devices were used for the dry solids blending and for wet massing, with a manual transfer step in between, as shown in part A of Figure 5. Following wet massing the entire batch was again manually granulated by transfer to an appropriate piece of equipment after which the granular material was further manually handled by being racked on a series of drying trays. After oven drying the entire batch was again manually removed from the trays and was dry sized by again being passed through a mechanical screening device. Thereafter, the entire batch was placed in a dry blender once again for incorporation of the lubricant, after which the batch was placed in drums or containers to be held for tablet compression. As can be seen in Figure 5A, the components of the batch or the entire batch was manually handled at least 10 or 11 times.

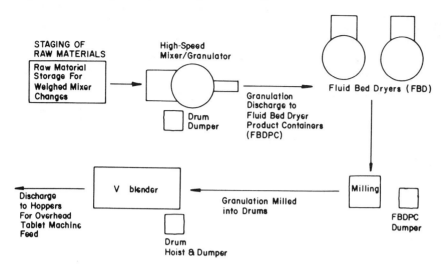

Figure 6 A general schematic of equipment used to redesign a tablet production facility.

With the development of specialized high-shear powder and mass mixers, and with the further development of fluid-bed dryers, the standard wet-granulation batch-processing operation as it is being conducted in the 1980s is shown in part B of Figure 5. The number of transfer steps has been reduced to three or four, the manual handling of the batch material has been greatly reduced, and the time of granulation manufacture has been cut from 2 days with an overnight drying step to as little as a few hours. This processing can be further illustrated by a hypothetical processing setup in Figure 6, and by the process flow chart for the production of Lasix in Figure 7.

New equipment is now being developed and gradually adapted by the pharmaceutical industry which handles all of the steps in granulation preparation in one piece of equipment. This is depicted in part C of Figure 5. It should also be pointed out that not only is handling of materials greatly reduced by the newer equipment used in the wet-granulation operation, but the new process equipment is also capable of producing granulation materials which have unique properties which could not previously be routinely produced. Granular particles with a near spherical shape can be routinely produced for they may be run under vacuum conditions that reportedly enhance the density and cohesiveness of the granular particles. Some of the newer equipment can also be used to apply protective coating to the particles during their manufacture. Some of these special applications are described in the sections which follow. The reduction of materials handling, which is obvious from Figure 5, as the process is currently practiced in the 1980s as compared to earlier times, is due in large measure to the development of equipment which can sequentially undertake a series of processing steps which earlier were accomplished by separate pieces of equipment. These new, multipurpose pieces of equipment, which are capable of combining virtually all of the steps in the wet-granulation process, are also described in the following sections.

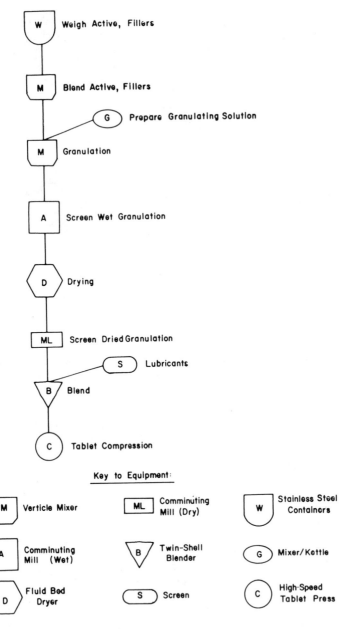

Figure 7   A process flow chart for the production of Lasix tablets.
(Courtesy of Hoechst-Roussel Pharmaceuticals, Somerville, New Jersey.)

CONTINUOUS-BATCH POWDER MIXING AND MASSING EQUIPMENT. The Littleford Lodige mixer (see Appendix) was one of the first high-shear powder blenders capable of rapidly blending pharmaceutical powders and wet massing within the same equipment. With some formulations the equipment may also be capable of producing agglomerated granular particles which are ready for fluid-bed or other drying methods without further processing. Figure 8 illustrates a conventional Lodige mixer and describes the various assemblies of the unit. The unit consists of the horizontal cylindrical shell equipped with a series of plow-shaped mixing tools and one or more high-speed blending chopper assemblies mounted at the rear of the mixer. For the addition of liquids, an injection tube terminating in one or more spray nozzles is provided. The nozzle(s) is located immediately above the chopper assembly.

In operation, the plow-shaped mixing tools revolve at variable speeds from about 100 to 240 rpm and maintain the contents of the mixer in an essentially fluidized condition. The plow device also provides a high-volume rate of transfer of material back and forth across the blender. When liquid granulating agents are added to dry powders the liquid enters the mixer under pressure through the liquid nozzle immediately above the chopper assembly or assemblies. Each chopper assembly consists of blades mounted in a tulip shape configuration rotating at 3600 rpm. As the liquid impinges on the powder in the area of the chopper it is immediately dispersed. By controlling the duration of the mixing cycle, the particle size of the granulation may be controlled. The choppers perform a secondary function in this type of high-shear powder blender. It will be noted on examination of part B of Figure 5 that the new processes involved in wet granulation may not include a sieving operation. When the chopper blades are operated during dry mixing dry lumps of powder are effectively dispersed. Consequently, it will often be found that sieving is no longer an essential prerequisite of powder blending when this type of equipment is employed.

Using this type of high-shear powder mixing equipment, complete mixing may be obtained in as little as 30−60 s. A temperature rise of 10−15° may be expected if dry blending is continued over a period of 5−10 min. When the Littleford Lodige blender is used for wet granulation the work which must be done by the mixer will increase as the powder mass becomes increasingly wet. This is often reflected in the readings on the ammeter of the equipment because the increased work will result in an amperage increase. Such readings may be very useful in helping to identify the proper end point for the wet-granulation process.

The equipment illustrated in Figure 8 employs air purge seals. One of the major difficulties in the operation of a high-shear powder mixer is powder making its way behind the seals and even contaminating the bearing assembly. This can lead to two difficulties: contamination of the next product with materials previously run in the blender and early failure of bearings and seals. A number of pharmaceutical manufacturers have found the air purge seal to be a useful device and an effective mechanism for overcoming this difficulty with this type of blender.

The Diosna mixer/granulator is another type of high-shear powder mixer and processor (Fig. 9). The mixer utilizes a bowl (1) mounted in the vertical position. The bowl is available in seven sizes between 25 and 100 L. The mixing bowl can be jacketed for temperature control. A high-speed mixer blade (2) revolves around the bottom of the bowl. The blade

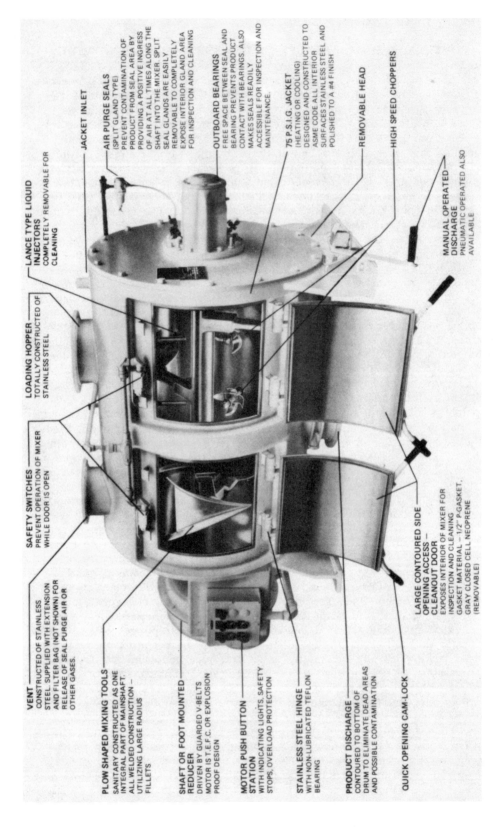

VENT
CONSTRUCTED OF STAINLESS
STEEL SUPPLIED WITH EXTENSION
AND FILTER BAG (NOT SHOWN) FOR
RELEASE OF SEAL PURGE AIR OR
OTHER GASES.

SAFETY SWITCHES
PREVENT OPERATION OF MIXER
WHILE DOOR IS OPEN

LANCE TYPE LIQUID
INJECTORS
COMPLETELY REMOVABLE FOR
CLEANING

LOADING HOPPER
TOTALLY CONSTRUCTED OF
STAINLESS STEEL

JACKET INLET

AIR PURGE SEALS
(SPLIT GLAND TYPE)
PREVENT CONTAMINATION OF
PRODUCT FROM SEAL AREA BY
PROVIDING A POSITIVE INGRESS
OF AIR AT ALL TIMES ALONG THE
SHAFT INTO THE MIXER. SPLIT
SEAL GLANDS ARE EASILY
REMOVABLE TO COMPLETELY
EXPOSE INTERIOR GLAND AREA
FOR INSPECTION AND CLEANING

OUTBOARD BEARINGS
FREE SPACE BETWEEN SEAL AND
BEARING PREVENTS PRODUCT
CONTACT WITH BEARINGS. ALSO
MAKES SEALS READILY
ACCESSIBLE FOR INSPECTION AND
MAINTENANCE.

75 P.S.I.G. JACKET
(HEATING OR COOLING)
DESIGNED AND CONSTRUCTED TO
ASME CODE ALL INTERIOR
SURFACES STAINLESS STEEL AND
POLISHED TO A #4 FINISH

REMOVABLE HEAD

HIGH SPEED CHOPPERS

MANUAL OPERATED
DISCHARGE
PNEUMATIC OPERATED ALSO
AVAILABLE

PLOW SHAPED MIXING TOOLS
SANITARY CONSTRUCTED AS ONE
INTEGRAL PART OF MAINSHAFT –
ALL WELDED CONSTRUCTION –
UTILIZING LARGE RADIUS
FILLETS

SHAFT OR FOOT MOUNTED
REDUCER
DRIVEN BY GUARDED V-BELTS
MOTOR IS T.E.F.C. OR EXPLOSION
PROOF DESIGN

MOTOR PUSH BUTTON
STATION
WITH INDICATING LIGHTS, SAFETY
STOPS, OVERLOAD PROTECTION

STAINLESS STEEL HINGE
WITH NON-LUBRICATED TEFLON
BEARING

PRODUCT DISCHARGE
CONTOURED TO BOTTOM OF
DRUM TO ELIMINATE DEAD AREAS
AND POSSIBLE CONTAMINATION

QUICK OPENING CAM-LOCK

LARGE CONTOURED SIDE
OPENING ACCESS –
CLEANOUT DOOR
EXPOSES INTERIOR OF MIXER FOR
INSPECTION AND CLEANING
GASKET MATERIAL – 1/2" P.GASKET,
GRAY CLOSED CELL NEOPRENE
(REMOVABLE)

Figure 8   Components of the Lodige high-shear mixer.   (Courtesy of Littleford Brothers, Florence, Kentucky.)

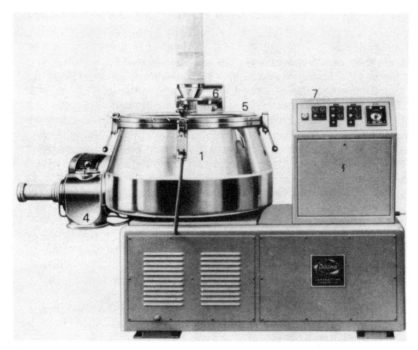

(A)

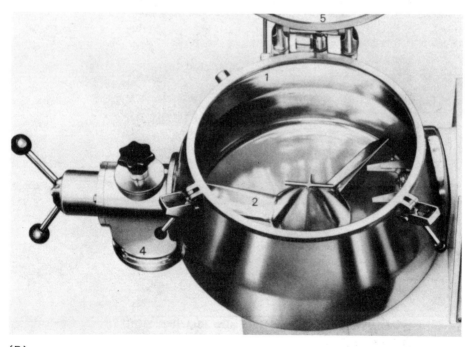

(B)

Figure 9 (A) The Diosna mixer-granulator, side view. (B) The Diosna mixer/granulator, top view. (Courtesy of Dierks & Sohne, Osnabruck, Germany.)

fits over the pin bar at the bottom of the mixing bowl which powers the blade. The blade is specially constructed to discourage material from getting under it. The speeds of the mixing blades vary with the size of the mixer. The tip speed, however, is kept at 3-4/10 m s^{-1} on low and 6-8/10 m s^{-1} on high. The mixer also contains a chopper blade (3) at either 1750 or 3500 rpm. The chopper functions as a lump and agglomerate reducer. A pneumatic discharge port (4) may be specially ordered for the unit to provide automatic discharge. The unit is provided with a lid (5) and the larger units employ a counterweight (6) to assist in raising and lowering the lid. The lid has three openings: one to accommodate a spray nozzle, a second larger opening for an air exhaust sleeve, and a third opening for a viewing port. The units are also equipped with an ammeter (7) which may be employed to determine the endpoint of granulation operations. Typical time sequences for the use of a Diosna mixer are as follows: mixing 2 min or less; granulating, 8 min or less; discharge, 1 min, with discharge capable of being preset when the pneumatic discharge system is in place.

Vosnek and Forbes [10] reported on the performance features of the Diosna. They compared granulations prepared by a traditional method as shown in part A of Figure 5 wherein a pony mixer was used for wet massing with granulations with the same product prepared in a Diosna mixer followed by fluid-bed drying. Figure 10 shows a comparison of particle size distribution of the two granulations. The Diosna equipment produced a granulation with a more normal particle size distribution with a smaller fraction of the granulation being 200 mesh or below (18 vs. 33%). The shape of the particles produced by the Diosna were also more

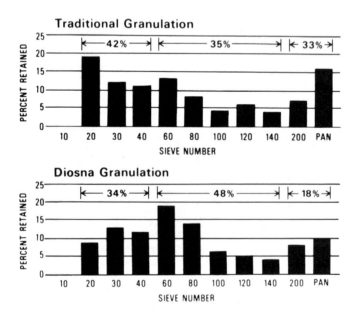

Figure 10 A comparison of the particle size distribution of a traditional and Diosna-produced granulation. (Courtesy of Eli Lilly and Company, Indianapolis, Indiana.)

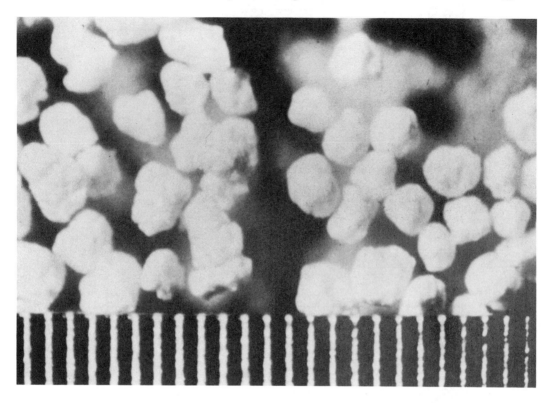

Figure 11   Photomicrographs of particles from a traditional and Diosna-produced granulation. (Courtesy of Eli Lilly and Company, Indianapolis, Indiana.)

spherical. This is illustrated in Figure 11, where the particles on the right side of the figure are from the Diosna, whereas those on the left are from the conventional wet granulation process. Physical comparisons of tablets prepared from granulations made using a range of granulating agents as prepared by the Diosna and by the traditional granulation equipment are shown in Table 2. The conclusion to be drawn from the table is that the tablets produced with the Diosna equipment using the streamlined manufacturing process were as good as and sometimes better than tablets made by the traditional wet-granulation process. The Lilly study summarized the advantages and disadvantages of the Diosna equipment and process as shown in Table 3. The relatively high cost of the equipment would be quickly offset by the efficiency and reduced handling involved in this streamlined production method. The advantages of the equipment obviously were thought to outweigh the disadvantages, since Lilly has used this Diosna equipment as their primary powder-mixing/processing equipment in their new dry products manufacturing facility (see Fig. 4). The available Diosna models with their vessel capacity and approximate working capacities are shown in Table 4.

Figure 12 describes the Littleford MGT mixer/granulator, which has been developed by this company to more specifically meet granulation needs.

Table 2 Physical Comparisons of Tablets Made from Diosna Versus Traditional Granulations

Die size (in)		Diosna			Traditional		
		Disintegration (min)	Friability (%)	Hardness (kg)	Disintegration (min)	Friability (%)	Hardness (kg)
7/32	Starch paste	3	0.49	1.25	2–6	0.27–0.57	0.22–1.37
	Starch, gelatinized powder, and water	5–6	0.25–1.42	0.97–1.42	2–8	0.25–0.75	1.40–2.97
1/4	Povidone	9	0.32	2.65	6–14	0.14–0.47	1.70–2.55
5/16	Starch paste	4	0.31	5.05	5–9	0.41–0.52	3.60–4.90
11/32	Starch-gelatin paste	7	0.05–0.25	3.52–4.32	5–13	0.15–0.20	3.75–4.85
3/8	Aqueous acacia solution and hydroalcoholic solvent	14	0.19	6.6	7–15	0.13–0.64	2.45–5.80
9/16	Hydroalcoholic solvent	5–10	0.22–0.45	6.00–11.1	8–14	0.32–0.75	6.30–12.37
3/4	Aqueous acacia solution and hydroalcoholic solvent	None	0.43–0.80	11.30–13.8	None	0.40–0.85	9.00–13.35
1/4 × 3/4	Starch paste	7–11	0.12–0.14	15.07–15.95	4–9	0.07–0.14	12.15–16+

Source: Courtesy of Eli Lilly and Company, Indianapolis, Indiana.

Table 3 Advantages and Disadvantages of High-Shear Mixer/Granulators

Advantages	Gravity loaded
	Unit formula maintained
	Homogeneously dry mixes quickly: color distribution is excellent; can eliminate premixes of addition by geometric progression
	Forms desired wet granules rapidly
	Less wetting, more rapid drying
	Self-discharging
	Improved coefficient of weight variation
	Improved content uniformity
	Relatively easy to clean
	Sanitary construction
	Mixing bowl may be jacketed
	Option to dry granulation with mixer
	Adequate safety devices
	Conforms to good manufacturing practices
Disadvantages	Relatively high cost
	Adding material directly is not convenient
	High noise level
	Temperature rise from head of friction
	Nonportable
	Must be raised to working height
	Foreign spare part

Table 4 Available Size of Diosna-Type Mixer/Granulator

Model no.	Mixing vessel capacity (L)	Approximate working capacity (L)
P-25	25	20
P-50	50	45
P-100	100	90
P-250	250	220
P-400	400	350
P-600	600	520
P-1000	1000	850
P-1600	1600	1350

Source: Courtesy of Eli Lilly and Company.

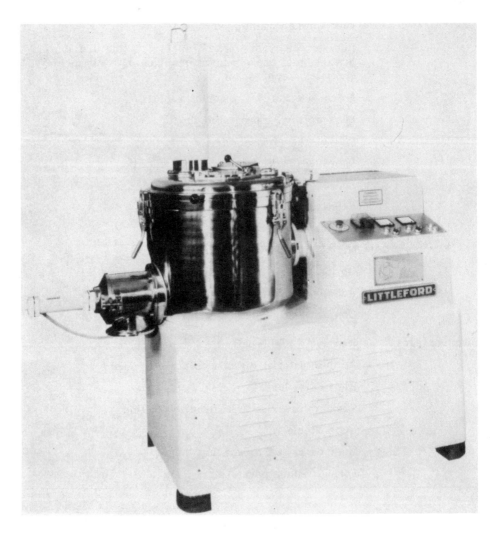

Figure 12   The Littleford MGT mixer/granulator.   (Courtesy of Littleford Brothers, Florence, Kentucky.)

For comparison, the horizontal configuration of the Lodige unit (see Fig. 8) seemingly has been rotated 90° to a vertical configuration, the drum assembly converted to a bowl assembly, and a discharge port added to facilitate the emptying and cleaning of the bowl. The principle of operation is, however, the same as that described previously for the Diosna mixer.

When working with a high-shear solids mixer in a production operation it may be convenient to mount the mixer in a position that will allow the placement of the bowl from a fluid bed cryer under the mixer to facilitate the materials transfer. This is illustrated in Figure 13 and in the Lilly facility (see Fig. 4). Most production fluid bed dryers have wheeled assemblies to facilitate materials transfer to and from the fluid bed unit.

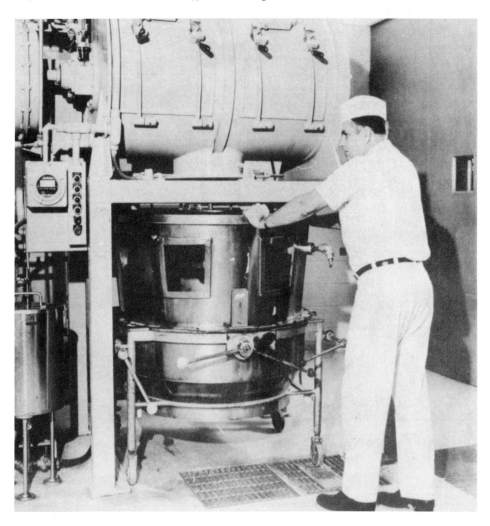

Figure 13   A fluid-bed dryer bowl positioned to directly receive the discharge from a Lodige mixer.   (Courtesy of Littleford Brothers, Florence, Kentucky.)

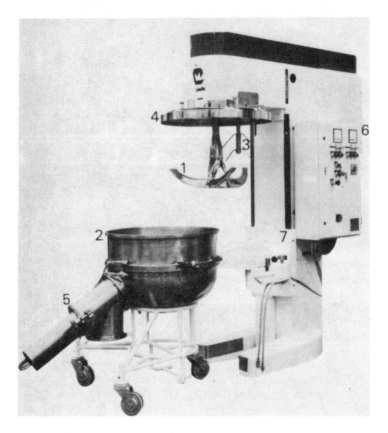

Figure 14   The Gral mixer/granulator. (Courtesy of Machines Collette,
Inc., Weheeling, Illinois.)

Since wet granular material may resist transfer by air conveyor systems
such as the Vacumax, the type of transfer provision shown in Figure 13
may be especially helpful. The need to raise the equipment to appropriate
working height in order to discharge directly into a bowl of a fluid-bed
dryer is not regarded as a major disadvantage, provided powder can be
conveniently charged into the unit when in a raised position.

Figure 14 illustrates the Gral mixer/granulator. Available from
Machines Collette, Inc., this equipment is a modification of the earlier
Gral industrial planetary mixers. The difference, however, between the
mixer/granulator and the standard planetary mixer is that the new unit
contains two mixing devices. A large mixing arm (1) is shaped to the
rounded configuration of the bowl (2) and provides the large-scale mixing
motion in the powder. A smaller chopper blade (3) enters off-center from
the mixing arm and is located above it. The larger mixing blade and a
secondary chopper blade system is, therefore, similar to the Lodige and
Diosna units previously described. The difference, however, is that the
Gral unit has the configuration of a planetary top-entering mixer. The
mixing bowl may be loaded at floor level and then raised to the mixing
position by the hydraulic bowl elevator cradle (7). The bowl is brought

into contact with a cover (4) providing a tight seal. An advantage of the unit is that it may be discharged by its hydraulic port (5), whereas in the raised position, offering sufficient space for a container to be placed beneath the discharged port. The entire mixer unit does not have to be elevated to provide this vertical discharge distance as is the case with the previously two mentioned high-shear mixers. As with the other high-shear mixers, all parts in contact with the product may be ordered in stainless steel. Fluid may be injected into the mixer bowl. The equipment is available with timer control (6). The Gral machines can also be supplied with explosion-proof as well as standard electrics. The equipment is available in five sizes ranging from 10 to 1200 L.

CONTINUOUS-BATCH MIXING, MASSING, GRANULATION, AND DRY-ING EQUIPMENT. The ideal equipment for the preparation of granulations by the wet-granulation process would be one unit which is capable of sequentially dry mixing, wet massing, agglomerating, drying, and sizing the material being processed, with no materials handling between steps. The only interruption in such a continuous-batch process might be to stop the unit in order to add the lubricant prior to discharging a final product ready for compression. This type of approach is indicated in part C of Figure 5. A number of equipment manufacturers and pharmaceutical scientists have been working toward this goal over the last several decades. However, it is only within the last several years that commercial equipment has become available for continuous-batch wet granulation in one unit.

Fluid-Bed Spray Granulators. The first equipment reported in the pharmaceutical literature to provide continuous-batch wet granulation was fluid-bed drying equipment which was modified by the addition of spray nozzles or fluid injectors to provide additional liquid-binding and adhesive agents to dry-powdered materials which were initially placed in the equipment. Scientists working in European pharmaceutical companies were the first to report on this approach [11–15]. However, several U.S. companies are employing fluid-bed spray granulators (see Appendix). Warner-Chilcott utilizes such a process in the manufacture of Pyridium tablets. With the active ingredient, phenazopyridine, being a powerful dye, the new process also benefits from the fact that the system is totally enclosed during the granulation stage [8]. Figure 15 presents a schematic cross section of such a fluid-bed spray granulator. The airflow necessary for fluidization of the powders is generated by a suction fan (2) mounted in the top portion of the unit which is directly driven by an electric motor. The air used for fluidization is heated to the desired temperature by an air heater (5), after first being drawn through prefilters to remove any impurities (6). The material to be processed is shown in the material container just below the spray inlet (1). The liquid granulating agent is pumped from its container (3) and is sprayed as a fine mist through a spray head (4) onto the fluidized powder. The wetted particles undergo agglomeration through particle–particle contacts. Exhaust filters (7) are mounted above the product retainer to retain dust and fine particles. After appropriate agglomeration is achieved, the spray operation is discontinued and the material is dried and discharged from the unit. Figure 16 provides a schematic view of the automatic fluid-bed spray-granulator system available from the Aeromatic Corporation, with its integrated materials-loading and -handling systems. The unit described in

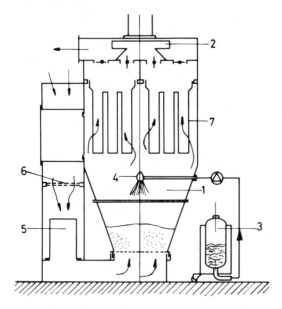

Figure 15　Schematic cross section of a fluid-bed spray granulator. (Courtesy of Aeromatic, Somerville, New Jersey.)

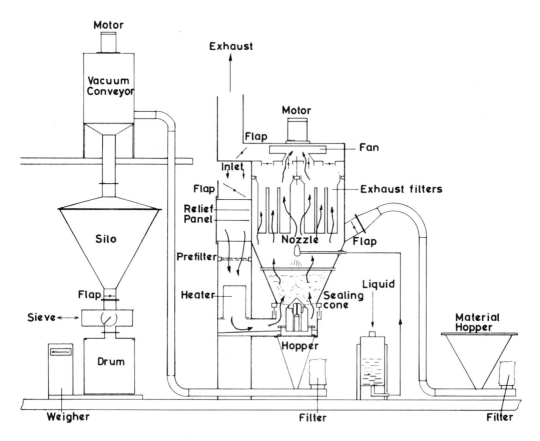

Figure 16　Schematic of an automatic fluid-bed spray granulator (Streba 150) with integrated materials loading and materials handling. (Courtesy of Aeromatic, Somerville, New Jersey.)

Figure 16 is reportedly capable of processing approximately 200 kg per batch. The advantages of such rapid wet massing, agglomeration, and drying within one unit are obviously attractive. Exclusive of equipment clean-up, the process may readily be sequentially completed within 60—90 min or less.

A number of pharmaceutical companies, both in Europe and in the United States, are utilizing fluid-bed processing as a rapid continuous-batch approach to wet granulation. However, there are a number of difficulties that exist for the process which may account for the fact that fluid-bed granulation processing has not been more widely accepted. Fluid-bed systems as currently available may not provide adequate mixing of powder components. Where potent drugs are employed in a fine state of particle size reduction, there will be a tendency of these materials to be separated from the powdered bed and collected on the filter of the unit. Thus, even if a separate powder-mixing operation is undertaken to produce adequate uniformity of drug distribution within the mix, thus de-mixing action must be considered in any attempt to process potent drugs in a fluid-bed spray granulator or when there is a considerable disparity in the particle size or density of the materials being processed. Unlike extrusion, wet screening, and the use of other more conventional mixing equipment, the forces of agglomeration which cause the particles to be brought together producing the agglomerates are relatively low in the fluid-bed spray granulator. Accordingly, not all materials may lend themselves to agglomeration in this continuous batch-processing equipment. Low-density and hydrophobic materials can be particularly troublesome. Another limitation of this type of equipment may be related to particles containing granulating agent on their surfaces which adhere to the filters of the equipment. This creates two problems: a reduction in the effective area of the filters, which may produce filter failure and a build up of pressure within the unit and other difficulties during the granulation operation, and problems connected with cleaning the unit following the granulation process.

All production-size fluid-bed dryer equipment should contain explosion relief panels. However, special attention should be given to safety precautions if organic solvents are used in the fluid-bed spray granulation process. A number of fatal accidents have occurred worldwide with the use of fluid-bed dryers, as have a number of less serious explosions in which only the installation was damaged or destroyed. Dust explosions can also occur in a fluid-bed dryer with dry materials. However, when working with solvents, especially those with flammable vapors, it might be wise to first check with the supplier of the equipment to review whether or not the operation is safe or advisable.

Other manufacturers of fluidized-bed drying equipment, such as Glatt Air Techniques, have developed specialized equipment to provide continuous-batch processing fluid-bed granulator capabilities. The number of scientific papers which have appeared in this field in recent years attests to the interest of the pharmaceutical industry in this continuous-batch processing approach. For example, investigators have studied the mixing of pharmaceutical raw materials in heterogeneous fluidized beds [11], the physical properties of granulations produced in a fluidized bed [12], the effect of fluidization conditions and the amount of liquid binder on properties of the granules formed [13], and the various process variables influencing the properties of the final granulation [14,15].

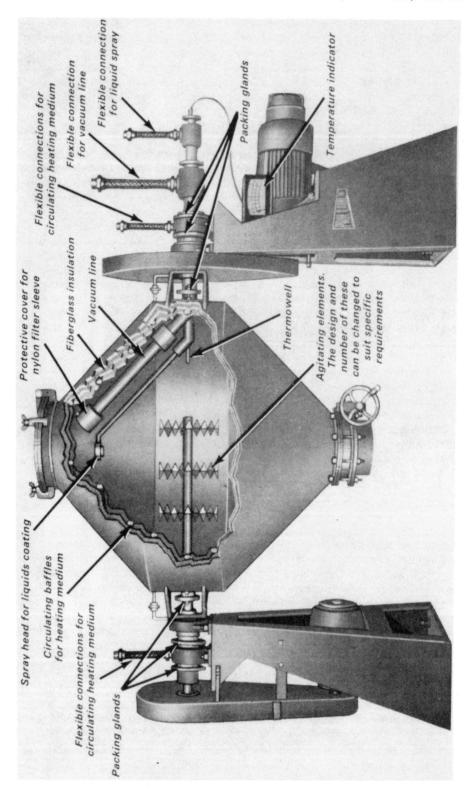

Figure 17 A cutaway view of a double-cone mixer/dryer processor. (Courtesy of Paul O. Abbe, Inc., Little Falls, New Jersey.)

Double-Cone and Twin-Shell Blenders with Liquid Feed and Vacuum-Drying Capabilities. A large number of manufacturers of both double-cone and twin-shell blenders have produced equipment modifications which provide the potential for sequencing the operations of powder mixing, wet massing, agglomeration, and drying. The specialized equipment typically includes a liquid feed through the trunion of the machine leading to a spray dispenser located above the axis of rotation of the unit, a vacuum inlet through the same or the opposing trunion leading to a vacuum intake port covered by a nylon or other appropriate fine-filter sleeve, also located above the axis of rotation and out of the direct path of powder motion, and agitating elements capable of rotation within the powder mass contained in the blender. In some cases, the blender will also be of a double-wall construction to provide circulation of a heating medium; in other cases the systems are designed to operate at room temperature and use vacuum as the sole source of water or liquid removal. Figure 17 provides a cutaway view of a double-cone mixer–dryer processor.

A number of pharmaceutical manufacturers have used this type of equipment for production manufacture of granulations (see Appendix). The equipment is commercially available and has been for a number of years. As in any vacuum-drying operation, equipment cost is high and drying costs are relatively high. Drying times will be considerably longer than is the case with the fluid bed granulator processor. The double-cone or twin-shell processor would, however, be considerably easier to clean. The attractiveness today of the double-cone or twin-shell mixer, granulator, and dryer as a continuous-batch processor of wet granulation products hinges on the use of nonaqueous granulating liquids. Standard auxiliary equipment is available to condense solvent vapors and provide substantially complete solvent recovery. This is important for two standpoints: solvent vapors are not discharged to the atmosphere, an environmental consideration, and efficient solvent recovery is achievable, an economic consideration. The Paul O. Abbe Company is a primary manufacturer of such double-cone equipment, whereas the Patterson-Kelley Company is a primary manufacturer of twin-shell equipment of this specialized type.

The Day-Nauta Mixer/Processor. The Nauta mixer (see Appendix) is one type of vertical screw mixer (Fig. 18). In this type of mixer, a screw assembly (2), is mounted in a conical chamber (1), with the screw lifting the powder to be blended from the bottom of the cone to the top. As such, it is a modification of an alternative to a double-cone blender which rotates about its axis to produce the tumbling of the particles within the cone. In the vertical screw mixer, the screw does the work to lift the powder in the cone and the cone does not rotate. In some vertical screw mixers, the screw assembly is fixed, whereas in others the screw assembly orbits around the vessel walls to ensure more uniform mixing throughout the entire bed. The Nauta mixer is in the latter category of vertical screw mixers. The Nauta mixer is manufactured in the United States by the Day Mixing Company, a division of LeBlond Inc., of Cincinnati, Ohio, under a license from Neutemix B. V., Haarlem, The Netherlands. In its original design, the Nauta mixer is not a mixer/granulator processor. However, engineers at the Day Mixing Company developed a modification of the Nauta mixer, as shown in Figure 18. This new vertical screw powder mixer granulation processor is described in U.S. Patent 3,775,863, and basically uses a source of hot, dry air (3), which is drawn through the wetted powder following powder mixing and the incorporation of the

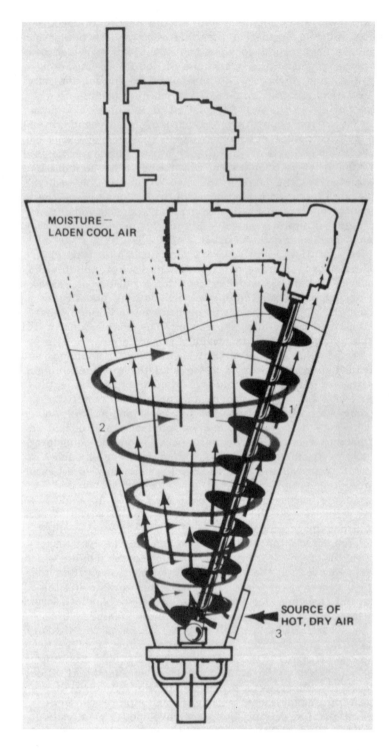

Figure 18   Schematic of the modified Day-Nata mixer for use with hot air
for drying. (Courtesy of Day Mixer, Cincinnati, Ohio.)

liquid granulating agent. There are several advantages of the Nauta
processor equipment over the two types of continuous-batch processor
granulators described in earlier parts of this section. Unlike the fluid-bed
dryer granulator, the Nauta mixer/processor is inherently a powder mixer
and is capable of producing very uniform powder mixtures which do not
demix. Unlike the double-cone and twin-shell blenders described in the
preceding section, the Nauta processor is not forced to rely on vacuum
for drying, but can use hot air. As noted previously, vacuum equipment
is inherently expensive to manufacture, operate, and maintain, and it is
also difficult to maintain close control of product temperatures in a vacuum
dryer, which may account for the long drying cycles necessary to achieve
the proper degree of dryness. Thus, the Day-Nauta mixer/processor would
appear to have the potential to overcome the two major disadvantages of
the earlier-described equipment, whereas having neither of these disadvantages itself.

The Day Company actually provides three methods of drying using the
Nauta equipment. In the first, hot air is introduced through a porous
plate, made of sintered metal, at the base of the cone. Air is supplied to
the inlet from an auxiliary system which can provide air over a temperature
range from ambient to about 400°F. The hot air passes up through the
product bed, which is kept in a state of agitation by the rotating screw/
orbital arm assembly, and exits at the top of the vessel. Since the
powder bed is in a constant state of motion, it is reported that hot spots
within the powder are avoided. Such air movement through the processor
is illustrated in Figure 18. The Nauta processor is also available as a
double-wall jacketed cone to provide direct-heat application to the shell of
the unit. It is reported that in some cases this method, coupled with the
use of hot air, is a more effective way of producing drying within the
conical unit.

A third drying system is also available which utilizes vacuum operation. This system has reportedly been made available by the company for
situations in which low drying temperatures are required or where the solvent vapors are to be recovered. The vacuum approach may also be useful when the material to be dried is oxygen sensitive, or when an unusual
fire or explosion hazard is present. Figure 19 describes the type of total
mixing – granulation – drying process system which the Day Company can
provide. The standard system has a production capacity of 1300 kg
(2280 lb) employing a processor (1) with 98 ft^3 per batch. A smaller,
400-kg unit is also available. Accessory equipment is available as shown
in Figure 19 to provide control over the granulation operation. A self-
powered lump breaker (2) may be mounted by the bottom of the cone to
break up lumps, to reduce caking, and to control better agglomeration
when liquid is being added to achieve granulation. The lump breaker may
eliminate the need to pass the product through a mill on the completion
of the drying/granulation process. Product temperature can be continuously monitored by the temperature monitor (3) as a method of following
the drying process as well as to control product temperature. A nuclear,
noncontact density gage (4) is located slightly above the thermometer to
allow continuous monitoring of product density, specific gravity, or percent solids during processing. This density information, together with
information on amount of fluid added and motor load, provides information
on the status of the agglomeration process. The unit also has a multi-
phase sampling system (7) to provide further process evaluation during

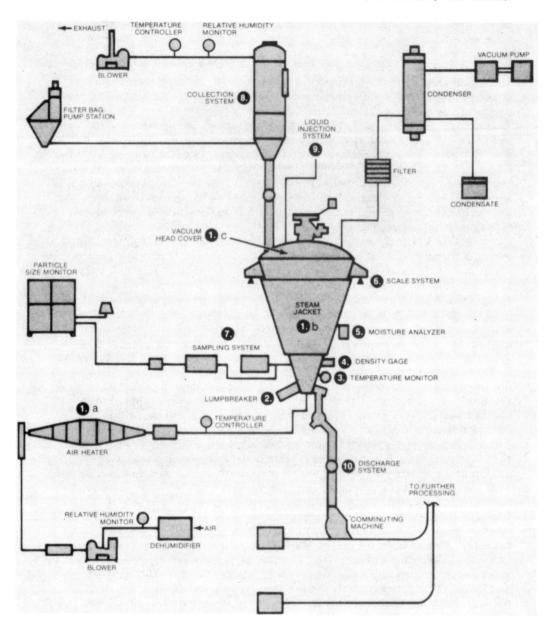

Figure 19   A total mixing-granulation-drying process system using the
Day-Nauta equipment.   (Courtesy of Day Mixing, Cincinnati, Ohio.)

manufacture. An infrared moisture analyzer (5) may also be located in the unit, as shown at the center of the cone for continuous monitoring of product moisture.

Shevlin [16] has done extensive research with the Day-Nauta processor and has reported the following advantages for the system: (1) lower investment than that required by other processors, (2) excellent product temperature control and uniformity, (3) freedom from product caking and lumping, (4) low maintenance cost, (5) ability to mix, granulate, dry, and package from one machine, (6) elimination of product handling, contamination, dusting, etc., (7) low operating cost, and (8) low labor required. Product loss during processing ranged from 1 to 2% and was typically due to the material drying on the bottom quarter of the screw where heat exposure was the greatest. Cleaning of the unit was accomplished by simply hosing the unit out with detergent and water and a final rinse. Working with an acetaminophen formulation and without the use of any external processing to control particle size, the author reported a dried granulation of satisfactory particle size.

SPECIALIZED GRANULATION EQUIPMENT. Roto Granulator. The Roto granulator (Fig. 20) is a one-step granulator consisting of (1) a jacketed and vacuum operating bowl where powders are granulated and dried (the bowl is t.lted at intervals); (2) a main impeller to mix, wet, and move the product during drying; (3) a chopper to affect the size of the granulates produced; and (4) a spray head for the introduction of binder solution. Some of the operating features include a hydraulic drive with continuous, precise regulated speed at all settings, an adjustable impeller clearance of up to 10 mm from the bottom of the vessel, a built-in filter on the lid, a telescopic chopper on the lid with variable-depth penetration control into the product, movement, reduced noise, and low maintenance costs. The Roto granulator is designed for pharmaceutical, food, and other granulation processes with GMP requirements considered in its design. Since the system operates under vacuum, the density of the granulation produced may be carefully controlled. Other considerations which cause improved granulation production include the ability to dry the product in the same bowl using vacuum, indirect heating (a jacketed bowl is used), chopper sizing, and good endpoint control. Key Industries indicates good granulation reproducibility based on a number of test runs. The Roto granulator may be used to produce granulations with water, organic solvents, steam, or melting of at least one of the components. This versatility is due to the fact that an efficient solvent-recovery device is used in the system. Some of the types of granulations that may be produced with the system include standard wet granulations, microgranulations, carrier-coated granulations, matrix systems, moisture-activated granulations, effervescent granulations, and melt-congealed mixtures because of the unique heat control system. The material produced in the Roto granulator is easily discharged and may be sized directly through any mechanical screening system if needed.

Another one-step granulation system is the Gral processor which is also capable of complete processing within the same bowl. It may also be

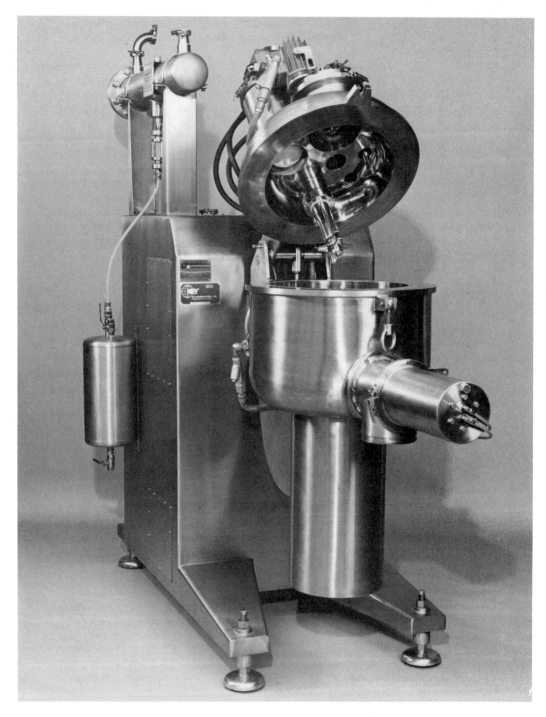

Figure 20   The Roto granulator. (Courtesy of Key Industries,
Englishtown, New Jersey.)

used for aqueous and nonaqueous solvent systems because of its solvent recovery systems. Both processors have the possibility of reducing the amount of floor space needed for granulation preparation which could reduce total capitol costs.

By imploding coating materials on existing granulations, coating within the unit reportedly is possible. In addition, by alternately imploding various drug and excipient materials, the equipment reportedly is capable of effectively separating incompatible drugs or of producing effervescent products of improved stability to moisture. Unfortunately, little scientific or technical information is available regarding products produced by this technique.

The Marumizer. The Marumerizer (Fig. 21) (see Appendix) is a special piece of granulation equipment originally developed in Japan and is distributed by the Luwa Corporation. It must be utilized in combination with an appropriate extruder such as the Xtruder (Fig. 22). Single or twin transport screws convey a damp, kneaded formulation from the feed hopper to the extrusion zone. A tapered rotor with longitudinal blades expels the material through a radial screen. The rod-shaped cylindrical segments are then transported to the Marumerizer. The Marumerizer incorporates three principal, precisely constructed components: a vertical cylinder with discharge port, a circular friction plate, and a variable-speed drive train which turns the plate. As the plate revolves the cylindrical segments of the product are fragmental and rolled into cylindrical or spherical shapes. The product is then dried and screened. The resulting product may then be tableted, coated, or otherwise processed. The diameter of the spheres that are formed will basically be the same as the diameter of the rod-shaped segments which are fed to the machine. Four models of the equipment are available, ranging in capacity from 1 L (10−30 L/h) to 50 L (500−1500 L/h). The process is not recommended for routine preparation of granulations for tableting, but is mentioned here as a specialized type of granulation equipment in which spherical particles may be required for the preparation of material for coating. Current research studies should expand the use of the equipment, especially in controlled-release systems or other applications.

C. Unit Operation Improvements

Wet Granulation Monitoring

The wet granulation of powders is a fundamental pharmaceutical technological process. Wet-granulation techniques are widely used in the pharmaceutical industry on the starting materials that are used to make tablets to achieve any one or all of a number of objectives. These objectives include improved flow; increased particle size; densification; uniform distribution of the active ingredient(s); production of uniform, spherical particles; production of hydrophilic surfaces; and increased compressibility [1−2]. The granulation that is formed during this process affects the characteristics of the finished tablets, including hardness, friability, capping tendency, disintegration, and dissolution. The process of granulation, however, is not well understood because of the many variables involved in the process. Attempts to obtain reproducible granulations and minimize lot-to-lot product variability have traditionally sought to control the

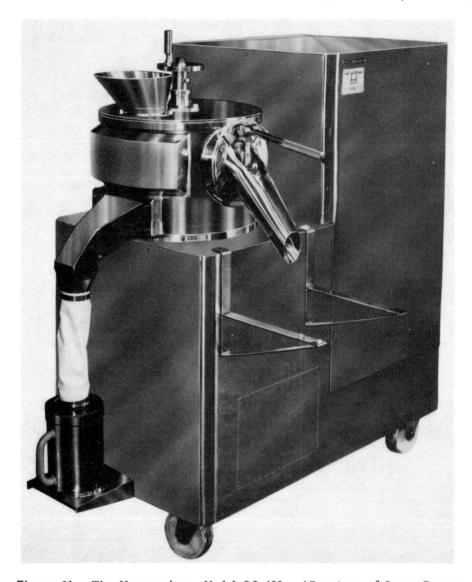

Figure 21   The Marumerizer, Model QJ-400.   (Courtesy of Luwa Corporation, Process Division.)

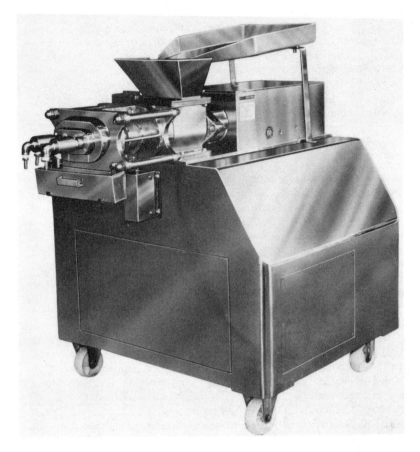

Figure 22   The Xtruder, Model EXDCS-100. (Courtesy of Luwa Corporation, Process Division.)

amount of granulation solution used and the total mixing time. However, control of these two variables has proved to be less than satisfactory at times.

The utilization of high-intensity mixers in the wet-granulation process dramatically reduces the total time required to reach or exceed a proper granulation end point. Therefore, the need of a better understanding and control of wet granulation has increased in recent years as the use of high-intensity mixers has increased. In recent years, more sophisticated techniques for monitoring the granulation process have been investigated. Power consumption [3–8], torque [9–11], rotation rate [12], and motor load analyzer [13] measurements are indirect methods of monitoring the granulation process. Bending moment [4], beam deflection [14], and probe vibrational analysis [15–16] techniques directly measure the density and frictional changes that occur during wet massing. Most recently, conductance [17] and capacitive-sensor [18–21] methods have been used and found to respond to moisture distribution and granule formation in high-intensity mixers.

While none of the systems studied have universal unity, all of the
various approaches have attempted to be responsive to the dynamic
variables of the process, be applicable to formulation research, and be
potentially useful in the control of manufacturing processes. The granulation monitoring system shows promise as a research tool for gaining insight into the granulation process and as a control system for obtaining
better reproduction of granulations and resultant tablets. The study of
the wet-granulation process remains an active research area [1-2,
22-26].

Tableting Improvements

Pharmaceutical tablet production improvements have also been made by improving the performance of a specific unit operation. The development of
high-speed tableting and capsule-filling machines has allowed many manufacturers to increase their tablet and capsule production output by replacing their older, much lower-capacity machines.

Since the introduction of high-speed rotary tablet presses tablet outputs are now possible in the range of 8000-12,000 tablets per minute.
Because of these high outputs, it has become advantageous, if not necessary, to consider automatic control and monitoring of tablet weight. One
of the early attempts to automatically monitor tablet production with an on-
line system for tablet press weight control was the Thomas Tablet Sentinel
(TTS). This unit utilizes commonly available strain gage technology.
Strain gages, appropriately placed on a tablet machine, monitor the strain
that is incurred during the tablet compression step on the machine.

When a tablet press is in good operating condition, is properly set up,
and the punch and die tooling has been properly standardized the amount
of pressure or compressional force developed at each station is dependent
upon the amount of powder that was contained in each corresponding die.
Measurement of this compressional force is thus an indirect method of
monitoring the tablet weights being produced by the machine, and if this
force could then be used to initiate an automatic weight adjustment, continuous monitoring of tablet production would be possible. The TTS system shown in Figure 23 is able to do such a task. The schematic of the
setup of the strain gages and weight adjustment servomotor mechanism is
shown in Figure 24. Figures 23 and 24 illustrate the latest monitoring
system which is known as the TTS-II. The TTS-II is a fully automatic,
on-line, electromechanical tablet weight-control system which is capable of
continuously monitoring and controlling weights of tablets as they are
being produced on a single- or double-rotary press. Figure 24 shows the
three elements of the TTS-II: (1) the sensing systems, (2) the weight
control system, and (3) the reject control system.

The control module may contain meters for monitoring tablets as they
are being produced within desired quality limits. The latest design also
includes a tablet-counting system, a defective tablet counter, and a printer
for recording when weight adjustments are made.   The TTS-II system
utilizes a sensing system of shield strain gages mounted on appropriate
pressure points on the machine. An electronic control system feeds power
to the strain gages and amplifies their output signal.

The third section of the TTS-II system consists of the weight-control
system, which functions according to signals received from the electronic
control portion of the system. Finally, an optional automatic reject-
control system is available which will reject the tablets that may drift out

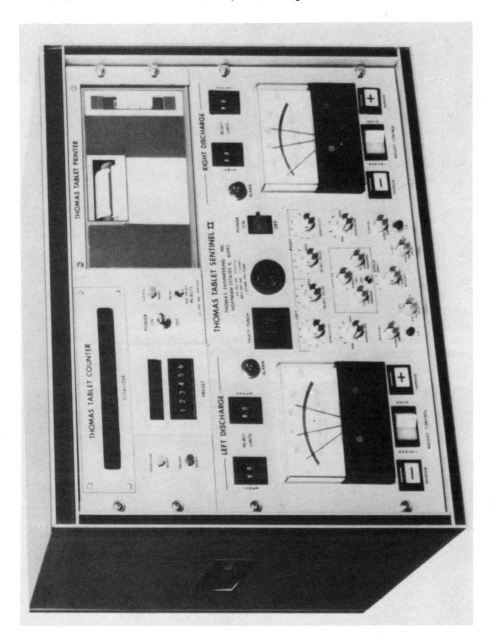

Figure 23 Thomas Tablet Sentinel II. (Courtesy of Thomas Engineering, Inc., Hoffman Estates, Illinois.)

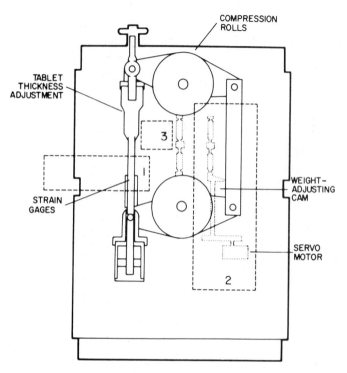

Figure 24   Schematic of the Thomas Tablet Sentinel force-monitoring system.   (Courtesy of Thomas Engineering, Hoffman Estates, Illinois.)

of specifications. The weight-control system is equipped with an audible signal to alert the operator when a machine drifts out of present limits as well as an automatic press shutdown after a chosen number of rejected tablets have been observed by the system.

The TTS-II unit can be used on a machine that is compressing up to 12,000 tablets per minute. If the rejection system is used, the maximum rate of tablet preparation is 8000 tablets per minute.

The printing unit records time and tablet count, and if tablets are rejected, the rejections appear in red print rather than the normal black print. Since there are no on-line weighing systems that are currently fast enough to monitor a high-speed tablet machine, this system is the most positive automatic controlling procedure for continuously monitoring the output of high-speed presses.

In order to meet further demands for maximum tablet press control, the TTS-III has been developed (Fig. 25). It was developed using proven tablet press monitoring concepts associated with advanced sampling and microprocessor technology. This system provides a flexible means to control tablet weight while monitoring tablet performance. Some of the function features of this new system include (1) maintaining compression forces within preset limits, (2) automated adjustment, (3) reading and setting fill depth, (4) activating reject dates, (5) stopping the press, (6) displaying compression force for each station in real time, (7) displaying press performance bar graph, (8) printing all CRT displays, and

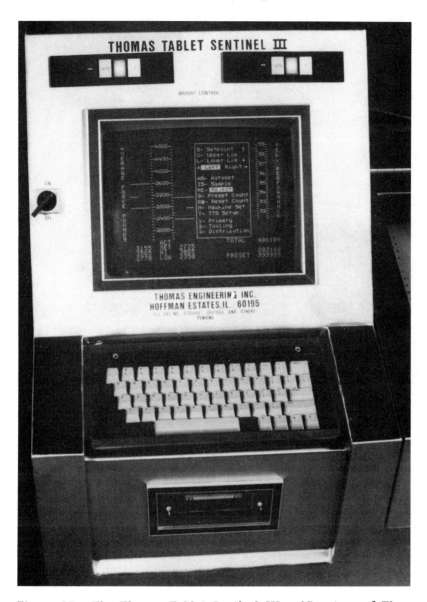

Figure 25 The Thomas Tablet Sentinel III. (Courtesy of Thomas Engineering, Inc., Hoffman Estates, Illinois.)

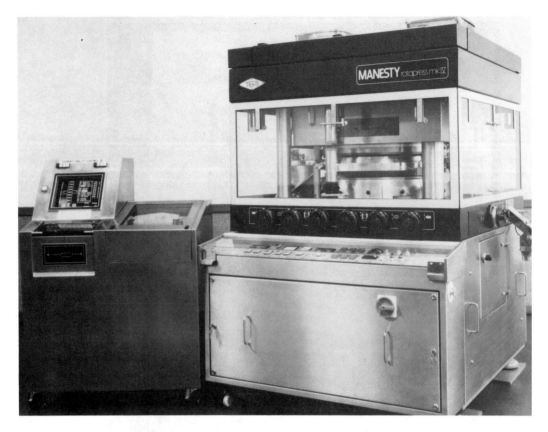

Figure 26   The TTS-III connected to a Manesty Mark IV Press.
(Courtesy of Thomas Engineering, Inc., Hoffman Estates, Illinois.)

(9) providing statistical data for machine performance analysis. Based on
these data, the TTS-III provides useful information on granulation uniformity and the amount of tableting variation due to tooling or granulation.
Figure 26 illustrates the use of the unit with a high-speed tablet press.

The use of computer technology to monitor rotary tablet presses has
been recently described [18]. Using a microprocessor, the Pharmakontroll
unit corrects automatically for weight variation, monitors mean and individual tablet values, controls the discard of faulty tablets, and may include
a quick-stop control that is put into operation when certain tolerances are
exceeded. This system also monitors for optimal speeds, helps to optimize
tool use, evaluates tableting data, records errors, and can conduct statistical evaluations during the run. It is said to assist in the operation of
a machine at maximum capacity without sacrificing speed or output. This
system also has the ability to provide hard copy printout for review after
a particular run has been completed.

Recently, the Korsch PH-800e automated tablet production system has
been described [18]. This is an update of the previously introduced
tablet-control program. The components include a PH-800e double rotary

tablet press, a Pharmakontroll 3 unit, a Pharmacheck unit, a weight/thickness/hardness unit, and a tablet-transfer system. Some of the operational features include continuous tablet weight verification, continuous tablet sorting, periodic quality control sampling, and fault diagnostics. It is anticipated that the total system will provide product optimization through real time adjustment.

Other improvements in tableting equipment might also include a recently introduced tablet press system (Fette Perfecta 2000 Cooltex) which enables the compression of systems at low temperature by connecting an appropriately constructed tablet press to a cooling unit. This cooling unit allows for the preparation by compression of suppositories, enzyme preparations, or other materials with thermosensitive active ingredients. The cooling unit, connected to a relatively high-speed press, can supply coolant so that $-6°C$ is attainable on the press. The press is enclosed to maintain the temperature on the die table. The cooling unit has been designed for continuous operation and remains fully effective throughout the tablet run. The liquid coolant is delivered to the areas of the tablet machines which would be in immediate contact with the sensitive material being compressed. The material is fed through a double-walled insulated feed hopper. This cool press should allow the production of many substances that are thermosensitive and provide the way for numerous new possible product entries.

It is anticipated that further innovations will be developed which will be directed to continuous monitoring of high-speed tablet presses as well as the introduction of new tablet machines for more efficient preparation of materials by compression.

Coating Process Improvement

For years the coating of tablets and pills was conducted in standard 42-in coating pans by coaters who would ladle a given volume of sugar syrup, or a mixture of syrup plus insoluble additives, onto the tumbling tablet bed at selected intervals. The tablets were then allowed to roll while warm air was applied for a period of time just necessary to dry the particular application of coating. This procedure was entirely operator dependent. In 1963, Lachman and Cooper [18] reported a programmed, automated, film-coating process which was frankly designed to remove the human factor in coating and to improve the uniformity of application of an enteric coating. Figure 27 illustrates the entire system. The important components for the improved technique include an airless spray system (1), a tape transmitter and programmer (2), suitable air controller valves (3), and a conventional exhaust air system (4). From this configuration it was possible to

1. Produce uniformly coated tablets as judged by their distintegration rates
2. Better produce reproducible tablets from batch-to-batch
3. Apply more coating to tablets per unit time
4. Decrease coating build up on the pan
5. Cut coating time by as much as one-half
6. Be able to train coaters faster because of the automated spray units
7. Adapt the method to water-soluble films and sugar coating

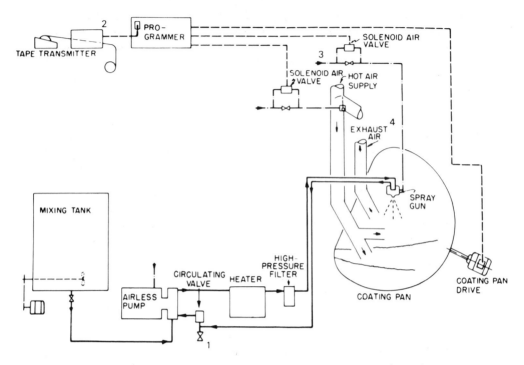

Figure 27   A schematic diagram of the design and equipment for the programmed automated coating operation.   ———, coating solution; — — — — —,
electrical line; — · — ·, compressed air.   (From Ref. 18, used with
permission.)

A significant finding in this early use of an automated approach to coating
was reportedly the greater uniformity of the coatings.

In the 1950s and 1960s many pharmaceutical companies began to in-
vestigate two equipment concepts which were to play a major role in the
subsequent automation of pharmaceutical coating processes: the employment of spray systems for the application of coatings, and the introduction of side-vented coating pans or other new coating systems (air-suspension coating).

SPRAY SYSTEMS AND CONTROL OF SPRAY CYCLES.   Two methods of
spraying coating solutions and dispersions were investigated: the so-called
airless and air-mix spray systems.   In the airless system, the coating fluid
is supplied to the spray nozzle at high pressure, where liquid pressure
alone induces atomization.   In air-mix spray systems, air under pressure
is mixed in an atomized chamber of the spray gun with the liquid to produce a mixed air–liquid spray.   It has been noted that relatively low-
pressure air-mix spray application is much slower, decreases coating
uniformity in the pan, and may produce tablets which are coated in a laminated manner [19].   Other conclusions were that airless spray was better
for sugar and solvent film coating, and that air spray was the best technique for aqueous coating.   Once spray systems were further developed
for a coating pan, automated studies were conducted to demonstrate that

this procedure could be used to sugar coat pharmaceutical tablets. In 1968, a method was developed to subcoat tablets by an automated system [20] and then used a conventional procedure to finish and polish. A programmed controller was used similar to that used by Lachman and Cooper [18], with provision to interrupt the process. The coatings that were applied by the airless spray procedure were considered to have a high degree of uniformity.

NEW COATING PANS OR CHAMBERS. One of the reasons for the evolution of new spray systems for pharmaceutical coatings was the design and development of several new vessels or techniques for the coating of pharmaceuticals. One of these techniques was the air-suspension procedure first developed by Wurster [21-23]. This procedure had the goal of removing the operator variable and approaching a more automated and controllable process. The air fluidization also provided much more rapid drying rates. One key to the success of air-suspension coating was the spray system that was available, accurate fluid pumping, and efficient methods for heating large volumes of air. Figure 28 is a schematic of a typical air-suspension coating system. All of the operating variables may now be

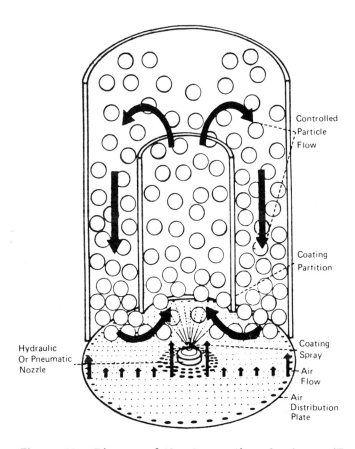

Figure 28   Diagram of Wurster coating chamber. (From G. Banker and C. Rhodes, *Modern Pharmaceutics*, Marcel Dekker, Inc., New York, 1979, p. 394.)

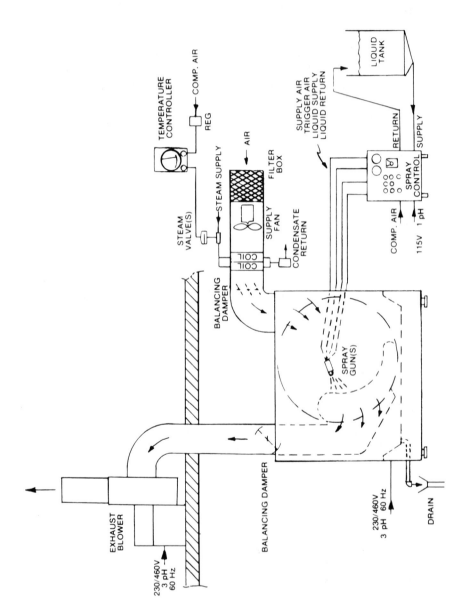

Figure 29 Typical Accela-Cota installation for aqueous or solvent film coating. (Courtesy of Thomas Engineering, Inc., Hoffman Estates, Illinois.)

programmed, so that the operator may load the coater, set the temperature, start the warm airflow, and then start the spray system. Based on
the requirements of the dosage form being coated (tablets, beads, or
small particles), the unit is set to coat for an appropriate preselected
period of time. This technique thus lends itself to the integration with a
miniprocessor, since all coating procedures are capable of being mechanically or electronically controlled. The air-suspension approach may be
effectively employed with either nonaqueous or aqueous film coating.

About the same time that air-suspension coating was being perfected,
another device was being investigated. This was a side-vented or perforated coating pan originally developed by Lilly and then sold as the
Accela-Cota by Thomas Engineering (Fig. 29). One of the major advantages of this equipment is the one-way flow of air through the tablet bed
and out the perforations of the pans. This greatly reduces or eliminates
the "bounce-back" of atomized spray and particle spray drying of the
spray droplets that occurs, especially with solvent-based coating, with the
conventional pans. It also benefits coating because the greater air flow
through the bed facilitates drying. Again, the key to the advance of this
new coating pan was the availability of suitable spray systems which would
provide the new spray requirements while allowing for automation and thus
programmable coating sequences within the coating unit. The side-vented
coating pan has been successfully used for continuous coating of films and
sugar systems [24]. It has been reported that by the selection of proper
viscosity sugar slurries, a complete sugar coat may be applied over an
8-h period. This must include such sequencing as spray, pause, and dry
cycles to allow for adequate sugar slurry spreading prior to drying. It
should be noted that the Pellegrini pan, which is not side vented, but
does have the capability of moving large amounts of air through the pan,
has been adapted to continuous sugar coating, and has also been used
with programmed control systems.

Automation and Coating

For the coating of tablets with sugar systems, it was recognized that it is
possible to spray, roll out the syrup, and dry. It is also known that this
sequence can be repeated to produce a suitable coating as long as an
adequate air supply is available and suitable spray systems can be used.
With these two elements in place, it is then possible to install timers,
mechanical or computer controllers, along with suitable solenoid valves, to
have a completely programmed system. In so doing an operation is developed that is capable of being readily validated, since all important
parameters must first be defined and then precisely controlled by the
automated system without the variability of human error. Once under
automated control, a validated process is easy to confirm with appropriate printout recording.

Associated with the concept of automation may be the desire to first
optimize a process, which would then ensure that the controlled process
is operating at its maximum efficiency. A side-vented, 48-in coating pan
has been used at Purdue University in the Industrial Pharmacy Laboratory
(Fig. 30) to study a number of coating variables. This pan is equipped
with the usual temperature-indicating dials and coating pan pressure dif-
ferential readout. However, it also includes the following features which
aid in the study of the coating process:

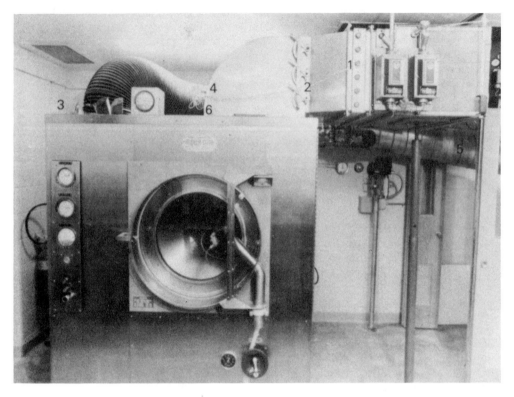

Figure 30   An instrumented 48-in Accela-Cota installation. (Courtesy of Industrial Pharmacy Laboratory, Purdue University, School of Pharmacy and Pharmacal Sciences, West Lafayette, Indiana.)

1. Variable heat input (1)
2. Variable air input (2)
3. Variable exit air control (3)
4. Measurement of dew point of input (4) or exit air (5)
5. Temperature detection for input (6) and exit air (7)
6. Chart recording of air velocity, input air temperature, and exit air temperature
7. Associated electronics with future microcomputer attachment capacity

With these measuring capabilities, studies have been conducted on bed load, baffling configuration, tablet shape, and spray-pattern configurations. The types of coating systems can be evaluated analytically with this setup. By measuring and being able to accurately control spray rates and conditions (spray angles, degrees of atomization, etc.), airflow rate through the pan, air temperature, and dew point into and from the pan it should be possible to optimize not only coat quality features, but coating and energy efficiency as well. As energy costs have risen rapidly, this latter consideration has become increasingly important. The optimization of the parameters involved with aqueous and sugar coating are currently being appropriately modeled and simulated, with the projected results being verified in the new installation.

Completely automated coating systems are now available for the control of both sugar- and film-coated products. An example of such a system is the Compu-Coat II. This is the second generation of a computerized coating system based on a new controller. This controller provides real time monitoring and control and documentation of the coating pan, air handler, and spray system while allowing complete back-up by an independent manual system. This system is available for use with the Accela-Cota pans in sizes of 24, 48, 60, and 66 in. The spray system is capable of handling sugar and film coatings. It is possible to network up to eight coating systems with a supervisor interface station, and to expand to 24 pans using a production monitoring unit. The software of the Compu-Coat system may control the coating formulations to be used, control process parameters, and respond to alarm conditions. As indicated earlier, the system is of a modular design and is adaptable to multipan use [25,26].

D. Increasing Role of Computer Process Control

Evolution and Growth

The digital computer control of processes, especially processes in the chemical industries, have been studied and used for approximately 25 years. By today's standards the original installations were slow and very space consuming. However, several successful computer-controlled processes were developed.

The evolution of the computer in process control systems can be seen in Figure 31. In the early stages of process control (Fig. 31a), instrumentation monitoring of a process, input (I) devices, such as meters, lights, recorders, etc., were mounted on a panel board to provide visual and sound input to an operator. The operator could control the process by manually activating devices on the panel, output (O) devices, such as switches and valves. Process control record keeping was also manually performed by the operator(s).

With the development of the computer, process control configurations as shown in Figure 31b, were used. At this point, computers were very large and very expensive. The computers were used to enhance the monitoring and alarm functions built into the panel board. Some predictive, calculation, and report-writing work was also done by the computer. However, the control of the process was still manually done by the operator. As computer technology improved, the size and cost of the computer decreased and actual computer control of the process was first initiated in this configuration by having the computer monitor specific set points on the panel board instrumentation. With the computer exerting some of the control functions, the inputs required for the operator and the manual activation required of the operator were reduced. Computer-generated records also increased.

The initial successes in computer applications to process control did not lead to a rapid growth in the computer process control field. Unfortunately, a lack of understanding of the necessity of a good project design, the size and cost of the first computers, and the lack of adequate I/O devices to link the process with the computer caused a great many frustrations on the part of both computer customers and computer suppliers. As a result, the larger computer companies concentrated their

52   *Peck, Anderson, and Banker*

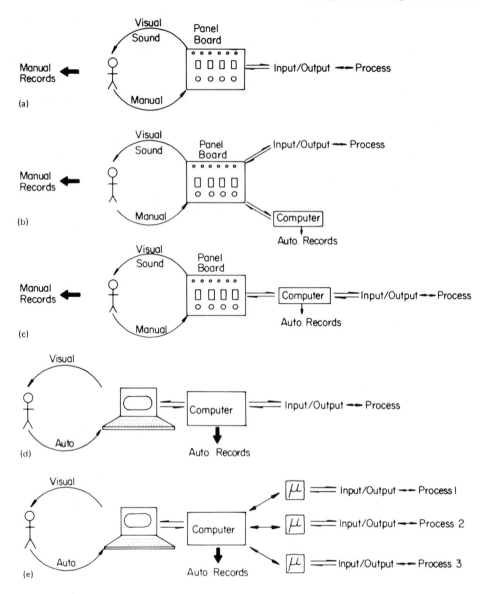

Figure 31   Process control systems.

efforts in the data-processing field, which requires little I/O equipment, and computer process control development was relegated to secondary importance.

At the outset of computer control design the first emphasis was to make the process fit the available computer devices. The "force-fit" approach resulted in computers being advertised and sold to the management function of companies who in turn then gave the computers to the engineering function to find an application. The computer purchase was generally done without an analysis of work to be done followed by the design of the best system. With this type of computerization approach failures occurred and the frustration between supplier and customer developed and added to the technical hurdles hampering the development of computer control of processes [25].

Interest in computer control of processes began to grow when the system-engineering approach to control design was used. In developing control designs, engineering groups began working with computer companies in an effort to design control devices to fit the processes as opposed to forcing processes to fit the devices. At the same time, major analog instrument manufacturers began to manufacture total I/O packages of computer hardware and software systems, enabling their products to be used for process control. Companies also began to develop the more powerful conversational software packages that enabled the process control engineers to use the languages without extensive professional programming aid.

Another prime factor in the growing interest in computer control is the current revolution in microelectronic technology [26]. In the early years of process control, the designs called for the use of electromechanical devices such as relays, timers, and solenoids in conjunction with analog instruments such as temperature- and pressure-monitoring devices. All of these components were mounted on large panel boards. The systems were rarely fully automatic and significant operator interaction was required, especially if the process went "out-of-spec."

At times, adding on to the control of a process was difficult simply because there was no more room on the panel board. As with any electromechanical system, wear and tear, dirt, and heat can take their toll if the devices are not carefully and frequently maintained [25].

Figure 31 illustrates the improved configuration for computer process control utilizing the increased capability of computers, their reduced size and cost, and the increased availability of I/O control devices. Because of the increased amount of control the computer was able to do, the amount of reports generated by the computer also increased. The panel board was essentially kept for visual display only; the operator received very little input, was required to take very little manual action, and made few written reports.

The development of solid-state electronic devices at first improved the reliability of process control by eliminating mechanical devices. As development continued, extensive flexibility in the process control could be developed into the controlling devices. In addition, since 1960 the cost of a computer divided by its computing power has dropped by a factor of more than 100 [27].

As computer technology developed, the devices for interfacing the operator and the computer developed to the point of eliminating the panel board (Fig. 31D). The televisionlike cathode ray tube (CRT) monitoring console expands the visual displays available to the operator, and what

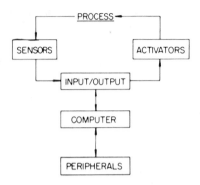

Figure 32   Basic devices required for a process control system.

little process control action is required by the operator can be made at the CRT monitoring console. The manual action and report writing by the operator are eliminated.

Basic Process Control Devices

The hardware required in computer process control can be divided into five basic components, and is illustrated schematically in Figure 32.

SENSORS. First of all, there must be devices to measure the variables of the process which must be considered in making control decisions. These devices are called sensors and are needed because a process computer cannot deal directly with the variables. For example, a computer cannot measure temperature directly. Therefore, a sensor must measure the temperature and convert (transduce) that information into an electrical signal for electronic use [28,29].

I/O DEVICES. The second basic device for computer process control is an I/O device. This device transforms the signals from the sensors into signals that are usable by the computer. In other words, the I/O device enables the computer to interface with the outside world. The I/O device must also be used to take signals from the computer and convert them into action via devices and instruments controlling the process.

COMPUTER. Programmable Controller. The third device is the computer itself. If the process to be controlled consists of numerous sequential (logical) steps, then the controlling device can be a first level computer device called a logic controller. A logic controller can replace the older relay-type control. As long as the process is purely logical, the controller will monitor the process step-by-step to the end and then go back and run the process over again in the exact same way. The programmable controller is the modern logic controller, making the purchase of relay logic systems nonadvantageous. Even though relay controllers are reliable, every change in the process has to be wired into the system by hand. With the modern controllers, a programming change in the controller itself can handle a process change [30].

Microcomputer. Unlike the logic control, which is a simple on/off type of control, the next level of control requires that measurements be taken during the process, such as pressures and temperatures, that an algorithm take those measurements and make some sort of decision, and that corrective action be implemented. This type of control is referred to as feedback control and is normally the system used in computer control systems. The computer device that can first be used in this type of situation is the microcomputer. The capacity of a microcomputer is such that a device can handle six to 12 feedback loops per process cycle.

Microcomputer systems are not very flexible unless the design engineers learn the particular machine language. Very few microcomputers operate in the higher level languages, such as FORTRAN, and microcomputers generally do not operate with a universal computer language. The basic language of each machine must be learned.

The flexibility of microcomputers is limited. If 10 processes require control, then 10 microcomputers in the plant could control them. However, the reality is that with time there could be four or five different microcomputer systems controlling the 10 processes, and therefore four or five different computer languages in use. The different languages add to the confusion when a process change takes place because consideration must now also be given to the compatibility of the languages in use.

The cost of the actual programmable controller and microcomputer devices is similar, but the microcomputer will cost more in terms of time to program.

Minicomputer. The number of feedback loops and the speed of the response times required in the loops determine the size of the computing machine needed. These factors determine when a control system design will require the minicomputer. Short response times and numerous loops require a minicomputer.

The distinction between microcomputers and minicomputers is very difficult. There are microcomputers that can outperform a minicomputer.

ACTIVATORS. The fourth basic component of a computer process control system is a set of process activators. Activator devices, such as electric solenoids, electric motors, and hydraulic valves, take the command signals from the computer via the I/O device and turn them into action in the process [28].

PERIPHERALS. The last basic set of process control components allows reports to be printed and information stored, information to be added to the control process or the process changed, and the system to be visually monitored. These devices are called peripherals, and the term comprises such items as disk storage devices, typewriters, printers, card readers, keyboards, and CRT screens.

Distributed Process Control Systems

DEVELOPMENT. The development of the microcomputer has made it possible to place the I/O monitoring and controlling device close to the point of use, which has allowed for a basic redesign of process control systems (see Fig. 31E). The control system can now be more sophisticated. Plant optimization and management information can be handled by a "host"

microcomputer while simultaneously monitoring the process-controlling microcomputers distributed throughout the entire process. This type of design
of computer process control is called distributed control.

Distributed control systems reduce installation costs by reducing the
amount of field wiring that must be done in the panel systems. The shorter cable runs of the distributed systems also help eliminate the electrical
interferences that often distort low-voltage electrical signals. The distributed system replaces the large panel board in favor of the much smaller
CRT display. Because of the low cost of microcomputers, each remote unit
can have an on-line backup unit which will continue the control function
should the first microcomputer fail, thus increasing the reliability of the
distributed system over the older systems. The repair of a distributed
microcomputer is relatively easy. In many cases, a device can be repaired
by the simple replacement of a printed circuit board [25,31].

To change to distributed systems has not come without criticism. Many
people feel that the distributed systems reduce the number of personnel
needed to monitor a control system below a safe limit and that in a situation of plant upset, several operators working simultaneously on a panel
board are better able to correct the situation than one person on a single
CRT. In addition, many people feel that it is a necessity that a panel
board showing the schematic of the process be used in the monitoring of
that process [31].

CONFIGURATIONS. There are two basic approaches to designing a
distributed control system: (1) the loop approach, and (2) the unit operation approach. In the loop approach, the individual computer is programmed to control a specific number of selected functions within the
process. Similarly, a single computer could be placed in control of a
single function in several process loops. With the unit operation approach,
the computer is in control of a single unit operation. The unit operation
approach has the advantage of being inherently modular and the control of
a process can be instituted in a stepwise manner. In other words, the
most critical operation of a process could possibly be controlled by computer first and the rest of the process added to the control system as
time and money allow.

The host minicomputer and the microcomputers it is monitoring can be
arranged in any one of a number of operational configurations. Figure 33
illustrates some of the configurations used in distributed process control.
In each configuration, if the host computer fails, the microcomputers can
continue their control functions. If any of the microcomputers fail, the
others can continue to communicate to the host computer and continue
their control functions [31].

The major obstacles to computer process control today are

1. The continued need for smaller computer devices with high
   capabilities
2. Better I/O interfacing devices
3. Better operator/machine interfacing devices

Process Control Organizations

Along with the development of computer process control design, hardware,
and software has come the development of several important related organizations that have enhanced, and can continue to enhance, its development:

(1) the control engineering functions in manufacturing companies, (2) major instrument- and equipment-manufacturing companies able to supply both equipment and related control devices, (3) process control groups within the major computer manufacturers, and (4) large engineering contractors specializing in the design and installation of computer control systems (Table 5) [26].

Application to Pharmaceutical Processing

Pharmaceutical manufacturing generally operates in a batch configuration with a series or sequence of steps. Most batch operations have a large number of simple steps that require the assistance of manufacturing personnel, and that assistance is not generally overly challenging. The automatic control of the sequential operation can in many situations improve the following areas:

1. Product throughput time
2. Consistency of acceptable product batch-to-batch
3. Compliance with OSHA and EPA regulations
4. Conservation of energy

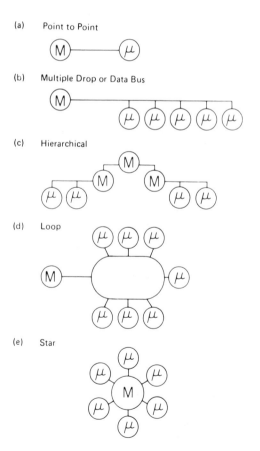

Figure 33   Distributed process control configurations.

Table 5   Suppliers of Computer Systems for Process Control

Bailey Controls 29801 Euclid Avenue Wickliffe, OH 44092	Kaye Instruments 15 DeAngelo Drive Bedford, MA 01730
Fisher Controls Co. 205 South Center Marshalltown, IA 50158	Reliance Electric Company Control Systems Division 350 West Wilson Bridge Road Worthington, OH 43085
Foxboro Company 120 Norfolk Street Foxboro, MA 02035	Taylor Instrument Company P.O. Box 110 Rochester, NY 14692
Honeywell, Inc. Process Management Systems Div. 2222 W. Peoria Avenue Phoenix, AZ 85029	

5. Reduction of labor
6. Flexibility to change the batch process control as the process changes
7. Stable plant operation with reduced operational errors and rejected product
8. Reliable control of the process

From the above list of advantages of automatic control it is obvious that the control system must (1) provide good performance characteristics, (2) maintain that performance over a long period of time, and (3) be easy to install, maintain, troubleshoot, and repair [30,32].

With the development of the microcromputer and distributed control design, several manufacturers of equipment that are used in the pharmaceutical industry are supplying microcomputers and controllers with their equipment. Not only does some of the equipment increase the efficiency of a process as described earlier, but the automatic controller increases the reliability of the operative control of the equipment and increases the ability of the machine to be interfaced into a computer controlled process. The individual control of a specific piece of equipment also offers the ability of automating a single-unit operation without automating the entire process. Table 6 gives a list of suppliers and their equipment that are so controlled.

Implementation of Computer Control

NATURE OF THE COMPUTER CONTROL PROJECT. Reducing the frustrations in implementing computer process control that were pointed out earlier in this section requires a high level of cooperation and communication between the various groups involved, especially between the function that wants the control and the group charged with designing and installing the control.

Table 6 Computer-Controlled Pharmaceutical Processing Equipment

Processing equipment	Developing company
Automatic particle inspection for ampuls and vials	Eisai USA, Inc.
Automatic tablet checker	Fuji Electric Co., Ltd.
Automatic tablet-coating system	Graco, Inc.
Automatic tablet sugar-coating module	Vector Corp.
Compu-Coat II coating system	Thomas Engineering
Dataplus 2000 control system	Glatt Air Techniques
Fette tableting presses	Raymond Automation
Fitzaire fluid-bed dryer	Fitpatrick Co.
Flo-Coater fluid-bed spray granulator	Vector Corp.
Fluidaire fluid air dryer	Fluidaire
Hata Rotary tableting presses	Elizabeth-Hata
Hi-Coater tablet-coating system	Vector Corp.
Pharmakontroll rotary press monitor	Emil Korsch oHG, Berlin
Thomas tablet sentinel	Thomas Engineering

The initial request or interest for some level of automatic process control will probably come from a research and development, production, or production support function within a company which thinks that a product can be produced better and/or quicker if computer control of the process were instituted.

Some engineering function of the company will then have the responsibility for putting the desires of the production request into operation.

The engineering function responsibility is to work with the process group to supply the mechanics of accomplishing the task required by the process group. The responsibility of the process group is to supply the engineering function with enough information about the process and the influences of the process on the quality of the product so that the engineering function can make the best decisions in securing the appropriate mechanics to accomplish the task.

THE IMPORTANCE OF COMMUNICATION. At the very outset of the control project design it is essential that communications be definite and clear. The first thing to realize is that in most companies the production and engineering functions speak different "languages."

The language problem stems from the fact that both the processing group and the engineering group use terms unique to their functions. The language probem can become worse when the topic of computers and the associated technologies are discussed. The vocabulary of data processing and process control is developing as fast as the technology it describes. The processing group should be aware of the engineering group's understanding of processing terminology. Likewise, the engineering group should be sensitive to a possible lack of understanding of engineering terminology within the processing group. Differences in terminology familiarity between groups should be minimized by education or communication style so that the communication between groups during the project can take place on a common level of understanding and be fully productive.

A short glossary of computer terms [33] has been included (Table 7) to exemplify the language problem that can exist and perhaps initiate a familiarization of "computerese."

The process group must first specify, in detail, how the process requiring change is now being run. The engineering function will reqgire such information as the equipment presently being used, the number of persons involved in the process, the exact details of each process step, and the effects of process steps on the final product quality.

The next information required is how the process needs to be changed. The process group does not need to indicate how the change will be accomplished, but should spell out in detail what changes are required in the old process.

Because of the data-processing capabilities of a computer, reports can be generated during the process that can be used to tell the process operator what is going on in the process. Data from such reports can be used for quality control records and other data could be used to make decisions. To eliminate the frustrations of future reprogramming, project cost overruns, specifying a computer with inadequate memory capacity, creating unhappy groups that cannot get the reports they want, the specifics of the reports to be generated during the process must be decided before the engineering group can specify the mechanics of the process control system. Such things as the type, number, frequency, and mode (pictures, listings, hard copy, black and white CRT, color CRT) of the reports need to be considered in detail and specified.

The report that details all of the process control objectives and requirements is sometimes referred to as the functional specification (funct spec). To reinforce the need for detail in writing this document, a good rule-of-thumb is to ask for every statement made: Can anyone assume anything in what has just been written? If assumptions can be made, then the statement is not detailed enough. If assumptions can be made, then the engineering function is forced to make decisions about a process that they probably know very little about, especially as it pertains to final product quality. Therefore, the people charged with writing the funct spec must take great pains to detail the process so that engineering does not make an erroneous assumption and jeopardize the quality of the final product.

With the funct spec in hand the engineering function can gain an understanding of the process and what is wanted, and can proceed to determine what equipment and technology is available or has to be invented to accomplish the goal established. The engineering function will also place a price tag on the project. If the cost of the control project is too great, the funct spec may be rewritten to scale down the size of the project and, hopefully, the cost.

The communication of the "needs" and the costs of satisfying those needs are often continued until the exact needs of the process group are

Table 7 Glossary of Computer Terms

Access time	The time needed to retrieve information from the computer.
Address	The number indicating where specific information is stored in the computer's memory
Architecture	A purely conceptual term signifying the fundamental design aspects of a computer system.
Batch processing	Literally, a batch of programs or data which has been accumulated in advance and is processed during a later computer run.
Binary	A number system based solely on ones and zeros (base 2).
Bit	The smallest information unit that a computer can recognize; 1 or 0.
Byte:	A byte is an arrangement of 8 bits.
Core memory	Using small magnetic doughnuts, or cores, as its storage element, core memory preceded semiconductor memory in the evolution of computer technology and is now largely obsolete.
CPU	(Central processing unit) The part of the computer that controls the interpretation and execution of the processing instructions.
CRT display	(Cathode ray tube) A televisionlike screen which may be used for viewing data while they are being entered into or retrieved from a computer.
Data	The raw information within a computer system.
Diagnostics	Programs for detecting and isolating a malfunction or mistake in the computer system; features that allow systems or equipment to self-test for flaws.
Digital circuits	Electronic circuits providing only two values as an output, one or zero, and nothing else.
Disk memory	Memory using rotating plates on which to store data and programs.
Downtime	The time during which a computer is not operating because of malfunctions, as opposed to the time during which it is functionally available but idle.
EDP	(Electronic data processing) The transformation of raw data into useful data by electronic equipment; sometimes referred to as ADP, or automatic data processing.
Floppy disk	A component similar to a 45 rpm record made of flexible material and used for storing computer data.

Table 7   (Continued)

GIGO	(Garbage in, garbage out) A shorthand expression meaning that if you put in incorrect or sloppy data, you will get incorrect or sloppy answers; originally contrived to establish that errors are always the user's fault, never the computer's.
Hard copy	Computer output recorded in permanent form, such as the paper copy produced by a printer.
Hardware	The physical components of the computer-processing system, for example, mechanical, magnetic, electrical, or electronic devices.
IC	(Integrated circuit) A digital electronic circuit or combination of circuits deposited on semiconductor material; the physical basis of a computer's intelligence and the key to the microelectronic revolution in computers.
Input	The data that is entered into the computer; the act of entering data.
Instruction	A group of bits that designates a specific computer operation.
Intelligent terminal	A typewriter with a television screen attached to it that can remember things, do calculations, type letters, communicate with other intelligent terminals, draw pictures, and even make decisions.
Interface	The juncture at which two computer entities meet and interact with each other; the process of causing two computer entities to intersect.
K	Equals 1024 bytes.
Language	A set of words and the rules for their use that is understood by the computer and operator alike for programming use.
Language, BASIC	An easy-to-use high-level programming language that is popular with the personal computer systems (Beginners All-Purpose Symbolic Instruction Code).
Language, COBOL	A high-level programming language widely used in business applications (Common Business Oriented Language).
Language, FORTRAN	A high-level programming language designed to facilitate scientific and engineering problem solving (Formula Translation).
Language, Machine	The language, patterns of ones and zeros, directly intelligible to a computer.
Mainframe	A large computer, as compared to minicomputers and microcomputers.
Memory	The selection of the computer where instructions and data are stored; synonymous with storage.

Table 7 (Continued)

Memory capacity	The maximum number of storage positions (bytes) in a computer memory.
Microcomputer	A small computer in which the CPU is an integrated circuit deposited on a silicon chip.
Minicomputer	A computer that is usually larger, more powerful, and costlier than a microcomputer but is not comparable to a mainframe in terms of productivity and range of functions.
Nibble	A nibble is an arrangement of 4 bits.
Output	The information generated by the computer.
Peripheral	A device, for example, a CRT or printer, used for storing data, entering it into or retrieving it from the computer system.
Program	A set of coded instructions directing a computer to perform a particular function.
Realtime	The immediate processing of data as it is entered into the computer.
Semiconductor	A material having an electrical conductivity between that of a metal and an insulator; it is used in the manufacture of solid state devices such as diodes, transistors, and the complex integrated circuits that make up computer digital circuits.
Software	A general term for computer programs, procedural rules and, sometimes, the documentation involved in the operation of a computer.
Storage	See Memory.
System	The computer and all its related components.
Terminal	A peripheral device through which information is entered into or extracted from the computer.
Throughput	A measure of the amount of work that can be accomplished by a computer during a given period of time.
Timesharing	The method that allows for many operators using separate terminals to use a computer simultaneously.
Turnaround time	The time between the initiation of a computer job and its completion.
Word	A group of bits that the computer treats as a single unit.
Word length	The number of bits in a computer word.
Word processor	An automatic typewriter, often equipped with a video display screen, on which it is possible to edit and rearrange text before having it printed.

refined to within budget constraints. The costs of the new control system must be justified by the improvements brought about by the new
process.

At this point in the project, the hardest and the most time-consuming
part has been completed. The remainder of the project, including specifying and ordering the actual control devices, writing and checking the
computer control programs, and installing and checking the system, becomes, in comparison, a minor part of the project providing the initial
background work has been done properly [31,32].

ROLE OF THE INDUSTRIAL PHARMACIST. In the introduction to this
chapter reference was made to the industrial pharmacist/scientist being
aware of certain areas from which process efficiencies could be developed
and, with such an awareness, being able to function with the engineering
group within a pharmaceutical firm to help improve the manufacturing
processes. As the development of computer process control grows and is
applied to pharmaceutical processes, the role of the pharmacist grows even
larger. The unique awareness of the impact and influence of a manufacturing process on the safety and efficacy of a final drug dosage form is
the sole reponsibility of the industrial pharmacist. In the age of computer
control the industrial pharmacist will have to know in detail how each unit
operation in the manufacture of a drug product can influence the final
drug product and what parameters within a unit operation are important
and should be monitored and controlled to produce reliable drugs. The
industrial pharmacist will play an important role in helping to develop the
increasing role of computer process control in the pharmaceutical industry.

IV. VALIDATION

Validation as a concept and a system of procedures came into being in the
pharmaceutical industry to ensure the sterility of parenteral and other
sterile products. Basically, the system involved placing sensors and
measuring devices in all the critical locations or recording sites within
sterilizers to accurately record temperature (or other conditions impacting
on the attainment of sterility) so that following a sterilization cycle with a
particular product, in a particular container, under full production conditions, examination of the records of the sterilization conditions would provide absolute assurance that sterilization was achieved in every product
unit so processed. Validation requires previously establishing, in such
sterilization applications, the permutations and combinations of conditions
(time, temperature, steam pressure, cycle conditions, etc.) which will
produce sterility with a very high degree of certainty. Thereafter, recorded data from each production sterilization run provide the documentation that all units within all regions of the sterilizer were exposed to conditions that have clearly been established and documented by careful previous experimentation to produce sterility.

Currently, validation concepts are being recognized for their value in
helping to assure the quality features of classes of drug products other
than sterile products. Validation procedures are being applied to solid
oral dosage forms and especially to compressed tablets. Validation is
most important in tablet products in which manufacturing process conditions are known to have the potential to affect important product quality

features, such as bioavailability. Thus, in the design of a new tablet product and its method of manufacture, or as the design of process for the manufacture of tablets is improved and evaluated, it will be necessary to consider the concept of validation. It is increasingly recognized that an adequate process for the pharmaceutical product is a validated process.

A definition currently in use by the Food and Drug Administration is: "A validated manufacturing process is one which has been proved to do what it is purported or represented to do. The proof of validation is obtained through the collection or evaluation of data preferably from the process and the developmental phase and continuing through into the production phase" [34]. While the FDA definition is for a validated manufacturing process, it suggests by reference to a developmental phase that validation involves more than the actual production process. Indeed this would be so for most tablet products.

Inherent in any discussion of validation is the assumption that the product involved is well understood and that the essential design parameters are under control. Validation, therefore, is not independent of product formulation. It is not enough to start thinking about validation when a formulation is turned over to a pilot plant or production group. It is essential that the development pharmacist or pharmaceutical scientist be knowledgeable not only in formulation and physical pharmacy, but also in pharmaceutical processing and manufacturing operations. Otherwise an experimental formula may be developed whereby the quality features of the product are very sensitive to the manufacturing conditions and variables routinely and normally encountered in practice, or involves such a large number of variables impacting on assorted quality features that validation becomes difficult or impossible.

There are pharmaceutical products currently being marketed that cannot be validated based on their design. Included in this group are some sustained-release products, which involve a sequence of steps whereby powdered drug is dusted on sugar beads with other mixed hydrophilic and hydrophobic powders, employing a "binder" of polymers, fats, waxes, and possibly shellac in a mixed solvent (sometimes including water plus organic solvents), followed by addition of a retard coating, again using fats, waxes, and polymers in varying stages of solution and dispersion. In such systems, simply controlling rates of powder addition, liquid binder addition, spray-gun conditions, and geometry in the coating pan, or other processing conditions will not lead to validation. When the binder and retard dispersions vary as to extent of polymer, fat, wax hydration/ solvation in each batch, and are not and cannot be controlled (a formulation factor), no degree of process manufacturing control can produce a controlled product. Furthermore, as the number of variables which can influence product quality increase (both process and formulation variables), the number of interaction effects capable of producing further (and often less predictable) effects increase in an exponential manner. Validation of such systems becomes a true nightmare.

Another design parameter that must be studied in development is the establishment of raw materials specifications. If raw materials specifications are inadequate, no amount of process validation can ensure a satisfactory product. Thus, an important responsibility of the development group is to determine that the physical and chemical specifications for all active and excipient materials have been adequately set. For example, where polymers are employed, have molecular weight, degree of substitution of chemical groups, and polymer grade, including purity, been adequately defined? Does the nature of the product or method of manufacture require special specifications for the drug or excipients (such as a particular particle size or particle size distribution for drugs which are to be directly compressed or which have dissolution or bioavailability problems)? Are special precautions required for a drug having chemical instability or reactivity potential (such as lower moisture content limits for excipients to be combined with a hydrolyzable drug)? Unless such formulation or drug-related variables, which can by themselves influence product quality features or do so by interacting with processing variables, are identified and appropriate specification limits set in place, no level of subsequent process control and validation can lead to a reproducible product.

Two approaches may be taken to determine the specifications that are adequate for raw materials after the need for such critical specifications has been identified. The first approach is to set the most rigid specification for that property that could reasonably be achieved. The advantage of this approach is that it is direct, reasonably simple, and requires minimal experimentation. The disadvantage is that this approach may represent overkill, and unnecessary costs or undue limitation of suppliers. The second approach involves conducting well-designed experiments to determine where the critical specification(s) should be set. Vary the specification in question for the raw material, employing the most rigid value that could reasonably be achieved as one specification, relax that specification for another sample of the material to a value that might be expected to be borderline, and use an intermediate specification for perhaps a third sample of the material. Make product of each raw material, employing manufacturing conditions in each case that would be expected to impact *least* favorably with the critical product quality features being examined. Review the data from the experiments and determine whether the most rigid specification is actually necessary, or whether the intermediate specification will suffice, or whether the least rigid specification is adequate. This approach is most useful when the development pharmacist has an accurate understanding of the product system in question and its ultimate, exact method of manufacture, and can project the range of processing variables the product may be subjected to and the effect of the direction of such process variations on the quality feature in question. Ideally, raw materials specifications will be appropriately set before a product is placed in production for process validation. When appropriate standards have not been established for raw materials specifications, and where such variation in raw materials is significantly impacting on product quality features, attempts to achieve process validation through control of the manufacturing operation can become an exercise in futility.

Experienced development and production personnel of most companies can recite case studies in which a new product could be made on a small scale in the laboratory but could not be reliably reproduced in production. A different type of frustration is expressed, depending on whether the account is told by the development person or by the production person. Production personnel have a powerful argument at their disposal against accepting any product and/or manufacturing procedure that defies or does not reasonably lend itself to validation. It is imperative that R&D and production groups work together to see that validation can be and is achieved.

As the validation concept is applied to pharmaceutical products of increasing complexity of design and manufacture, it is very clear that validation must be initiated at a very early stage in the design of any product, not only from the traditional "process" orientation, but also from a "product" orientation. Based on this philosophy, validation may be defined as a systematic approach to ensuring product quality, by identifying process variables that influence product quality features, in order to establish processing methods and the necessary control of these methods, which when followed will assure meeting all product quality specifications after assuming that the formulation is reasonable and that the raw material specifications are adequate.

A. Validation Priorities

Perhaps the initial step in validation is to consider which product most requires a full validation treatment and which least. Validation efforts could be centered on processes that involve a company's largest selling and most commercially important products. Products containing drug(s) with a very low dose, chemical instability, low solubility or poor wetting properties, which can lead to content uniformity, stability, or bioavailability problems; products with a history of production problems, often bordering on being unacceptable, or which unaccountably produce occasional lots that are unacceptable or borderline; sustained or controlled release products whose processes are not under control should have a high validation priority. In other words, the initial validation effort could be focused to provide the greatest beneficial effect.

Another approach to validation priority setting is to review the documentation and data currently available on present products and start validating those products which can be done the quickest and easiest. For example, a product that has a moderate dose (perhaps 25 to 150 or 200 mg) of a very soluble, stable drug, which is readily compressible and has no bioavailability or other problems, and which has been made for years by direct compression, with no history of a defective batch, while readily meeting all product specifications, might be easily validated with historic data. This approach can be advantageous in that validation concepts are learned with the easier projects before more complex validations are undertaken.

B. Steps in Validation

Step 1

Identify all the quality features and specifications which will or do define product quality and acceptability, final product as well as in-process specifications (see Table 8 for examples of in-process product specifications as well as process control parameters).

The first step in validation is thus to be certain that specifications have been appropriately set to define the primary product quality features and to establish their limits of acceptability. Specifications may be set on intermediate materials as well as on the finished product. For example, a variety of specifications may be placed on the powder mixture or granulation, in addition to the specifications which are placed on the final tablet

Table 8   Unit Operations and Possible Control Tests Associated with the Manufacture of a Wet-Granulated Compressed Tablet

Process variable	Purpose	Test parameters
Screening	Ensure a set particle size of raw material	1. Mesh analysis 2. Bulk volume
Mixing	Homogeneous mixture	1. Mesh analysis 2. Chemical content uniformity analysis 3. Yield reconciliations
Granulating	Convert powders to granules having suitable flow and compressive properties	1. Weight per subpart 2. Amount of granulating agent per subpart 3. Endpoint of batch 4. Mixing time 5. Granule size (wet)
Drying (oven)	Reduce moisture content to proper level for compression	1. Weight per tray 2. Thickness per tray 3. Relative humidity of air 4. Velocity of air 5. Time 6. Loss on drying 7. Yield reconciliation
Size reduction	Size reduction	1. Bulk volume 2. Flow 3. Mesh analysis 4. Yield reconciliation 5. Loss on drying
Compression	Manufacture of compressed tablet	1. Weight/10 tablets 2. Hardness 3. Thickness 4. Appearance 5. Disintegration 6. Dissolution 7. Weight variation 8. Content uniformity 9. Friability 10. Compressional force 11. Tablets per minute 12. Yield reconciliation 13. Karl Fischer/loss on drying

product. It is important that the list of specifications be sufficiently full and complete to assure full compendial, new drug application (NDA), or company standards. Not all product specifications come under validation treatment. Some product specifications bear on purity and generally are not influenced by processing; they bear on raw material quality and specifications. Other quality features may not be sensitive to processing condition variations and thus may not be included in the validation treatment or are of minor concern in such treatment. An example might be a tablet which is formulated such that compressional force, under any projected range of compressive loads, has no significant influence on tablet disintegration or drug dissolution rate.

Quality features for tablets have been addressed throughout the chapters in this series of books and will not be repeated here, other than to note that they should usually include, as a minimum for an oral uncoated tablet, weight variation, content uniformity, hardness, friability, disintegration-dissolution specifications, and size uniformity.

Identification of critical product quality features for tablet products must be treated as a separate undertaking for each and every product. No standard or master approach exists. For example, not all tablet products have fr.ability problems. In fact, the great majority do not, and friability may then be discounted as a feature in the validation program. Rate of drug dissolution, as it relates to the rate and completeness of bioavailability, and assurance of consistency of bioavailability from lot to lot may be of great concern for some tablet products and of little or minor concern for others.

Dissolution might reasonably be expected to be of great concern in situations of potential bioavailability, such as with a very slightly soluble acidic drug moiety which has an intermediate to large dose and is only well absorbed in the upper gastrointestinal tract. In such a case, great attention must be paid to such factors as methods of wet massing, how binders are incorporated in the product, wet massing times, or the granulation method employed, rate of compression, consistency of feeding granulation to the dies, compressive force, particle size and particle size control, methods of incorporating disintegrants, and other factors depending on the method of tablet manufacture. On the other hand, the assured achievement of content uniformity in such a large-dose product, through an extensive validation program, might be totally unnecessary or of minimal concern.

The concerns of product quality might be just the reverse with a low dose of a highly soluble amine drug which is well absorbed along the gastrointestinal tract. Bioavailability assurance through validation might be completely unnecessary and pointless, but in comparison to the acidic high-dose drug previously described, content uniformity may now become the primary concern and focus of the validation efforts. In other situations, validation of both bioavailability and content uniformity goals might be warranted and in some situations neither of these quality features is of major concern because they are readily achieved under all conceivable permutations and combinations of processing conditions that could be imagined for the product.

The situations given above are intended to point out that the critical quality features are matters to be identified for each and every product. These critical quality features may depend on the pharmacokinetic properties of the drug (including but not limited to where and how the drug is absorbed), physical chemical properties of the drug, drug dose, and chemical stability of the drug.

Step 2

Review product performance against the proposed specifications. After describing the quality features which must be achieved in the product and the minimum acceptable values for each such feature, the specifications developed for that product should be reviewed and agreed upon as being appropriate and reasonable by knowledgeable people in research and development, production, and quality assurance.

Another point that might be reviewed in this step is whether or not the product in question has sets of specifications which constitute possibly critical "competing objectives." Nearly all tablet products do have competing objectives. For example, if during the manufacture of a hard, nonfriable, nondusting uncoated tablet these quality features are enhanced, then the rapid tablet disintegration and drug dissolution release rate quality features would be expected to degrade and even become unacceptable.

Another type of competing objectives circumstance is encountered with insoluble antacids. Most insoluble antacids exist as very fine powders which have very poor compressibility. Their effectiveness is related to their fine particle size and large surface, which is directly related to their ability to neutralize gastric acid. Any steps which are taken to facilitate compression by enhancing particle consolidation may be expected to reduce the activity of such antacids.

Thus, processing procedures such as precompression, increased punch dwell time, increased pressure, or procedures used to increase granule bonding cannot benefit both sets of quality features simultaneously because these processing effects will produce competing effects on the two sets of quality features, no matter how the processing effects are controlled. Fortunately, through proper formulation such competing objectives are not difficult to handle for most drugs. However, when the occasional drug comes along with such traits as a large dose, low solubility, poor wetting, borderline bioavailability, *and* poor compression properties, the fact that one is dealing with competing objectives cannot be ignored, and should be carefully considered in the design of the validation protocol.

Step 3

Identify the methodology, processes, and pieces of equipment that are or will be used in the manufacture of the product(s).

Once the product quality and acceptability standards have been established in steps 1 and 2, the process that manufactures the product must be thoroughly identified. If a tablet is made by direct compression, the process will differ significantly in the unit operations involved as compared with wet granulation. Not only must the processes that impact directly on the manufacture of the product be identified but those systems that support the process and thereby have an indirect impact on the process must be identified. Table 9 lists some of the associated systems that support tablet production and could have an impact on tablet validation considerations.

Table 9   Support Systems Associated with
the Manufacture of Pharmaceutical Solid
Dosage Forms

Heating, ventilation, air conditioning (HVAC)

Periodic maintenance systems

Water systems

Compressed gas systems (air)

Cleaning systems

Vacuum systems

Electrical

Drainage

Dispensing of raw material

Paperwork systems

Personnel training

Computer process control

Special environmental protection systems

Step 4

Identify the potentially relevant and critical process variables. The information base for this step in the total product validation is the list of
specifications and limits for the quality features which have been placed on
the product, together with the basic manufacturing process, formulation,
and raw materials specifications which were previously set. A knowledgeable development pharmacist can usually look at the product specifications
and manufacturing method, and predict the process variables and process
steps which will have the greatest potential for impacting on the particular
specifications for the product. The processing steps and control of these
steps which are expected to impact most directly on primary product objectives, such as bioavailability or drug dissolution rate, should receive
the closest attention. Examples of the types of processing variables which
should be considered for particular product specifications are binder concentration, granule density, optimal mixing time, mill settings, and others.

Step 5

Conduct the process validation experiments. Before validation experiments
can be performed, the various pieces of equipment used in the different
unit operations of the process must be certified to operate as they were
designed to. In addition, any auxiliary equipment operation-monitoring

instruments such as ammeters, wattmeters, rpm indicators, chart recorders, and temperature indicators must be in working condition and calibrated. While equipment certification should be a responsibility of a company's engineering function, those involved in the validation project must be sure that the certification is performed to ensure that the equipment used in the validation studies will function reliably.

The next step is to undertake well-designed and controlled experiments to establish the influence of the processing variables and combinations of variables on the quality features of the product. A variety of approaches can be taken, from full mathematical/statistical optimization, with the system actually being modeled, to a relatively few determinations for a drug having no bioavailability or manufacturing problems. Validation in the latter case may simply involve the documentation of current process controls and a historic review of the product's acceptance test records.

When the validation project becomes more complex, such as where competing objectives exist, or where cause and effect relationships are not obvious, the following general approach is suggested in order to develop a validation protocol.

1. Establish preliminary limits on each processing procedure, above and below which you never expect to go in practice. In some cases it will be possible to set an exact single specification for a processing procedure, such as a given mixing time. In other cases a range will be required and it should be set as noted above. A range should be used when an exact condition cannot be achieved, as in the volumes of granulating agent used, wet-massing times, tablet machine and coating pan speeds, coating weights, temperatures, or airflow rates. When such processing conditions are expected to impact on quality features, and where exact control is not feasible, project or determine the maximum range that might be reasonably expected to be encountered in practice (remember, future production runs must be inside these ranges or the product will be "outside validation").

2. Examine the listing of limits from the preceding step in light of the most critical product quality features you are to achieve. Select the processing variables *and combination of variables* along with their respective limits which you would expect to impact *least* favorably on these quality features and make the product under those conditions. Examine to see if any extremes of the above processing conditions or combination of extremes of processing conditions place the product outside the acceptance specifications for any parameter.

Step 6

Review, monitor, and revalidate as needed. Once a process has been validated it is necessary to continuously monitor the parameters controlling the process. If instruments are used they must be calibrated on a routine basis. Equipment must receive periodic maintenance so that performance does not change. Care must also be taken that no part of the process is changed. A process change, improvement or otherwise, must be revalidated. Constant review of all specifications, product and process, is also necessary to enable the specifications to be "tightened" or "broadened" to enhance the total validated system.

ACKNOWLEDGMENT

Special acknowledgment to Mr. Ken Main, P.E., Division Electrical Engineer, Aluminum Company of America, Alcoa, Tennessee, for his help and insight in the development of the computer process control section.

APPENDIX: LIST OF MANUFACTURERS

Mixer/Granulator

Drydispenser
  Jaygo, Inc.
  199 Seventh Avenue
  Hawthorne, NJ   07506

Diosna
  Dierks and Sohne
  45 Osnabruck
  Sandbachstrasse 1
  West Germany

Lodige Mixer/Granulator
MGT Vertical Mixer/Granulator
  Littleford Brothers, Inc.
  15 Empire Drive
  Florence, Kentucky   41042

Fielder Mixer/Granulator
  Raymond Automation Co.
  508 Westport Avenue
  Norwalk, Connecticut   06856

Gral Mixer/Granulator
  Maines Collette, Inc.
  P.O. Box 818
  Wheeling, IL   60090

Fluid-Bed Granulator/Dryer

Aeromatic
  198 Route 206 South
  Somerville, NJ   08876

Glatt
  Glatt Air Techniques, Inc.
  260 West Broadway
  New York, NY   10013

Freund
  Vector Corp.
  675 44th Street
  Marion, Iowa   52302

Double-Cone and Twin-Shell

Blenders with liquid feed and
vacuum drying capabilities

Double Cone Rota-Cone
  Paul O. Abbe
  146 Center Avenue
  Little Falls, NJ   07424

Twin Shell Processor
  The Patterson-Kelley Co., Inc.
  Process Equipment Division
  East Stroudsburg, PA   18301

Nauta Mixer
  Day Mixing Co.
  Cincinnati, Ohio   45212

L/D Series Blender
  Gemco, Inc.
  301 Smalley Avenue
  Middlesex, NJ   08846

Specialized Granulation Equipment

Roto Granulator
  Key International, Inc.
  480 Route 9
  Englishtown, NJ   07726

Marumerizer
  Luwa Corporation
  4433 Chesapeake Drive
  P.O. Box 16348
  Charlotte, NC   28216

REFERENCES

1. Sigman, D. A., *Drug Cos. Ind.*, *125*(5):84 (1979).
2. Beckley, J. N. and Bathgate, T. A., *Drug Cos. Ind.*, *125*(4):54 (1979).
3. Schuessler, O. P., *Pharmaceutical Plant Design in Today's Regulatory Climate.* Paper presented before the Pharmaceutical Processing Symposium, American Institute of Chemical Engineers, 88th National Meeting, Philadelphia, June 10, 1980.
4. Morrissey, J. T., *Renovation of a Pharmaceutical Facility.* Paper presented before the Pharmaceutical Processing Symposium, American Institute of Chemical Engineers, 88th National Meeting, Philadelphia, June 10, 1980.
5. Snyder, H., *Automated Production Procedures in Drug Manufacturing.* Paper presented before the First Annual Conference on Quality Programs and Government Regulations, Arlington, Virginia, April 12, 1976, Automated Process Controls and GMPs Workshop.
6. Greene, J. H., *Production Control Systems and Decisions.* Irwin, Homewood, Illinois, 1965, p. 257.
7. Dickinson, J., *Pharm. Technol.*, *2*(2):41 (1978).
8. Snyder, H. T., Battista, J. V., and Michelson, J., *Development and Technology of a Semi-Automated Continuous Extrusion Process for the Preparation of a Tablet Granulation.* Paper presented before the Industrial Pharmacy Section, 113th Annual Meeting, American Pharmaceutical Association, Dallas, April 15–29, 1966.
9. Kamman, J. P., *Pharmaceutical Plant Design for GMP and Process Efficiency.* Paper presented before the Pharmaceutical Processing Symposium, Annual Meeting, American Institute of Chemical Engineers, New York, November 17, 1977.
10. Vosnek, K. J. and Forbes, R. A., *Diosna-Granulating with Wet Particle Size Control.* Paper presented before the 69th Annual Meeting of the American Institute of Chemical Engineers, Chicago, December 2, 1976.
11. Thurn, U., Soliva, M., and Speiser, P., *Drugs Made in Germany*, *14*:12 (1971).
12. Ormos, Z. and Hung, J., *Ind. Chem.*, *1*:207 (1972).
13. Ormos, Z., Pataki, K., Osukas, B., and Hung, J., *Ind. Chem.*, *1*:307 (1973).
14. Davies, W. L. and Gloor, W. T., *J. Pharm. Sci.*, *60*:1869 (1971).
15. Rouiller, M., Gurny, R., and Doelker, E., *Pharm. Acta Technol.*, *21*(2) (1975).
16. Shevlin, E. J., *Pharm. Technol.*, *2*(3):56–59 (1978).
17. Schwartz, J. B., *Drug Dev. Ind. Phar.*, *14*(14):2071–2090 (1988).
18. *Korsch PH-800e Automated Tablet Production System Bulletin*, Korsch Tableting, Inc., Somerville, New Jersey, 1989.
19. Kristensen, H. G. and Schaefer, T., *Drug Dev. Ind. Phar.*, *13*(4,5):803–872 (1987).
20. Hunter, B. M. and Ganderton, D., *J. Pharm. Pharmacol.*, *25*(Suppl.):71P–78P (1983).
21. Lindberg, N. O., Leander, L., Wenngren, L., Heigesen, H., and Reenstierna, B., *Acta Pharm. Suecica*, *11*:603–620 (1974).

22. Leuenberger, H., Bier, H. P., and Sucker, H. B., *Pharm. Technol.*, 3(6):61−68 (1979).
23. Leuenberger, H., *Pharm. Acta Helv.*, 57:72−82 (1982).
24. Ritala, M., Jungensen, O., Holm, P., Schaefer, T., and Kristensen, H. G., *Drug Dev. Ind. Phar.*, 12(11−13):1685−1700 (1986).
25. *Compu-Coat II Bulletin*, Thomas Engineering, Inc., Hoffman Estates, Illinois, 1986.
26. Jean Y. LeFloc'h, *Automation and Networling of Coating Systems*, Thomas Engineering, Inc., Hoffman Estates, Illinois, April 1987.
27. Ritala, M., Holm, P., Schaefer, T., and Kristensen, H. G., *Drug Dev. Ind. Phar.*, 14(8):1041−1060 (1988).
28. Travers, D. N., Rogerson, A. G., and Jones, T. M., *J. Pharm. Pharmacol.*, 27(Suppl.):3P (1975).
29. Lindberg, N. O., Leander, L., and Reenstierna, B., *Drug Dev. Ind. Pharm.*, 8:775−782 (1982).
30. Ghanta, S. R., Srinivas, R., and Rhodes, C. T., *Drug Dev. Ind. Pharm.*, 10:305−311 (1984).
31. Lindberg, N. O. and Jonsson, C., *Drug Dev. Ind. Pharm.*, 9: 959−970 (1983).
32. Timko, R. J., Barrett, J. S., McHugh, P. A., Chen, S. T., and Rosenberg, X. X., *Drug Dev. Ind. Pharm.*, 13(3):405−435 (1987).
33. Kay, D. and Record, P. C., *Mfg. Chemist*, 48(9):45−46 (1978).
34. Staniforth, J. N. and Quincey, S. M., *Int. J. Pharm.*, 32: 177−185 (1986).
35. Staniforth, J. N., Walker, S., and Flanders, P., *Int. J. Pharm.*, 32:277−280 (1986).
36. Spring, M. S., *Drug Dev. Ind. Pharm.*, 9:1507−1512 (1983).
37. Fry, W. C., Stagner, W. C., and Wichman, K. C., *J. Pharm. Sci.*, 73:420−421 (1984).
38. Fry, W. C., Stanger, W. C., Wu, P. P., and Wichman, K. C., *Computer-Interfaced Capacitive Sensor for Monitoring the Granulation Process. I: Granulation Monitor Design and Application* (C. E. Capes, ed.), Proceedings of the 4th International Symposium on Agglomeration, June 2−5, Toronto, Ontario, Canada, Book Crafters, Chelsea, Michigan, 1985, pp. 497−501.
39. Fry, W. C., Wu, P. P., Wichman, K. C., and Stanger, W. C., *Granulation Monitoring*. In Proceedings of Pharm. Tech. Conference '85. Aster Publishing Corp., Springfield, Oregon, 1985, pp. 358−367.
40. Fry, W. C., Wu, P. P., Stanger, W. C., Wichman, K. C., and Anderson, N. R., *Pharm. Technol.*, 11(10):30 (1987).
41. Alleva, D. S. and Schwartz, J. B., *Drug Dev. Ind. Phar.*, 12(4): 471−487 (1986).
42. Holm, P., *Drug Dev. Ind. Phar.*, 13(9−11):1675−1701 (1987).
43. Pemon, J. P. and Schwartz, J. B., *Drug Dev. Ind. Phar.*, 13(1): 1−14 (1987).
44. Chowhan, Z. T., *Pharm. Technol.*, 12(2):26−44 (1988).
45. El-Gindy, N. A., Samaha, M. W., and El-Maradny, H. A., *Drug Dev. Ind. Phar.*, 14(7):977−1005 (1988).
46. Korsch, W., *Pharm. Technol.*, 5(4):62 (1981).
47. Lachman, L. and Cooper, J., *J. Pharm. Sci.*, 52:490 (1963).

48. Berfield, D., *Pharm. Technol.*, *1*(40):53 (1977).
49. Krause, G. and Iorio, T., *J. Pharm. Sci.*, *57*:1223 (1968).
50. Wurster, D., U.S. Patent 2,648,609, 1953.
51. Wurster, D., U.S. Patent 2,799,241, 1957.
52. Wurster, D., *J. Am. Pharm. Assoc., Sci. Ed.*, *48*:451 (1959).
53. Bulletin 303-873, Graco, Inc., 1977.
54. Skrokov, M. R. (ed.). In *Mini- and Microcomputer Control in Industrial Processes*. Van Nostrand Reinhold, New York, 1980, pp. 1–58.
55. Noyce, R. N., *Sci. Am.*, *237*(3):63 (1977).
56. Terman, L. H., *Sci. Am.*, *237*(3):163 (1977).
57. Hunter, R. P. *Automated Process Control Systems Concepts and Hardware*. Prentice-Hall, Englewood Cliffs, New Jersey, 1978, pp. 15–110, 305–335.
58. Foster, D. *Automation in Practice*. McGraw-Hill, London, 1968, pp. 48–54.
59. Leitner, M. and Cocheo, M. S. In *Mini- and Microcomputer Control in Industrial Processes* (M. R. Skrokov, ed.). Van Nostrand Reinhold, New York, 1980, pp. 128–163.
60. Thor, M. G. In *Mini- and Microcomputer Control in Industrial Processes* (M. R. Skrokov, ed.). Van Nostrand Reinhold, New York, 1980, pp. 212–219.
61. Copeland, J. R. *Microcomputers and Programmable Controllers for Process Control*. Center for Professional Advancement, East Brunswick, New Jersey, 1979.
62. Renner, K. M., *Pharm. Technol.*, *9*(12):24 (1985).
63. Gopal, C., *Pharm. Technol.*, *13*(4):20 (1989).
64. Grosswirth, M., *Output*, *1*(1):33 (1980).
65. Byers, T. E., *Manufacturing Process Validation: A Systematic Approach to Quality Assurance*. Paper presented at the Management Conference for the Pharmaceutical Industry, Purdue University, West Lafayette, Indiana, September 13–15, 1978.

2

Coating of Pharmaceutical Solid-Dosage Forms

Stuart C. Porter and Charles H. Bruno

Colorcon, West Point, Pennsylvania

I. INTRODUCTION

The application of coatings to the surface of pharmaceutical solid-dosage forms, especially tablets, has been practiced for over 150 years.

Although such a process is often applied to a dosage form that is functionally complete, and thus may cause us to reflect on the need for incurring the additional expense, it is evident that the continued use of coating processes in pharmaceutical production remains very popular. Such popularity relates to the many benefits obtained when a dosage form is coated, which include:

Improved esthetic qualities of the product
Masking of unpleasant taste and odor
Enabling the product to be more easily swallowed by the patient
Facilitating handling, particularly in high-speed filling/packaging
   lines
Improving product stability
Modifying drug-release characteristics

Over the course of time, coating processes have developed from the art of earlier years to those that are more technologically advanced and controlled such that compliance with good manufacturing practices (GMPs) is facilitated. The design of new equipment, the development of new coating materials, and the recognition of the impact of applied coatings on subsequent release of drug from the dosage form have all contributed to improved products.

Changes that have occurred in coating processes reflect a desire to:

Consistently obtain a finished product of high and reproducible
   quality
Achieve processes in which the economics are maximized, particularly
   with respect to process times and equipment utilization

While the methods for applying coatings to solid-dosage forms are
varied, and some are described elsewhere in this book, this chapter will
focus on the processes of sugar coating and film coating, and will discuss
these processes with respect to:

Raw materials
Application techniques
Potential problems
Available coating equipment

II. SUGAR COATING

A. Introduction

The process of sugar coating, which has its origins in the confectionery
industry, is perhaps one of the oldest pharmaceutical processes still in
existence.

Although in recent years modernization of the process with respect to
panning equipment and automation has taken place, sugar coating is still
considered to be more of an art rather than a science.

While methods (and materials) for coatings date back over 1000 years
(early Islam makes reference to pill coatings based on mucillage of
psyllium seeds), the current pharmaceutical process of sugar coating
originated in the middle of the nineteenth century when sugar as a raw
material became plentiful, and the forerunner of modern panning equipment was invented.

Although the tendency is to produce pharmaceutical coating pans from
stainless steel, early pans were made from copper because drying was effected by means of an externally applied heat source. Current thinking,
even with conventional pans, is to dry the coated tablets with a supply
of heated air and to extract the moisture and dust-laden air from the
vicinity of the pan.

Although the sugar-coating process has experienced declining popularity in the United States, it is still retained by many companies worldwide, since many advantages can be realized, including:

Raw materials are inexpensive and readily available
Raw materials are widely accepted with few regulatory problems (with
   the exception of perhaps colors)
Inexpensive, simple equipment can be used
Sugar-coated products are esthetically pleasing and have wide con-
   sumer acceptability
The process is generally not as critical (as film coating) and recovery
   (or rework) procedures are more readily accomplished

However, in spite of the relative simplicity of the sugar-coating process, it does have some potential shortcomings, for example:

The size and weight of the finished product results in increased packaging and shipping costs

The brittleness of the coatings renders the coated tablets susceptible to potential damage if mishandled

The achievement of high esthetic quality often requires the services of highly skilled coating operators

The final gloss is achieved by a polishing step which can make imprinting difficult

The inherent complexity (from the standpoint of the variety of procedures and formulations used) of the process makes automation more difficult

In spite of these difficulties, many companies have made excellent use of modern process technology (including automation), so that the requirements of current GMPs, including documentation, are readily achieved with a high degree of reproducibility in the quality and performance of the finished product.

B. Raw Materials Used in Sugar Coating

As expected, the major ingredient used is sugar (sucrose), although this may be substituted by other materials (such as sorbitol) for low calorie/diabetic products (typically in the candy industry). Sugar-coating formulations are for the most part aqueous.

The sugar-coating process consists of various steps, each designed to achieve a particular function. Consequently, a variety of additives may be incorporated into each type of formulation. Examples of such additives are:

Fillers (calcium carbonate, talc, titanium dioxide)
Colorants (dyes, aluminum lakes, iron oxides, titanium dioxide)
Film formers (acacia, gelatin, cellulose derivatives)
Antiadhesives (talc)
Flavors
Surfactants (as wetting agents and dispersion aids)

Although most of the coating formulations used in the sugar-coating process are applied as liquids, some (e.g., dusting powders) are applied dry.

A typical sugar-coating process encompasses five stages:

1. Sealing
2. Subcoating
3. Grossing
4. Color coating
5. Polishing

While each of these stages is varied, the common feature throughout is that the process requires repeated applications of coating liquid, each application followed by a period during which the tablets are allowed to tumble freely to allow complete distribution of the coating materials, and finally, a drying period when moisture is removed from the coating prior to the next application.

Sealing

Most of the coating formulations used in the sugar-coating process are aqueous, whereas tablet cores are typically porous, highly absorbent, and formulated to disintegrate rapidly when they make contact with water. Consequently, if these cores are not appropriately protected at the outset, ultimate product stability (both physical and chemical) can be seriously compromised. The purpose of sealing is to offer this initial protection, and to prevent some tablet core ingredients from migrating into the coating, and ultimately spoiling the appearance of the final product.

Sealing is accomplished by the application of a polymer-based coating (either by ladle or spray techniques) to the surfaces of the tablet cores. Examples of polymers that might be used include shellac, zein, hydroxypropyl methylcellulose (HPMC), polyvinyl acetate phthalate (PVAP), and cellulose acetate phthalate (CAP). These are typically dissolved (at a 15–30% w/w concentration) in an appropriate organic solvent, preferably one of the denatured ethanol products.

While use of shellac has been universal, this polymer can cause problems. One problem results from the fact that shellac can polymerize on storage, causing the solubility characteristics of the coating to change. This problem can either be minimized by incorporating PVP into the shellac formulation [1] or by using one of the other, more stable polymers (such as PVAP).

When using any of the water-insoluble polymers as the basis for a seal-coat formulation, it is important to apply only the minimum quantity of coating needed to give the appropriate protection; otherwise drug-release characteristics may well be affected.

When the seal coat is applied by a ladle technique, detackifiers, such as talc, are often used to minimize the risk of "twinning" or clumping. Overzealous use of talc should be avoided, however, otherwise it might be difficult for the subsequent sugar coat to bond to the surface of the seal coat.

Finally, if the final product is to have enteric properties, this result is usually achieved by using one of the enteric polymers (such as PVAP or CAP) as the basis for the seal coat and ensuring that sufficient coating material is applied.

Subcoating

Subcoating is the first major step of the sugar-coating process and provides the means for rounding off the tablet edges and building up the core weight. It also provides the foundation for the remainder of the sugar-coating process, with any weakness in the final sugar coat often being attributable to weaknesses in the subcoat.

In order to facilitate this buildup, subcoating formulations almost always contain high levels of fillers such as talc, calcium carbonate, calcium sulfate, kaolin, and titanium dioxide. In addition, auxiliary film formers such as acacia, gelatin, or one of the cellulose derivatives may

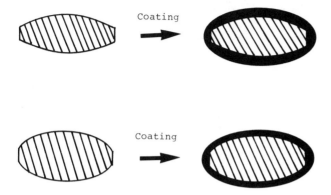

Figure 1 Schematic of examples of acceptable tablet-core shapes for sugar coating.

also be included in order to improve the structural integrity of the coating.

It is important during subcoating to get effective coverage of the coating material over the tablet corners and on the edges if a quality result is to be achieved. To this end, selection of appropriate tablet shapes is important. Certainly, tablet shapes which minimize the corners (such as tablets compacted on deep concave punches or dual radius punches), as shown in Figure 1, can aid in effective coverage. Additionally, it is necessary to minimize tablet edge thickness, otherwise twinning will be more prevalent and incomplete edge coverage (by the coating) is likely to occur (Fig. 2).

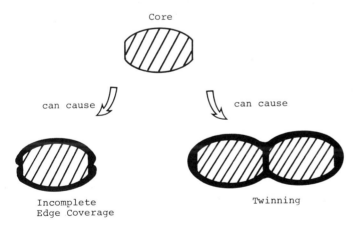

Figure 2 Schematic example of poor tablet core shape for sugar coating. (The twinning problem illustrated is more prevalent when using capsule-shaped tablets.)

Table 1   Examples of Formulations Used in the Lamination Subcoating
Process

		I	II
Binder solutions	Gelatin	3.3% w/w	6.0% w/w
	Gum acacia	8.7	8.0
	Sucrose	55.3	45.0
	Distilled water	32.7	41.0
Dusting powders	Calcium carbonate	40.0% w/w	–
	Titanium dioxide	5.0	1.0
	Talc (asbestos free)	25.0	61.0
	Sucrose (powdered)	28.0	38.0
	Gum acacia	2.0	–

Two main approaches to the process of subcoating are often practiced,
depending on whether a lamination technique or a suspension subcoat
formulation is used. Each has its distinct features and advantages.

LAMINATION PROCESS. The lamination process is perhaps the older
of the two techniques used, and involves alternate applications of binder
solutions and dusting powder until the required level of coating is achieved.
While materials and formulations for binder solutions and dusting powders
are varied, some typical formulations are shown in Table 1.

When using the lamination technique it is important to ensure that a
careful balance is achieved between the relative amounts of binder solution
and dusting powders used. Underutilization of dusting powders increases
the risk of sticking and twinning, whereas overdusting can create tablets
that have brittle coatings.

While achievement of quality results with the lamination process typically requires employment of skilled operators, there is no doubt that this
type of process can permit rapid buildup of the coating.

On the downside, the lamination process can be messy, more difficult
to use by less-skilled operators, and more difficult to automate.

SUSPENSION SUBCOATING PROCESS. In simple terms, suspension
subcoating formulations result from combining the binder and powder
formulations used in the more traditional lamination process. Examples of
a typical formulation are shown in Table 2.

Use of the suspension subcoating approach reduces the complexity of
the process, allowing it to be used effectively by less-experienced operators, and ultimately facilitates automation of the process.

Table 2 Examples of Suspension Subcoating Formulations

	I	II
Sucrose	40.0% w/w	58.25% w/w
Calcium carbonate	20.0	18.45
Talc (asbestos free)	12.0	–
Titanium dioxide	1.0	1.00
Gum acacia	2.0	–
Gelatin (120 bloom)	–	0.01
Distilled water	25.0	22.29

Grossing (or Smoothing)

In order to manufacture a quality sugar-coated product, it is imperative that the surface of the coating be smooth and free from irregularities prior to application of the color coat.

While the requisite smoothness may be achieved during the application of the subcoat, it is not unusual to find that further smoothing (prior to color coating) is necessary. Depending on the degree of smoothing required, the smoothing coating may simply consist of a 70% sucrose syrup, often containing titanium dioxide as an opacifier/whitening agent, and possibly tinted with other colorants to provide a good base for subsequent application of the color coat.

If a substantial amount of smoothing is required, as in the case in which the subcoat tablets have a pitted surface, other additives (such as talc, calcium carbonate, corn starch) may be used in low concentrations to hasten the smoothing process.

Color Coating

Many would agree that color coating is one of the most important steps in the sugar-coating process because of the immediate visual impact that is associated with overall quality.

Use of appropriate colorants, which are dissolved or dispersed in the coating syrup, allows the desired color to be achieved. Two basic approaches to coloring sugar-coating syrups exist, each giving rise to differing coating techniques. These two approaches involve the use of either water-soluble dyes or water-insoluble pigments.

Prior to the 1950s, soluble dyes were used extensively to achieve the desired color. This technique was handled by an experienced coater, who had acquired his skill over many years of work experience. Much of the color coating required 2 or 3 days, and unless handled properly, resulted in tablets that were nonuniform in color or mottled, since the soluble dye can migrate to the surface during drying. Additionally, color reproducibility from batch-to-batch was not predictable, and light sensitivity with subsequent fading was also a problem when using dyes.

The use of insoluble, certified lakes has virtually replaced the soluble dye in pharmaceutical tablet coating. Lakes have several advantages; namely, color migration on drying is eliminated, since lakes are insoluble, light stability is improved, mottled tablets are a rare occurrence, and coating time is substantially shortened. While lakes are insoluble, they are not totally opaque. Consequently, coloring properties can be optimized by combining lakes with opacifiers such as titanium dioxide. The most efficient process for color coating involves the use of predispersed, opacified lake suspensions. By varying the ratios of lake and opacifier, various shades can be produced.

DYE-COATING PROCESS. The features of a typical sugar-coating process that utilizes water-soluble dyes as colorants include:

Sequential application of coating syrups containing specific dye concentrations (typically, as coating progresses, dye concentrations in the syrup may be increased until the target color is achieved)

Addition of a quantity of colored syrup (at each stage) that is sufficient to just wet the *total* tablet surface, followed by gentle drying to achieve requisite smoothness and prevent color migration

Employment of relatively low concentrations of colorant (necessary to achieve final color uniformity), resulting in a requirement to make anywhere up to 50 separate color syrup applications (particularly for dark colors)

There is no doubt that in the hands of a skilled operator the quality of sugar-coated tablets that employ the dye-coating method are difficult to match (this is particularly true from the standpoint of "cleanliness," depth, and "brilliance" of the final color).

However, such a process is not without its difficulties, namely:

Color migration problems (resulting from either underdrying or too rapid a drying) are commonplace.

Color variability, across the surface of individual tablets, which occurs as the result of unevenness of the subcoat layer and transparency of the color coat.

Tablet-to-tablet color variability which may result because the transparent coloring system has not been uniformly distributed.

Batch-to-batch color variation which is likely to occur because of variability in the total quantity of color applications made, or as a result of small differences in amount of colorant weighed out for each batch (water-soluble dyes produce very intense colors and a little goes a long way).

The process is time consuming (because of the slow drying required and the need to make so many individual color applications).

PIGMENT-COATING PROCESS. Pigments have demonstrable advantages over water-soluble dyes, two important ones being:

1. Lack of solubility in aqueous media (which eliminates color migration on drying)
2. Superior light stability

However, because pigments are discrete, insoluble particles, careful attention must be paid to the pigment-dispersion process. Hence, the popularity of commercially available pigment-dispersion concentrates.

Some of the major characteristics of sugar-coating formulations and processes when pigment colorant systems are used include:

Use of a single-color concentration throughout the color-coating process, thus making it easier to achieve the target end color (in order to obtain a different color, it is necessary to vary the ratios of the lake pigments with respect to the opacifier, titanium dioxide)

Achievement of batch color uniformity after only a few applications of colored syrup (often color development is complete after eight to 10 applications, and the remaining five to seven applications are simply used to smooth off the tablet surface)

Reduced drying times resulting from the fact that the insoluble colorants do not migrate on drying, and thus can be dried more rapidly

Overall shortened color-coating process as a result of reduced number of color applications and shortened drying times

One should, however, be aware of what some might construe to be disadvantages with pigment coloring systems and the associated coating process:

Colorants derived from pigments (especially when lakes are used in combination with titanium dioxide) are generally not as bright or clean-looking as those obtained with soluble colorants.

If the pigment color-coating process is rushed, it is relatively easy to produce rough tablets that are difficult to polish.

There is a need to ensure that pigments are effectively dispersed in the coating syrup (certainly, pigment color concentrates eliminate this problem), otherwise color "specking" might be a problem.

Since most pigment coloring systems contain lakes (which are typically acidic), it is inadvisable to keep coating systems hot for any length of time once the color has been added; otherwise excessive amounts of invert sugar will be formed.

With the exception of the first of these problems, all the others can easily be avoided, and thus advantages of the pigment coating process tend to prevail, making it the process of choice.

Summarizing these advantages, they are:

Greater ability to get a uniform color on the surface of each tablet
Greater batch-to-batch color uniformity
Significant reduction in thickness of the color coat
Significant reduction in processing time

Polishing (Glossing)

Since freshly color-coated tablets are typically dull (i.e., they have a matte surface finish), it is necessary to polish them in some way to achieve the gloss that is typical of finished sugar-coated tablets.

While methods to achieve a desirable gloss tend to vary considerably, it is generally recommended that tablets should be trayed overnight (prior to polishing) to ensure that they are sufficiently dry. Excessively high moisture levels in tablets submitted for polishing will:

Make achievement of a good gloss difficult
Increase the risk of "blooming" and "sweating" over longer periods of time

Glossing or polishing can be carried out in various types of equipment (e.g., canvas- or wax-lined pans), including that used for applying the sugar coating itself (which is more typical in automated processes).
Polishing systems that may be used include:

Organic-solvent-based solutions of waxes (beeswax, carnauba wax, candelilla wax)
Alcoholic slurries of waxes
Finely powdered mixtures of dry waxes
Pharmaceutical glazes (typically alcohol solutions of various forms of shellac, often containing additional waxes)

Printing

If sugar-coated tablets are to be further identified with a product name, dosage strength, or company name or logo, this has to be accomplished by means of a printing process.
Typically, such printing involves the application of a pharmaceutical branding ink to the coated tablet surface by means of a printing process known as offset rotogravure.
Sugar-coated tablets may be printed either before or after polishing, with each approach having its advantages and disadvantages. Printing prior to polishing enables the ink to adhere more strongly to the tablet surface, but any legend may subsequently be removed by either friction or as a result of contact with organic solvents during the polishing process. Printing after polishing avoids the problem of print rub-off during polishing, but branding inks do not always adhere well to the waxed tablet surface. Adhesion of printing inks can be enhanced by application (prior to printing) of a modified shellac, preprint base solution.

C. Application Techniques

Application of sugar coatings to pharmaceutical tablets has long been considered one that requires a significant amount of skill on the part of the operator. While this philosophy has a lot of truth in it, and while it is certainly difficult for untrained operators to achieve quality results, the employment of special techniques (such as the use of suspension subcoat formulations and coatings colored with proprietary pigment dispersions) makes quality results achievable even for less-skilled operators.
While many different types of coating formulation (Sec. II.B) will be applied during the coating process, similarities in application exist for each of them.
The basic application procedure in each case involves three steps in sequence:

1. Application of an appropriate volume (sufficient to completely cover the surface of every tablet in the batch) of coating liquid to a cascading bed of tablets
2. Distribution of the coating liquid uniformly across the surface of each tablet in the batch
3. Drying of the coating liquid once uniform distribution is achieved

Specific details of actual procedures adopted may vary from company-to-company. However, the ultimate goal in each case is to ensure that the coating is uniformly distributed throughout the batch. Although this goal may be facilitated by the manner in which the coating liquid is applied, and by manual stirring of the wet tablets to help eliminate "dead spots" (regions in the tablet bed that are difficult to reach with the coating liquid), the main mechanism for distribution of the coating liquid relates to the shearing action that occurs as tablets cascade over one another.

For the greatest period of time, sugar-coating liquids were applied manually by allowing premeasured quantities of coating liquid to be poured across the moving tablet bed. In recent times, there has been a greater reliance on mechanical dosing techniques, involving the use of spray guns or dosing "sparges" (Fig. 3).

One of the major misconceptions concerning the use of mechanical dosing techniques, particularly spray guns, is that they can exert a major influence on uniformity of distribution of the sugar-coating liquid. Again, it is important to emphasize that the main factor controlling distribution of the coating liquid relates to contact between the cascading tablets, and transfer of liquid from one tablet to another as the result of this contact. Thus, particularly when using spray guns, it is not necessary to finely atomize the coating liquid in order to ensure effective distribution of that liquid. Indeed, excessive atomization can cause "fogging" where much of the coating liquid can end up on the walls of the pan rather than on the tablets. Consequently, many advocates for the use of spray guns simply allow the liquid to stream from the nozzle. For this reason, use of a device similar to that shown in Figure 3 can be equally effective and less expensive than using spray guns.

Summarizing, since coating uniformity is achieved as the result of tablet-to-tablet transfer of liquid coating material, it is not necessary for each tablet to pass through the zone of application (which is a necessity in the film-coating process). Factors which influence coating uniformity in the sugar-coating process are that:

The coating material remains fluid until it is spread across the surface of every tablet in the batch.

Sufficient volume of coating liquid is applied to ensure that every tablet in the batch is capable of being wetted (thus liquid volumes may have to be changed as the process progresses in order to reflect changes in tablet size and drying conditions).

The coating pan exhibits good mixing characteristics, particularly so that dead spots are avoided (many coating pans of conventional design, i.e., the traditional pear-shaped design, may have to be modified by inclusion of mixing baffles, otherwise mixing may have to be augmented by manual stirring of the tablets by the operator).

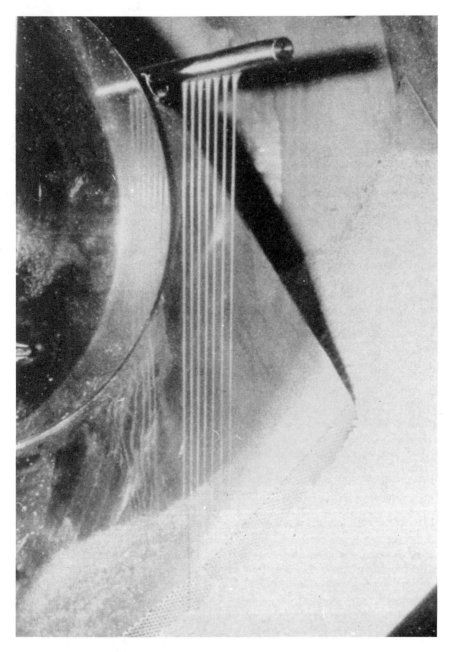

Figure 3   Figure showing a dosing sparge for sugar coating.

D. Problems in Sugar Coating

In any coating process, a variety of problems may arise. Often such problems may be related to formulation issues that have been compounded by those associated with processing.

Problems with Tablet Core Robustness

The attritional effects of any coating process on tablet cores is well understood. Consequently, tablet cores must be sufficiently robust to resist the stress to which they will be exposed during coating.

With this in mind, particular attention must be paid to important tablet physical properties such as hardness (diametral crushing strength), friability, and lamination tendency. Failure to address these issues is likely to result in a situation in which tablet fragmentation occurs during the coating process.

Tablet fragmentation is not only a problem from the standpoint that the broken tablets will obviously not be saleable (and thus would have to be inspected out), but additionally, the broken fragments may typically become "glued" (because of the adhesive nature of the coating fluids) to the surface of undamaged tablets (Fig. 4); thus spoiling a significant portion of the batch.

Quality Problems with Finished Tablets

CHIPPING OF COATINGS. Sugar coatings are inherently brittle and thus prone to chipping if mishandled. Addition of small quantities of polymers (such as cellulosics, polyvinyl pyrrolidone, acacia, or gelatin) to one or more of the various coating formulations often helps to improve structural integrity, and thus reduces chipping problems.

Excessive use of insoluble fillers and pigments tends to increase the brittleness of sugar coatings, and thus should be avoided where possible.

CRACKING OF THE COATING. Tablet cores that expand, either during or after coating, are likely to cause the coating to crack (Fig. 5). Such expansion may result from moisture absorption by the tablet core, or may be caused by stress-relaxation of the core after compaction (a phenomenon which is known to occur, for example, with ibuprofen). Moisture sorption can be minimized by appropriate use of a seal coat, whereas expansion due to postcompaction stress relaxation can be resolved by extending the time between the compaction event and commencement of sugar coating.

NONDRYING COATINGS. Inability to dry sugar coatings properly, especially those based on sucrose, is often an indicator that excessive levels (greater than 5%) of invert sugar is present. Inversion of sucrose is exacerbated by keeping sucrose syrups at elevated temperatures under acidic conditions for extended periods of time. Such conditions occur when sugar-coating solutions containing aluminum lakes are kept hot for too long, or such sugar-coating formulations are constantly being reheated to redissolve sugar that is beginning to crystallize out.

TWINNING (OR BUILDUP OF MULTIPLES). By their very nature, sugar-coating formulations are very sticky, particularly as they begin to

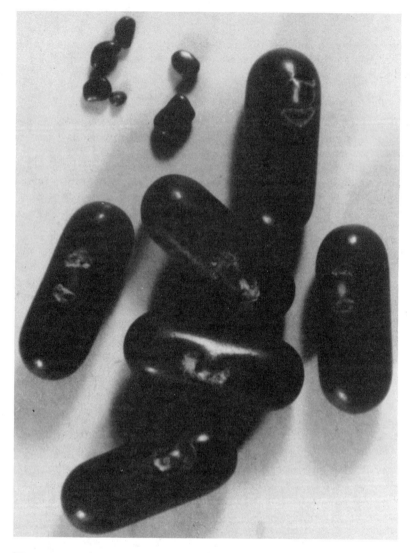

Figure 4   Figure showing how broken tablets can ruin a whole batch of product in sugar coating.

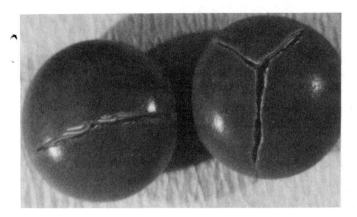

Figure 5   Sugar-coated tablets with cracked coating.

dry, and allow adjacent tablets to stick together. Buildup of multiples
really becomes a problem when the tablets being coated have flat surfaces
(as shown in Fig. 2) which can easily come into contact with one another.
This can be particularly troublesome with high-dose, capsule-shaped
tablets that have high edge walls. Appropriate choice in tablet punch design can be effectively used to minimize the problem.

UNEVEN COLOR. Because it has a major impact on final tablet appearance, the color-coating stage of the sugar-coating process is critical
to ultimate tablet quality.

Uneven distribution of color, particularly with the darker colors, is
often visually apparent, and thus a major cause of batch rejection. Many
factors may contribute to this type of problem, including:

Poor distribution of coating liquids during application. This may be
    caused by poor mixing of tablets in the coating process, or failure
    to add sufficient liquid to coat completely the surface of every
    tablet in the batch.
Color migration of water-soluble dyes while the coating is drying.
Unevenness of the surface of the subcoat when using dye-colored
    coatings. This unevenness causes a variation in thickness of the
    transparent color layer that is perceived as different color
    intensities.
"Washing back" of pigment-colored color coatings. While pigments do
    not migrate on drying, if excessive quantities of coating liquid are
    applied during the coloring process, there is a tendency for the
    previously applied (and dried) color layers to be redissolved and
    distributed nonuniformly; thus giving rise to nonuniform appear-
    ance. This problem is particularly noticeable for formulations pre-
    dominantly colored with aluminum lakes where the level of opacify-
    ing pigments (such as titanium dioxide) is low (i.e., dark colors).
Excessive drying between color applications. This can cause erosion
    of the color layer and contributes to unevenness in the color coat.

"BLOOMING" AND "SWEATING." Residual moisture (in finished sugar-coated tablets) can often be a problem. Over a period of time, this moisture can diffuse out and affect the quality of the product. Moderate levels of moisture egress cause the polish of the product to take on a fogged appearance, a phenomenon often termed blooming. At higher levels (of moisture egress), the moisture may appear like beads of perspiration on the tablet surface. This second phenomenon, often called sweating, can be much more serious, since tablets stored in closed containers will ultimately stick together.

Obtaining appropriate levels of moisture in the sugar coating is conducive to good polish characteristics (polishing can be difficult if the tablets are too dry) and avoidance of sweating and blooming. Thus, great care has to be taken with the drying stage at the end of each application of coating liquid as well as to selection of appropriate racking/drying of tablets prior to polishing.

"MARBLING." One of the secrets to achieving a high-quality, sugar-coated product is to ensure that color is uniformly distributed in the color layer, and at the same time at the end of the application of the color coating that a smooth coating surface (prior to polishing) is obtained.

Failure to achieve the requisite smoothness often results in a marbled appearance on polishing. This problem occurs as the result of the collection of wax in the small surface depressions (Fig. 6) of a rough coating and is particularly evident with darker colors.

Recovery of Reject Sugar-Coated Tablets

Owing to the amount of material applied as a coating in the sugar-coating process, it is not appropriate to grind up reject sugar-coated tablets for recompaction. One potentially viable recovery procedure (although one not without its difficulties because of handling problems) is to wash off the sugar coating by carefully dipping the coated tablets (held on a screen)

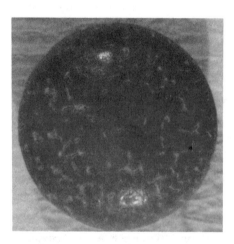

Figure 6 Figure showing marbled appearance on the surface of sugar-coated tablets resulting from wax buildup during polishing of rough tablets.

into a water bath until sufficient coating is removed such that on subsequent refinishing, the desired quality is achievable. Once the requisite quantity of coating is removed, the tablets can be dried by tumbling in a coating pan under a warm air stream (50°C). Such a procedure must obviously be validated to ensure that overall product quality is not compromised for the sake of improving visual quality.

III. FILM COATING

A. Introduction

Film coating is quite a complex process that draws on technologies associated with polymer chemistry, industrial adhesives and paints, and chemical engineering. The process of film coating can be simplified to represent one that involves the application of thin (in the range of $20-200$ μm), polymer-based coatings to an appropriate substrate (tablets, beads, granules, capsules, drug powders, and crystals) under conditions that permit:

Balance between, and control of, the coating liquid addition rate and drying process

Uniformity of distribution of the coating liquid across the surface of product being coated

Optimization of the quality (both visual and functional) of the final coated product

While film coatings can be applied by manual ladling techniques, they now almost always utilize a spray-atomization technique.

In the spray-application process, bulk coating liquids are finely atomized and delivered in such a state that droplets (of coating liquid) retain sufficient fluidity to wet the surface of the product being coated, spread out, and coalesce to form a film. Because of the highly adhesive (or "tacky") nature of partially dried droplets, it is imperative that the droplets of coating liquid dry almost instantaneously the moment they contact the surface of the substrate; otherwise sticking and picking will occur. Hence, there is a need to strike an appropriate balance between liquid application rate and the drying process. A simplified schematic of the film-coating process is shown in Figure 7.

Because of the rapid drying that typically takes place during the application of film coatings, uniformity of distribution of the coating is controlled both by uniformity of application of the coating liquid (i.e., the number of spray guns used, types of spray patterns used, and fineness of atomization of coating liquid) and the uniformity of mixing (controlled by pan speed, baffle design, tablet size and shape) of the product being coated. Unlike sugar coating, it is not desirable in film coating to have partially dry coating material being transferred from one tablet to another, since this would create imperfections in the coating that would be readily evident at the end of the coating process. However, this does not mean that the tumbling action (of tablets, etc.) in a coating process has no effect on ultimate coating structure. On the contrary, Rowe [2] has described how the high shear developed at the tablet surface (as the result of the mutual rubbing together of adjacent tablets) can promote sufficient flow of the coating (which induces a leveling effect) to achieve better cohesion within the film.

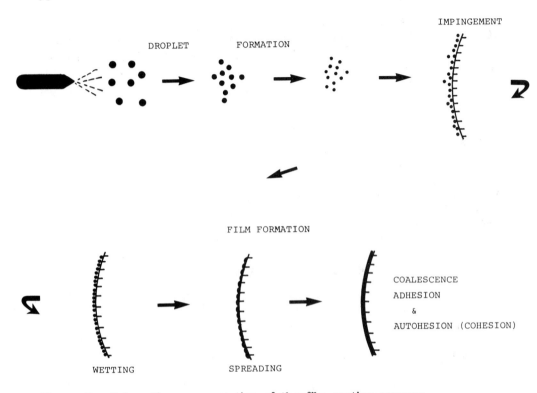

Figure 7   Schematic representation of the film-coating process.

Most current film-coating processes are considered to be continuous; that is, application of coating liquid continues uninterrupted until all the coating material has been applied. However, it is perhaps more appropriate to consider film coating as a discontinuous process, since each tablet (or granule, etc.) receives only a small fraction of its total coating each time it passes through the spray zone. Thus, film coatings are generally built up as a series of layers one upon another so that the final coating may structurally be far from homogeneous (Fig. 8).

Film coating has supplanted sugar coating as the method of choice for coating pharmaceutical solid-dosage forms, even though many people consider the elegance of the sugar-coated product to be superior. The major advantages of film coating (that have made this the preferred process) include:

Substantial reduction in quantity of coating applied (2−4% for film coating, compared with 50−100% for sugar coating)

Faster processing times

Improvement in process efficiency and output

Greater flexibility in optimizing formulations as a result of the availability of a wide range of coating materials and systems

A simplified process (compared to sugar coating) that facilitates automation

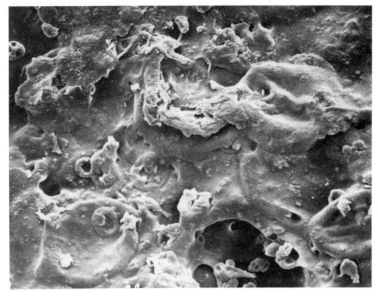

(a)

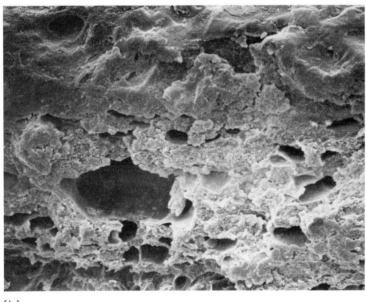

(b)

Figure 8 Scanning electron micrographs of film-coated tablets to show heterogeneous film structure. (a) Surface view, ×1000 and (b) transverse section through coating, ×1000.

Ability to be applied to a wide range of pharmaceutical products (e.g., tablets, capsules, granules, nonpareils, powders, drug crystals)

It is important to note, however, that in the early days of film coating, processing relied heavily on converting existing sugar-coating pans (which were conventional in design) by appropriate addition of air-handling and spraying equipment. Such conversions were relatively unsophisticated, and created processes where drying efficiencies were adequate at best. Consequently, to ensure that the conversion from sugar coating to film coating was successful, volatile organic solvents had to be used to help offset the deficiencies in drying capacity that the conventional processing pans exhibited.

Over the years, as film coating has grown in popularity, use of organic solvents (with their associated flammability, toxicity, and environmental pollution hazards) has proven somewhat limiting. Fortunately, significant improvements in processing equipment have facilitated the introduction of aqueous-based coating formulations. The result is that aqueous film-coating processes are used preferentially by a majority of manufacturers (of film-coated products). A useful review of aqueous coating systems has been given by McGinity [3].

Types of Film Coatings Used

The applications for use of film coatings are quite diverse. While such applications require some functionality of the coating formulation, it is not uncommon to see film coatings described as either functional or nonfunctional. Functionality in this context relates specifically to an ability to modify drug-release characteristics. Nonfunctional (or conventional) film coatings are typically reserved for situations in which it is necessary to improve product appearance, ease of swallowing, and product stability, and for taste masking. Functional film coatings are used when drug-release characteristics need to be modified, and are represented by enteric coatings and sustained- (or controlled-) release coatings.

Factors Affecting the Quality of Film Coatings

Film coating is a process in which the results obtained are attributable to the complex interaction of numerous factors. Application of a statistical design approach [4-6] (in both formulation and process development) can play a significant role in the optimization of the whole process. Additional optimization of process conditions can be achieved by employment of an appropriate thermodynamic model (such as that proposed by Ebey) [7]. Such an approach may be necessary when designing an automated coating process. These thermodynamic models can also be used to identify critical processing variables in the aqueous process where the margin for error may be low.

In order to better understand those factors that influence the quality (both visual and functional) of the finished coated product, it is necessary to examine the factors that have an effect on:

Interaction between the core material (substrate) and the applied coating

The drying process
The uniformity of distribution of the coating

Some of these important factors are highlighted in Tables 3 – 5.

Mechanisms of Film Formation for Film-Coating Systems

In the early days, pharmaceutical film-coating formulations consisted of solutions of polymers (and other additives) in organic solvents or organic-solvent mixtures. As utilization of the film-coating process became more common, and as regulatory pressures relating to health, safety, and protection of the environment have grown, a transition to using aqueous solutions of polymers has occurred. More recently, availability of aqueous polymeric dispersions (commonly called latices or pseudolatices) has attracted interest, particularly for situations in which the final dried coating needs to be water insoluble (as with modified-release products).

Clearly, modern film-coating practices require that coatings be formed from either polymeric solutions or polymeric dispersions. Since these coating systems are initially liquids, the coating process involves the conversion of a liquid into a "dry solid." However, polymers used in film coating are, for the most part, amorphous, and thus the term dry solid can be misleading. In order to clarify this situation, one can consider that:

A solid film is one which will not flow significantly under those forces to which it is subjected at the time of observation [18].
A practical definition [19] of a dry film is one that will resist blocking when two coated surfaces (e.g., two coated tablets) are brought into contact, for 2 seconds, under a pressure of 14 kPa (20 psi).
Such block resistance occurs when the viscosity of the coating exceeds 10^7 Pa.s (10^8 P).
A viscosity conducive to such blocking occurs when, according to the relationship proposed by Williams et al. [20], a coating is exposed to temperature conditions approximately 20°C above its glass-transition temperature (T_g).

Since pharmaceutical film-coating processes may now employ polymeric solutions (organic-solvent based or aqueous) or aqueous polymeric dispersions, the formulator and process engineer must be very much aware of how such coatings form films in order to be sure that appropriate formulation additives and process conditions are employed to achieve consistent, quality results.

FORMULATION OF FILMS FROM POLYMERIC SOLUTIONS. The film-forming process, and internal structure of the final dried coating, will very much depend upon the rate of solvent evaporation. Rate of solvent evaporation will in turn be controlled by the latent heat of vaporization of that solvent and the drying conditions provided in the process.

Film formation generally comprises:

Initial rapid evaporation of solvent from the atomized droplets of coating liquid, causing an increase in polymer concentration (and, hence, viscosity) and contraction in volume of the droplets

Table 3 Factors Influencing Interaction Between Substrate and Coating

Factor	Has influence on
1. Tablet core	
Ingredients	Wetting by coating liquid Adhesion of dry film [8]
Porosity	Adhesion of dry film [9]
Surface roughness	Wetting by coating liquid Spreading of coating liquid across surface Roughness of coating [10]
2. Coating liquid	
Solids content	Roughness of dry coating [5] Coating liquid viscosity [11]
Viscosity	Spreading of coating liquid across surface of substrate Coalescence of droplets of coating liquid into a continuous film
Surface tension	Wetting of surface of substrate by coating liquid Spreading of coating liquid across surface of substrate Coalescence of droplets of coating liquid into a continuous film
3. Drying process	
Drying rate	Viscosity of coating liquid at time of contact with surface of substrate Structure of dried coating
Heat	Development of internal stress within film (and effect on adhesion and cohesion) [12] Mechanical properties of coating (and effect on defects) [13]

Table 4　Factors Influencing the Drying Process

Factor	Has influence on
1. Spray equipment	
Nozzle design	Fineness of atomization of coating liquid [5,11] (and thus evaporation rate of solvent/vehicle)
Atomizing air (for air-spray nozzles)	Fineness of atomization of coating liquid [5,11] (and thus evaporation rate of solvent/vehicle)
Number of spray guns used	Uniform distribution of coating liquid
	Avoidance of localized overwetting
2. Drying conditions	
Air flow Temperature Humidity	Rate at which solvent/vehicle *can* be removed from the coating liquid
	Product temperature
3. Spray rate	
Nozzle design Number of spray guns Pumping system	Rate at which solvent/vehicle *needs* to be removed from coating liquid
	Product temperature
4. Solids content of coating liquid	Quantity of solvent/vehicle that *must* be removed from coating liquid

Further loss of solvent from the film (that is, coalescing on the surface
　　of the dosage form) at a slower rate which is now controlled by
　　the rate of diffusion of solvent through the polymer matrix
Immobilization of the polymer molecules at the "solidification point"
Further gradual solvent loss from the film at a very much reduced
　　rate

Solvent loss from the film coating will be continuous but at an ever-
decreasing rate. Solvent loss from the polymer matrix is governed by
the amount of space between the polymer molecules (usually termed the
free volume). As solvent loss progresses, the glass-transition temperature
of the polymer film *increases* and free volume *decreases*. Ultimately, free
volume becomes so small that further solvent loss is so restricted that total
removal of solvent from the coating becomes almost impossible. Indeed,
total solvent removal requires heating the film to a temperature significantly above the glass-transition temperature of the solvent-free polymer

Table 5   Factors Influencing Uniformity of Distribution of Coating

Factor	Has influence on
1. Spray equipment	
Nozzle design	Fineness of atomization of coating liquid [5, 11]
	Area over which coating liquid is applied
Atomizing air	Fineness of atomization of coating liquid [14]
Number of spray guns	Area over which coating liquid is applied [14, 15]
	Length of coating process [15]
2. Drying conditions	

Airflow
   Temperature }
   Humidity
	Efficiency of coating process (i.e., amount of coating that ends up on core material)

3. Spray rate	Length of coating process
	Amount of coating liquid that is deposited on substrate at each pass through spray zone
	Amount of coating that is lost during process [16]
4. Solids content of coating liquid	Amount of coating liquid that is deposited on substrate at each pass through spray zone [15]
	Length of coating process [15]
	Smoothness of dried coating [15]
5. Pan speed or fluidizing air velocity	Uniformity of mixing [15, 17]
	Amount of coating liquid that is deposited on substrate at each pass through spray zone
	Loss of coating due to attritional effects
6. Baffles (in coating pans)	Uniformity of mixing

[21]. Since the glass-transition temperature of hydroxypropyl methylcellulose has been reported to be in the range of 170–180°C [22], it is easy to
understand how impractical it would be to try and produce solvent-free
film coatings with this commonly used polymer.

One final note concerning film formation from polymeric solutions, solvent loss (from the coating) that occurs beyond the solidification point
creates shrinkage stresses that contribute to the internal stress within the
coating, a factor which is related to some of the mechanical problems that
are observed with film coatings applied to pharmaceutical solid-dosage
forms [23].

FORMATION OF FILMS FROM AQUEOUS POLYMERIC DISPERSIONS.
Film formation from aqueous polymeric dispersions requires the coalescence
of polymer particles into a continuous film. Drying of such a system
(i.e., the removal of water) is often quite rapid, whereas coalescence can
be a much slower process, extending into weeks and months if appropriate
formulation and processing parameters are not used.

The actual mechanism of film formation from an aqueous polymeric dispersion is quite complex, and many competing theories exist to explain the
process. A review of this process has been given by Bindshaedler et al.
[24].

In simplified terms, this process involves:

Rapid evaporation of water, causing the particles of dispersed polymer
    to be brought into close contact with one another
Development of pressures (associated with capillary forces within the
    structure) that overcome repulsive forces between particles and
    cause deformation of the polymer particles
Gradual coalescence of the polymer particles as a result of viscous flow
    and movement of polymer molecules across the interfaces between
    particles

This process of film formation is very sensitive to process conditions
used during film coating. The coalescence of the latex particles will be
very much dependent on free volume (which influences the movement of
polymer molecules between individual latex particles). Consequently,
aqueous polymeric dispersions must be processed at temperatures in excess
of the glass-transition temperature of the polymer (or plasticized polymer
in the case of, e.g., ethylcellulose). However, referring back to earlier
discussion on what constitutes a dry film, it is apparent that "blocking"
of coated product becomes a problem at temperatures in excess of 20°C
above the glass-transition temperature. Thus, the optimum processing
conditions for aqueous polymeric dispersions occur over a narrow range of
temperatures. This explains why tackiness is a common problem cited when
film coating with such aqueous dispersions.

The subject of morphological changes that occur in latex films has been
discussed by Bradford and Vanderhoff [25].

Ingredients Used in Film Coating

The first film-coated product was introduced to the market in late 1953
[26]. At that time, film-coating formulations consisted of an extensive
list of ingredients, including film formers, plasticizers, colorants, surfactants, flavors, glossing agents, and solvents. Since that time such

Table 6   Important Features of Film Coatings

Feature	Has impact on
1. Mechanical properties	Visual quality of coating
	Resistance to damage on handling
	Barrier properties of coating
	Drug-release characteristics from modified-release products
	Taste-masking efficiency
2. Permeability characteristics	Barrier properties of coating
	Product stability
	Drug-release characteristics from modified-release products
	Taste-masking efficiency
3. Coating solution viscosity	Spraying characteristics
	Interaction with substrate
	Visual quality of coating
4. Hiding power	Visual quality
	Quantity of coating needed for uniform appearance
	Stability of photo-labile actives

formulations have been refined and simplified, so that a typical formulation contains polymer, plasticizer, colorant, and solvent (or vehicle).

Film coating permits much more flexibility in choice of ingredients than does sugar coating, and allows the properties of the coating formulation to be tailored specifically to the needs of the dosage form being coated.

Certain features of the film-coating formulation are important, however, if the benefits described at the beginning of this chapter are to be realized. These features (and their impact) are described in Table 6, and will be very much affected by the ingredients used in the formulation.

POLYMERS. In the majority of film-coating formulations, the polymer is the major ingredient. Consequently, this material will have the greatest impact on the final properties of the coating.

Polymers are not, however, well-defined entities. A multiplicity of differing chemical types are available, each in turn often having various grades (as determined by viscosity or molecular weight). Finally, for a particular grade of one chemical type, batch-to-batch variation often occurs as a result of the polydisperse nature of polymers. When selecting

Table 7   Effect of Polymer Molecular Weight on Coating Properties

Property	Effect of increasing polymer molecular weight
1. Tensile strength	Increases
2. Elastic modulus	Increases (i.e., coating becomes *less* elastic)
3. Film adhesion	Decreases
4. Solution viscosity	Significantly increases
5. Film permeability	Typically unaffected, unless the structural (mechanical) properties improve as molecular weight of the polymer increases

a polymer for film coating, it is thus necessary to define this material in terms of chemical structure, molecular weight, and molecular weight distribution. While a particular grade of polymer is often defined (by its manufacturer) by a viscosity rating (determined by measuring the viscosity of the polymer at some definite concentration in an appropriate solvent), it is often better to submit this type of material to gel permeation (or size exclusion) chromatography, whereby average molecular weight, molecular weight distribution, and polydispersity can be determined.

The molecular weight characteristics of the polymer have a significant effect on coating properties, as shown in Table 7.

PLASTICIZERS. Most of the polymers that are used in pharmaceutical film coatings are amorphous in nature. One characteristic of these polymers is that as the temperature is lowered, a point known as the glass-transition temperature (T_g) is reached, below which there is a critical cessation of molecular motion on the local scale. Under these temperature conditions, the polymer exhibits many of the properties of inorganic glasses, including toughness, hardness, stiffness, and brittleness. For this reason, the glass-transition temperature is often described as one below which a polymer is brittle, and above which it is flexible. This definition is, at times, a little simplistic, and so a better definition of glass-transition temperature is that temperature above which there is an increase in the temperature coefficient of expansion [20].

Because the glass-transition temperatures of many of the polymers used in film coating are in excess of the temperature conditions experienced in the typical coating process, it is often necessary to modify the properties of the polymer. This modification allows the final coating to better withstand the conditions to which it will be subjected in the typical coating process. An appropriate modification involves the process of plasticization.

Plasticizers reduce the glass-transition temperature of amorphous polymers and impart flexibility. The basic requirements to be met by a plasticizer are permanence and compatibility. Permanence dictates that the plasticizer has a low vapor pressure and low diffusion rate within the polymeric film, a requirement that favors high molecular weight plasticizers. Compatibility, on the other hand, demands that the plasticizer be miscible with the polymer and exhibit similar intermolecular forces to those present within the polymer.

It is not uncommon to see reference made to two types of plasticization. The first is internal plasticization, and refers to the situation in which chemical changes are made within the structure of the polymer itself, as with copolymers (exemplified by many of the acrylic polymers systems used in film coating). The second, termed external plasticization, occurs when an external additive (the plasticizer) is combined in admixture with the polymer.

Effective plasticization is critical when using aqueous polymeric dispersions in order to ensure that sufficient free volume exists at normal processing temperatures to facilitate coalescence of the polymeric particles into a continuous film.

Since the plasticizer by its interaction with the polymer affects the intermolecular bonding between polymer chains, it is only to be expected that this additive will change the properties of the coating (Table 8). In these cases, although well-defined quantitative effects can be demonstrated, the magnitude of the effect is very much dependent on the compatibility, or degree of interaction, of the plasticizer with the polymer. Methods for determining the interaction between film-coating polymers and appropriate plasticizers have been described by Sakellariou et al. [29] and Entwistle and Rowe [22]. Plasticizers, by their very nature, are not universal, since selection is very much determined by which polymer is being used.

COLORANTS. Colorants are included in many film-coating formulations to improve the appearance and visual identification of the coated product. Certain types of colorant (as will be discussed later in this section) can provide other physical benefits.

As described under sugar coating (Sec. II), various types of approved colorants exist that can be used in film coating. While a detailed review of colorants that can be used in pharmaceutical dosage forms has been

Table 8   Effects of Plasticizers on the Properties of Film Coatings

Property	Effect of increasing plasticizer concentration
1. Tensile strength	Decreased [27]
2. Elastic modulus	Decreased
3. Film adhesion	May be increased, but results often variable [27]
4. Solution viscosity	Increased, and magnitude of effect dependent on molecular weight of plasticizer [11]
5. Film permeability	Can be increased [27] or decreased [28], depending on chemical nature of plasticizer
6. Glass-transition temperature	Decreased, but magnitude of effect dependent on compatibility with polymer [29]

given elsewhere [30], it is appropriate to briefly review here those types that may be used in film coating. Such colorants include:

Water-soluble dyes (e.g., FD&C Yellow #5 and FD&C Blue #2)
Aluminum lakes (of FD&C water-soluble dyes)
Other lakes (e.g., D&C Red #6)
Inorganic pigments (e.g., titanium dioxide, iron oxides, calcium sulfate, calcium carbonate)
"Natural" colorants (e.g., riboflavin, tumeric oleoresin, carmine 40)

Unlike sugar coating, film coating had its origins as a nonaqueous process. Consequently, with few exceptions, most formulators preferred to use pigments as colorants in their film-coating formulations. While the more recent introduction of aqueous technology has opened the door to using water-soluble colorants, use of pigments has persisted owing to the advantages shown by this form of colorant, including:

Ability to increase solids content of coating solution without dramatically affecting viscosity [11] (particularly advantageous in aqueous film coating)
Ability to improve the moisture barrier properties of film coatings [27]

Pigments consist, however, of discrete particles, and thus a substantial effort is required to ensure that they are well dispersed in the coating liquid. Such dispersion will be inadequate if dry pigment is simply added to the coating liquid with the aid of a low-shear stirrer (e.g., a Lightnin' mixer). Inadequate pigment dispersion leads to coating defects, as discussed by Porter [31] and Rowe [32]. Particle size of the pigment within the film (a parameter often related to efficiency in the dispersion process) will also affect perceived color [32] and may influence the surface roughness of the coating [33].

Since colorants are mostly added to a film-coating formulation for their visual effects, it is important to understand the physical behavior of colorants in a polymer film. As pigments are used almost exclusively as colorants in film coatings, further reference in this section to colorants will be restricted to pigments.

When coloring a film coating not only is it important to create a given visual effect, but also to ensure that the appearance is as uniform as possible throughout the particular batch of coated product, and consistent from batch-to-batch.

Such uniformity is facilitated when the colorant chosen is able to effectively mask the appearance of the substrate without requiring the use of excessive quantities of colorant (which could increase the risk of physical defects in the coated product) or applying excessive quantities of coating (which impacts total cost of the process). This ability to mask the substrate is often described in terms of hiding power or opacity of the colored coating. These characteristics of the coating are often related to contrast ratio, a term defined as the ratio of the Y tristmulus value for a film measured over a black background (i.e., Yb) to the similar value measured over a white background (Yw). Thus

$$\text{Contrast ratio} = \frac{Yb}{Yw} \times 100$$

Colored films having contrast ratios close to 100 exhibit excellent hiding power, whereas those having values close to zero are almost transparent (and thus have poor hiding power). Since contrast ratio is also affected by film thickness, determinations (and comparisons) must always be made on films of equal thickness.

Rowe [35] has listed the contrast ratios for coatings containing various colorants. From his comparison, it is evident that the better results are obtained for films containing certain inorganic pigments (e.g., titanium dioxide and iron oxides), or those that absorb the higher wavelengths of visible light (e.g., FD&C Blue #2). These results can be explained by the theories of light, which predict that hiding power will be influenced by:

Light reflected at the polymer/pigment interface, which is influenced by differences in the respective refractive indices of the polymer and pigment [35]
Quantity (and wavelength) of light absorbed by the colorant

Understanding these basic principles may help the formulator optimize a particular coating formulation, especially with respect to the concentration of colorant required, and the quantity of coating needed to develop a uniform appearance. Some optimal results in this respect have been described by Porter and Saraceni [15].

While it is important to understand the physical behavior of colorants, one should not lose sight of the impact that pigments can have on other physical characteristics of the coating. Some of these effects are listed in Table 9.

SOLVENTS. While choice of an appropriate solvent deserves careful attention, the rise in importance of aqueous film coating has virtually eliminated solvent selection from the formulation process. Nonetheless, certain types of film coatings and film-coating processes require that some organic

Table 9   Effects of Pigments on the Properties of Film Coatings

Property	Effect of increasing pigment concentration
1. Tensile strength	Decreased (effect may be minimized by effective pigment dispersion)
2. Elastic modulus	Increased [36]
3. Film adhesion	Little effect [27]
4. Solution viscosity	Increased, but not substantially [11]
5. Film permeability	Decreased [27], unless critical pigment volume concentration is exceeded
6. Hiding power	Increased, but magnitude of effect dependent on refractive index of pigment, and light absorbed by pigment [34]

Table 10   Common Solvents Used in Film Coating

Class	Examples
1. Water	–
2. Alcohols	Methanol
	Ethanol
	Isopropanol
3. Esters	Ethyl acetate
	Ethyl lactate
4. Ketones	Acetone
5. Chlorinated hydrocarbons	Methylene chloride
	1:1:1 Trichloroethane

solvents still be used. Thus, to a limited extent, selection of an appropriate solvent may still be necessary.

A list of some of the more common solvents that have been used in film coating is shown in Table 10.

When selecting a particular solvent or solvent blend there are several factors that must be considered. The first prerequisite is the ability to form a solution with the polymer of choice. In this respect, it is often difficult to determine whether true solutions are formed or whether they are mainly macromolecular "dispersions." Banker [37] stated that optimal polymer solution will yield the maximum polymer chain extension, producing films having the greatest cohesive strength and thus the best mechanical properties.

One method for determining interactions between the polymer and solvent, and aiding in selecting the most suitable solvent for a given polymer, is to use the solubility parameter approach. This approach is based on the theoretical treatment of the familiar free energy equation as proposed by Hildebrand and Scott [38] and is expressed in this way:

$$\Delta H_m = V_m \left[\left(\frac{\Delta E_1}{V_1} \right)^{1/2} - \left(\frac{\Delta E_2}{V_2} \right)^{1/2} \right]^2 \phi_1 \phi_2$$

where ΔH_m = overall heat of mixing

V_m = total volume of the mixture

ΔE = energy of vaporization of either component 1 or 2

ϕ = volume fraction of either component 1 or 2

The expression $(\Delta E)/V$ is often termed the cohesive energy density, written δ^2, where δ is the solubility parameter and is equivalent to $([\Delta E]/V)^{1/2}$ in the above equation. If $\delta_1 = \delta_2$, then $\Delta H_m = 0$. Thus, in the free-energy equation

$$\Delta F = \Delta H_m - T \Delta S$$

where ΔF is the free-energy change, T is absolute temperature, and ΔS is the entropy of mixing. The free energy is now dependent on the mixing entropy. As there is a large increase in the entropy when a polymer dissolves, the set of circumstances thus far described ensures that there will be miscibility between the solvent and polymer.

Kent and Rowe [39] used the solubility parameter approach in evaluating the solubility of ethylcellulose in various solvents for film coating. They determined the intrinsic viscosities of several grades of ethylcellulose in a range of solvents of known solubility parameters utilizing the equations derived by Rubin and Wagner [40]. They graphically evaluated the effect of solvent solubility parameter on intrinsic viscosity for a range of solvents classified either as (1) poorly hydrogen bonded, (2) moderately hydrogen bonded, or (3) strongly hydrogen bonded, and determined both the best class of solvent to use and the optimum solvent solubility parameter. Thus, this approach can be used to determine the best solvent for the polymer from a thermodynamic standpoint. The technique can also be used for optimizing solvent blends, the individual components of which may or may not themselves be thermodynamically good solvents.

Before dissolution can take place the solvent must penetrate the polymer mass. Once this has occurred, a swollen gel will form which rapidly disintegrates to form a solution. The rate of solution is facilitated by small solvent molecules which diffuse rapidly into the polymer mass. Unfortunately, thermodynamically good solvents are not always kinetically good ones, and vice versa; thus, a compromise may be necessary.

An additional function of the solvent system is to ensure a controlled deposition of the polymer onto the surface of the substrate. If a good coherent and adherent film coat is to be obtained, the volatility of the solvent system is an important factor. In the final formulation, the selected solvent system usually represents a compromise between thermodynamic, kinetic, and volatility factors and results in a solvent blend being used.

After all formulation factors have been resolved, attention must be paid to the changes in solvent ratios that can occur during the application process. This will cause no problem if all components of the blend, or the least volatile component, are good solvents for the polymer. However, if this is not the case, the solvent–polymer thermodynamic balance changes as evaporation progresses. The polymer can thus be precipitated before a cohesive film is formed. Alternatively, the solubility of the polymer in the remaining solvent may not be sufficient to ensure that the optimum film properties will be obtained. In this situation, it is essential to use a constant-boiling or azeotropic solvent mixture whose composition does not change on evaporation.

B. Conventional Film Coatings

The greatest area of application for film coatings is that where the coating is mainly designed to improve product appearance, perhaps improve stability and ease of ingestion of the dosage form, but not alter drug-release characteristics from that dosage form.

From this description, it is apparent that esthetics are of paramount importance, and consequently are likely to influence selection of the raw materials to be used in the formulation. This selection is often based on factors that affect the mechanical properties (such as tensile strength, elasticity, and adhesion) of the coating, allow the smoothest, glossiest coatings to be obtained, and produce coatings that readily dissolve in the human gastrointestinal tract.

Conventional film coating is also the area where aqueous technology has gained the highest acceptance. Thus, with few exceptions, most ingredients are selected for their solubility in water (this is especially true for polymers).

Polymers

Common polymers used in conventional film coating are listed in Table 11.

The most popular class of polymers used in conventional film coating are cellulosics, many of which have good organic-solvent and aqueous solubility, thus facilitating the transition to aqueous film coating. Of these cellulosics, ethylcellulose is not water soluble, and was originally used as a film modifier in admixtures with hydroxypropyl methylcellulose (HPMC) in organic-solvent-based formulations. To a limited extent, this blending process has continued in aqueous film coating. In this case, aqueous solutions of HPMC are mixed with aqueous dispersions of ethylcellulose. However, except when one needs to produce special barrier

Table 11 Polymers Used in Conventional Film-Coating Formulations

Class	Examples
1. Cellulosics	Hydroxypropyl methylcellulose
	Hydroxypropylcellulose
	Hydroxyethylcellulose
	Methylhydroxyethylcellulose
	Methylcellulose
	Ethylcellulose
	Sodium carboxymethylcellulose
2. Vinyls	Polyvinyl pyrrolidone
3. Glycols	Polyethylene glycols
4. Acrylics	Dimethylaminoethyl methacrylate-methylacrylate acid ester copolymer
	Ethylacrylate-methylmethacrylate copolymer

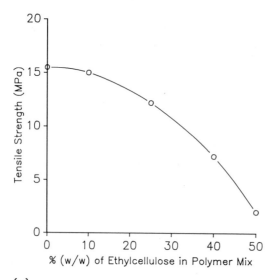

(a)

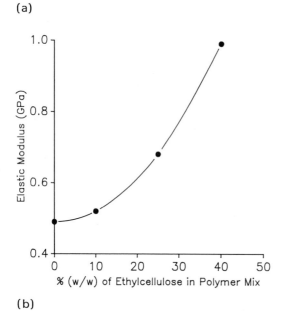

(b)

Figure 9   Effect of combining an aqueous solution of hydroxypropyl-methylcellulose (Methocel E 5) with an aqueous latex of ethylcellulose (Aquacoat) on free-film properties.   (a) Tensile strength and (b) elastic modulus.

coatings (where aqueous solubility of the coating is intentionally reduced), this practice is questionable, since the addition of the dispersed polymer (ethylcellulose) can significantly impair the mechanical ability of the water-soluble polymer (e.g., hydroxypropyl methylcellulose) (Fig. 9), without gaining any major advantage that cannot be realized with a more conventional formulation approach.

Polymers such as polyvinylpyrrolidone and polyethylene glycols have not been popular as the major polymer in film-coating formulations. Polyvinylpyrrolidone films are brittle and hygroscopic, whereas polyethylene glycol films are waxy, hygroscopic, and soften readily at only moderately elevated temperatures. The lower molecular weight grades of polyethylene glycol tend to be more appropriately used as plasticizers in aqueous film coating.

While enjoying more popularity in Europe, the acrylics are not extensively employed in the United States. Dimethylaminoethyl methacrylate-methacrylic acid ester copolymer has some unique characteristics in that it is soluble in water at only low pH, making it particularly attractive for taste masking. Unfortunately, its use is restricted in organic-solvent-based formulations. Ethyl acrylate-methyl methacrylate copolymers, also water insoluble, are available as aqueous latex-coating systems.

Although film-coating formulations vary tremendously, depending on the preferences of the formulator and the needs of the dosage form to be coated, use of either HPMC or hydroxypropyl cellulose (HPC) has become a standard in the pharmaceutical industry. Hydroxypropyl methylcellulose films have superior tensile properties, whereas HPC films tend to be more elastic (i.e., exhibit lower elastic moduli) and possess better adhesive properties (Fig. 10). Since each of these polymers is available in several grades, the common practice is to use the lower molecular weight grades of each in aqueous film coating in order to optimize the properties of coating solutions with respect to solids content and solution viscosity.

Plasticizers

Those plasticizers commonly used in conventional film coating are shown in Table 12. As discussed previously, the choice of plasticizer may to some extent be determined by the polymer used, since a strong interaction between the plasticizer and polymer is required if the plasticizer is to be effective.

With aqueous film-coating formulations, the general preference is to use water-soluble plasticizers, since this approach helps to facilitate interaction between the polymer and plasticizer. For this reason, plasticizers such as glycerol, propylene glycol, the polyethylene glycols, and triacetin are often used with aqueous formulations.

Entwistle and Rowe [22] and Sakellariou et al. [29] have published extensively on the interaction of water-soluble plasticizers with hydroxypropyl methylcellulose. Their results suggest that the polyetheylene glycols are the most effective plasticizers for this cellulosic polymer, with effectiveness being *inversely* proportional to the molecular weight of the polyethylene glycol chosen.

While these water-soluble materials are effective as plasticizers in their own right, some consideration must be given to the fact that being somewhat hygroscopic, they help retain moisture which augments the plasticizing effect.

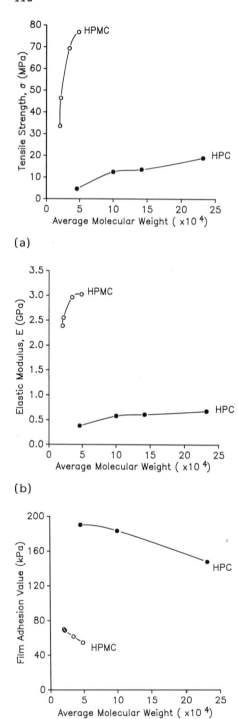

Figure 10   Effect of polymer molecular weight on mechanical properties of
film coatings.   (a) Tensile strength, (b) elastic modulus, and (c) film
adhesion.

Table 12 Common Plasticizers Used in Conventional Film Coating

Class	Examples
1. Polyhydric alcohols	Propylene glycol
	Glycerol
	Polyethylene glycols
2. Acetate esters	Glyceryl triacetate (Triacetin)
	Triethyl citrate
	Acetyl· triethyl citrate
3. Phthalate esters	Diethylphthalate
4. Glycerides	Acetylated monoglycerides
5. Oils	Castor oil
	Mineral oil

Use of triacetin as a plasticizer in aqueous formulations, although less popular, may have certain advantages when trying to improve the moisture-barrier properties of the film coating. This effect has recently been confirmed by data presented by Johnson et al. [41].

Colorants

Any of the approved colorants discussed earlier would be suitable for use in conventional film coatings, although preference is usually shown for insoluble colorants (pigments).

C. Modified-Release Film Coatings

Film-coating techniques can be effectively used to modify the release of the active ingredient from a pharmaceutical solid-dosage form.

While modern pharmaceutical technology makes possible the design of dosage forms that exhibit modified time of release or rate of release (or both) of the active ingredient, a plethora of terminology (relating to these kinds of dosage forms) exists that confuses formulators, prescribers, and consumers alike.

The *United States Pharmacopeia/National Formulary* (USP/NF) has simplified this terminology somewhat by defining a modified-release dosage form as one in which "the drug-release characteristics of time course and/or location are chosen to accomplish therapeutic or convenience objectives not offered by conventional dosage forms. . . ."

Under this umbrella definition, the USP/NF recognizes two types of modified-release dosage form:

1. Extended release: One that permits at least a twofold reduction in dosing frequency as compared to the situation in which the drug is presented as a conventional dosage form (extended-release dosage forms are often called sustained-release or controlled-release dosage forms)
2. Delayed release: One that releases the active ingredient at some time other than promptly after administration (an enteric-coated product is an example of this type of dosage form)

Enteric Film Coatings

By definition, enteric coatings are those which remain intact in the stomach (and exhibit low permeability to gastric fluids), but break down readily once the dosage form reaches the small intestine. The prime uses of such coatings are:

To maintain the activity of drugs that are unstable when exposed to the gastric milieu (e.g., erythromycin and pancreatin)

To minimize either nausea or bleeding that occurs with those drugs that irritate the gastric mucosa (e.g., aspirin and certain steroids)

Early approaches to preparing enteric-dosage forms involved treating gelatin capsules with formalin or coating tablets with shellac. Both of these approaches were unreliable, since the solubility of the membrane (which is responsible for the enteric effect) can be unpredictable. Modern enteric coatings are usually formulated with synthetic polymers that contain ionizable functional groups that render the polymer water soluble at a specific pH value. Such polymers are often referred to as polyacids.

Examples of commonly used enteric-coating polymers (including those introduced more recently) are listed in Table 13. Since many of these polymers are esters, they may be subject to degradation (as a result of hydrolysis) when exposed to conditions of elevated temperature and humidity. Such hydrolysis can result in a substantial change in enteric properties.

While many of the polymers shown in Table 13 have been used for many years in enteric-coating formulations, the special aqueous-solubility requirements for an enteric polymer have delayed thr routine employment of *aqueous* enteric-coating technology. More recently, various systems of aqueous enteric coating have been introduced, and examples are shown in Table 14. As these examples suggest, many of the coating systems exist as dry powders, with the coating liquid being prepared shortly before use by dispersing (or dissolving) the polymer in water. The reason for supplying many enteric coating systems as dry powders is to avoid problems of poor stability (due to hydrolysis) when these polymers are exposed to water for extended periods.

Very little information (one exception being that for PVAP) [42] is given regarding the stability of many of these polymers once converted into aqueous dispersions.

The performance of enteric-coated dosage forms has often been open to question. Certainly, much of the uncertainty can be related to the earlier common use of "natural" polymers (such as shellac) and simplistic coating procedures. The use of synthetic, predictable polymers and the adoption

Table 13 Examples of Enteric-Coating Polymers

Polymer	Comments
Cellulose acetate phthalate (CAP)	Subject to hydrolysis (high)[b]
Cellulose acetate trimellitate (CAT)	Subject to hydrolysis[b]
Polyvinyl acetate phthalate (PVAP)	Subject to hydrolysis (low)[b]
Hydroxypropyl methylcellulose phthalate (HP)	Subject to hydrolysis (medium)[b]
Hydroxypropyl methylcellulose acetate succinate (HPMCAS)	Subject to hydrolysis (low)[b]
Poly (ME-EA) 1:1[a]	—
Poly (MA-MMA) 1:1[a]	Relatively high dissolution pH
Poly (MA-MMA) 1:2[a]	Relatively high dissolution pH

[a]MA, methacrylic acid; EA, ethylacrylate; MMA, methyl methacrylate.

[b]When exposed to conditions of elevated temperature and humidity.

of modern processing technology should have done much to dispel these concerns. However, problems still exist today. Unfortunately, many of the factors that can dramatically effect the performance of enteric coatings have long gone unrecognized. Ozturk et al. [43] recently presented information on some of the important factors that can influence the behavior of enteric coatings. These factors include:

The nature of the drug in the dosage form (the presence of aspirin, for example, can greatly influence dissolution of the coating).
The quantity of coating applied (application of excessive quantities of coating can substantially delay release of drug from the dosage form).
The presence of imperfections in the coating (fissures or "pick" marks will destroy the integrity of the coating).
The dissolution pH of the polymer used in the coating.
The effect of in vitro test conditions (dissolution of the coating, and ultimate drug release, can be affected dramatically by the pH and ionic strength of the test solutions and the agitation rate).

Finally, while most enteric product are in tablet form, it has been demonstrated that enteric-coated tablets are influenced significantly by gastrointestinal (GI) transit. Focus has thus begun to shift toward using enteric-coated pellets or granules, which can give greater reproducibility [44] (with respect to release and absorption of drug).

Sustained-Release, or Controlled-Release,
Film Coatings

Film-coating techniques to produce sustained-release dosage forms have been utilized since the late 1940s, when SmithKline used a pan-coating

Table 14 Examples of Aqueous Enteric-Coating Systems

Product	Form	Polymer	Comments
Eudragit L 30 D	Latex dispersion	Poly (ME-EA) 1:1[a]	System essentially contains only the polymer
Eudragit L-100-55	Spray-dried latex	Poly (ME-EA) 1:1[a]	Requires dispersing in water with addition of alkali
			System only contains polymer
HP-F	Dry powder	HP	Requires dispersing in water
			System only contains polymer
Coateric	Dry powder	PVAP	Complete system
			Requires dispersing in water with addition of ammonia
Aquateric	Spray-dried pseudolatex	CAP	System essentially contains only polymer
			Requires dispersing in water
HPMCAS	Dry powder	HPMCAS	System contains only polymer
			Requires dispersing in water
CAP	Dry powder	CAP	System contains only polymer
			Requires dissolving in water with aid of alkali (ammonia)
CAT	Dry powder	CAT	System contains only polymer
			Requires dissolving in water with aid of alkali (ammonia)

[a]MA, methacrylic acid; EA, ethacrylic acid.

Table 15   Examples of Coating Materials Used in Sustained-Release
Film-Coating Formulations

Coating material	Membrane characteristics
Fats and waxes (e.g., beeswax, carnauba wax, cetyl alcohol, cetylstearyl alcohol)	Permeable and erodible
Shellac	Permeable and soluble (at high pH)
Zein	Permeable and soluble (at high pH)
Ethylcellulose	Permeable
Cellulose esters (e.g., acetate)	Semipermeable
Silicone elastomers	Permeable (when PEG added)
Acrylic esters	Permeable

process to apply various mixtures of fats and waxes (dissolved in organic
solvents) to drug-loaded beads. Since that time, a variety of materials
and coating processes have been used for the same purpose. Drug release from such sustained-release products is moderated by the film coating which acts as a membrane that allows infusion of GI fluids and the
outward diffusion of dissolved drug. In some instances, the release
process may be augmented by a coating that slowly dissolves (e.g.,
shellac), or is subject to digestion by enzymes (e.g., fats and waxes).

As with enteric coatings, most formulators today prefer to use synthetic polymers that have more predictable properties. A list of many of
the coating materials used in sustained-release film coatings is shown in
Table 15.

Various pharmaceutical forms may be used as substrates for sustained-
release film coatings. These may generally be classified as:

Tablets
Multiparticulates (e.g., drug-loaded beads, granules, crystals,
    powders, drug/ion-exchange resin complexes)

While both general types of substrates are in current use, the preference now shows a trend toward multiparticulate systems which are perceived to have advantages such as minimization of risk of dose dumping
(should membrane rupture occur) and optimization of GI transit.

Although multiparticulates (especially drug-loaded beads) were once
commonly film coated in pans, the wide variety of multiparticulate systems
coated today often requires specialized processing techniques that involve
the use of fluid-bed coating equipment.

As with other types of film coating, great interest has been shown in
using aqueous-coating technology for sustained-release products. Although aqueous coating systems capable of producing sustained-release
film coatings were first introduced in the early 1970s, aqueous sustained-
release film coating is still not yet widely practiced. Such coating systems

Table 16   Examples of Aqueous Polymeric Dispersions for Sustained-Release Film Coating

Material	Polymer	Comments
1. Surelease	Ethylcellulose	Aqueous polymeric dispersion contains requisite plasticizers Addition of lake colorants should be avoided because of alkalinity of dispersion
2. Aquacoat	Ethylcellulose	Pseudolatex dispersion Requires addition of plasticizers to facilitate film coalescence
3. Eudragit NE 30 D	Poly(ethylacrylate-methyl methacrylate) 2:1	Latex dispersion No plasticizers required unless improved film flexibility is desired
4. Eudragit RL 30 D	Poly(ethylacrylate-methyl methacrylate)triethyl ammonioethyl methacrylate chloride 1:2:0.2	Aqueous polymeric dispersion No plasticizers required unless improved film flexibility is desired
5. Eudragit RS 30 D	Poly(ethylacrylate-methyl methacrylate)triethyl ammonioethyl methacrylate chloride 1:2:0.1	Aqueous polymeric dispersion No plasticizers required unless improved film flexibility is desired
6. —	Silicone elastomer	Requires addition of PEG

typically consist of aqueous dispersions of water-insoluble polymers (Table 16) which form films by a process of coalescence of submicron polymer particles. This process can be greatly affected by conditions used in the coating process, and variable results (as they relate to ultimate drug-release characteristics) can often be attributed more to lack of control over the coating process (or choice of inappropriate processing parameters) rather than to any variability in the aqueous dispersion used.

A useful description of the use of aqueous sustained-release film-coating systems has been given elsewhere [3].

Irrespective of the coating materials or types of coating systems used, most formulators prefer to prepare simple membranes that modify drug release by diffusion. Some rather unique approaches, however, have also

Table 17   Factors Influencing Drug Release from a Sustained-Release
Film-Coated Dosage Form

Parameter	Influenced by
1. Surface area	Size, size distribution, and surface topography of material being coated
2. Diffusion coefficient	Formulation of film coating
	Structure of coating
	Nature of drug
3. Drug-concentration gradient across membrane	Initial drug loading
	Drug content inside the membrane at any intermediate time
	Agitation rate (which influences drug concentration on outside of membrane)
4. Membrane thickness	Size, size distribution, and surface topography of material being coated
	Quantity of coating material applied (related to theoretical quantity of coating to be applied, and coating efficiency)

been used that result in the creation of incomplete film coatings. One
such approach is exemplified by the simple osmotic pump in which a delivery orifice is formed in the otherwise intact film coating by means of
laser drilling [45]. Alternatively, a microporous membrane may be formed
by the inclusion within the film structure of various water-soluble, powdered
ingredients that may subsequently be leached out so as to enhance drug
release. This approach has been described by, among others, Lindholm
and Juslin [46].

Sustained-release dosage forms from which drug release is moderated
by an applied film coating are often called reservoir systems. Drug release from such systems can often be described by application of Fick's
first law of diffusion [47].

The rate of drug release through the membrane is *directly* proportional
to surface area, diffusion coefficient, drug solubility in and drug concentration gradient across the membrane, and inversely proportional to membrane thickness. Factors which have an impact on these parameters are
listed in Table 17.

With respect to drug-release characteristics, variable results may ensue
through inability to effectively control many of these influencing factors.
For example:

Variations (from batch-to-batch) in size and shape of the core material
(to be coated) would certainly cause variations in surface area and
coating thickness.

Variations in coating structure may well result from variable processing
conditions that cause picking or spray drying (particularly with
organic-solvent-based coating solutions) and incomplete coalescence
with aqueous polymeric dispersions, and general variation in
process efficiencies (which influence uniformity of distribution,
and overall quantity applied, of the coating material)

D. Application Techniques in Film Coating

As in sugar coating, film-coating liquids can be applied either by manual
ladling techniques or by means of spray atomization. However, in recent
years, manual ladling procedures have waned in popularity and are not
extensively practiced today. Some pigmented, shellac-based film-coating
systems are available that facilitate ladle application, and the technique
may also be used for applying certain types of enteric coatings and sustained-release coatings based on shellac.

Far more popular are techniques that utilize the spray-atomization
process, which allows coating liquids to be applied in a much more controlled and reproducible manner. This precision is especially important
when applying aqueous-coating formulations where liquid delivery and distribution must be carefully matched to the drying conditions developed in
the process.

Three basic types of spray-atomization processes (which will be described in more detail later in this chapter) are:

1. Airless spray techniques: Because of high delivery rates, these
   are typically reserved for production-scale film-coating processes
   where organic-solvent-based coating liquids are to be applied.
2. Air-spray techniques: Typically used in small-scale coating
   processes and all those involving aqueous-coating systems.
3. Ultrasonic spray techniques: Still considered to be experimental
   techniques owing to certain limitations imposed by the rheology of
   the coating liquids.

E. Problems in Film Coating

Film coating, as with sugar coating, is a process that subjects the product
being coated to a significant amount of stress. Unavoidable attritional effects demand that both the product being coated and the coating itself be
formulated with appropriate mechanical properties if problems associated
with fragmentation (of the cores) and erosion (of the cores and coating)
are to be avoided.

The replacement of organic solvents with water (as either solvent or
vehicle) has also increased the complexity of the process. Water has a
significantly higher latent heat of vaporization (than the previously used
organic solvents), and thus greater attention must be paid to monitoring
(and preferably controlling) the drying conditions in the aqueous process.

Finally, the interaction between a film coating and its substrate is extremely complex. Core characteristics such as porosity, surface rugosity,
and surface energy can hinder or enhance wetting by the coating liquid.
Viscosity and surface tension of the coating liquid are also factors that
influence the inital wetting process (of the substrate by the coating liquid).

For this reason, aqueous-coating formulations are more likely to experience wetting (and ultimate adhesion) problems than their organic-solvent-based counterparts. The interaction between coating and substrate is also likely to be influenced by stresses that form within the coating. Such stresses are related to [48]:

Shrinkage phenomena that develop as the coating dries

Expansion/contraction of both coating and substrate as they are subjected to heating and cooling cycles in the process

Other core-expansion factors (such as swelling due to moisture absorption)

These factors can affect both the integrity of the film itself and adhesion of the film to the substrate.

It is thus apparent that significant potential exists for problems to develop either during the film-coating process, or once the process has been completed. Consequently, it is important that appropriate attention be paid to formulation of the core material, selection of coating ingredients, and design of the coating process. Such attention is of paramount importance if subsequent major changes (in either formulations or process conditions) are to be avoided at a time when these changes might be severely limited by regulatory constraints.

Many of the problems which are, unfortunately, all too common in film coating are illustrated in Figure 11.

Picking

Picking results when, for example, the coating on two adjacent tablets is not sufficiently dry before contact between them occurs. Because the partially dried coating can be extremely tacky, once the two tablets make contact they adhere to one another only to break apart later (under the influence of attrition) once the coating has dried. The result is shown in Figure 11A. In extreme cases, tablets with flat faces or flat edges (as with capsule-shaped tablets that have thick side walls) may become permanently glued together so that twinning (or the buildup of multiples) occurs

Overwetting typically occurs when the spray rate is excessive for the drying conditions in the process. Localized overwetting often results when an insufficient number of spray guns is used such that the application of coating liquid is concentrated too much in one region of the tablet bed (rather than being spread out so as to take full advantage of the drying process). Localized overwetting may also occur with some multiple-gun set-ups when one nozzle becomes blocked, causing all the coating liquid to be channeled to the remaining guns.

Finally, certain types of coating formulations (e.g., those based on hydroxypropylcellulose, many of the enteric-coating formulations, and several of the acrylic aqueous latex-coating systems) are inherently tackier during application, and are thus more likely to create the conditions under which picking occurs.

"Orange Peel" (Roughness)

For a successful film-coating process, it is critical that the droplets of coating liquid dry (at least to the point of being tack-free) very soon after they make contact with the surface of the product being coated.

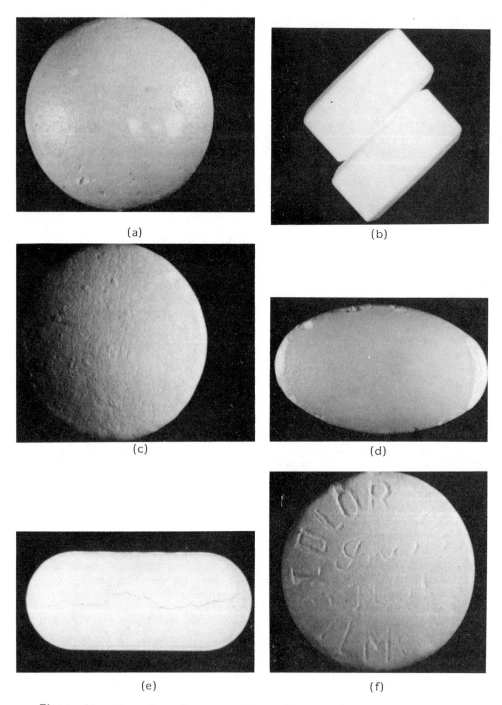

Figure 11 Examples of common film-coating problems. (a) Picking,
(b) twinning, (c) orange peel roughness, (d) edge erosion, (e) film
cracking, (f) logo bridging, and (g) film splitting and peeling.

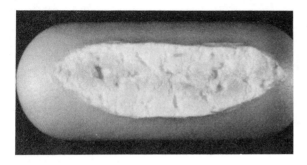

(g)

Consequently, almost all film-coated tablets exhibit a characteristic known as orange peel (so-called because of a resemblance to the skin of an orange). Optimized coating processes will allow this characteristic to be kept to a minimum such that it is not readily visible to the naked eye. Certain process conditions, however, are likely to cause this inherent roughness to become visible (as shown in Fig. 11C). Such process conditions include low spray rates coupled with excessive drying conditions (high processing temperatures and airflows) and use of excessive atomizing air pressures (for air-spray systems) which accentuate premature drying of the droplets of coating liquid.

The problem may also be compounded by attempting to spray coating liquids with excessively high viscosities such that optimal automization is difficult to achieve.

Edge Wear (Chipping)

The attritional effects in the typical film-coating process cannot be over-stated. Because tablet edges are often exposed most to these attritional effects, fracture at this point is not uncommon and results in parts of the tablet surface being exposed (see Fig. 11D). Causes of this problem include:

Tablet cores having high friability values
Worn tablet punches (that produce "flashing" on the tablet edges)
Minor lamination problems (with the tablet cores) that exacerbate edge-
    erosion problems
Brittle film coatings that offer insufficient protection to tablet edges

Film Cracking

Cracking of film coatings occurs when the internal stress (that develops within the coating on drying) exceeds the tensile strength of that coating. Cracking may be manifested in many ways and can be catastrophic (or major) in nature (see Fig. 11E).

Although such problems may under many circumstances be purely cosmetic, cohesive failure of the coating certainly detracts from many of the functional qualities of the coating. These problems are, of course, totally unacceptable for products where the applied coating is a major factor in modifying drug-release characteristics.

While cohesive failure is often associated with brittleness of the coating, the problem is certainly exacerbated by thermal expansion effects, particularly when significant differences exist between the thermal-expansion coefficients for the core and coating, respectively [49,50].

Bridging of Logos (Intagliations)

Internal stress is also a major causative factor in logo bridging (see Fig. 11F). This phenomenon occurs when a component of the internal stress becomes sufficiently high so as to cause partial or complete detachment of the coating (from the substrate) in the region of the logo. As a result of such detachment, the film is able to "shorten," and thus partially relieve the stress within the film. In doing so, legibility of the logo can be significantly reduced. Typically, this type of problem becomes progressively worse as more coating is gradually applied during the process.

Solutions to bridging involve improving film adhesion and/or reducing stress within the film, and usually require some reformation of either the tablet core or the coating. In addition, appropriate design of tablet punches (especially with respect to the logo) may help to alleviate the problem, whereas adjustment of process conditions may also prove beneficial [51,52].

Film Peeling

On occasion (particularly during application of aqueous-coating formulations), if cohesive failure (cracking) of the coating occurs, that coating may subsequently peel back from the surface of the substrate (see Fig. 11G). While both cohesive and adhesive failure are implicated here (both phenomena being linked to internal stress), appropriate solutions typically involve addressing the initial cracking problem by increasing the mechanical strength of the coating.

In-Filling of Logos

While visually similar to bridging, in-filling of logos typically occurs [53] during the spray application of aerated aqueous film-coating solutions. When a foamy coating solution impinges on a regular part of the tablet surface it will, under the shear forces generated, form a film with "normal" characteristics. However, those droplets of coating liquid that reside in the logo, being protected from the shear forces at the surface, gradually dry to form a solid foam that eventually obliterates the legend.

While some degree of aeration is not uncommon with many aqueous-coating solutions, when the viscosity of these solutions is too high, dissipation of the foam (on standing) does not occur. Thus, the coating liquid that is sprayed on during the coating process will still be extremely aerated.

Recovery of Film-Coated Tablets

Unlike with sugar-coated tablets, film-coated tablets cannot be readily recovered (should a batch be rejected) by simply washing off the coating.

Recovery of film-coated tablets thus typically involves milling of the tablets to produce "granules" that can be introduced (at a predetermined level) into other batches of compression mix (of the same product). Depending on the fracture characteristics of the tablets, and to some extent the adhesion of the coating to the tablet surface, the milling process may cause the coating to flake off so that it can be removed from the tablet core material by sieving.

Usually, however, a portion of the coating will remain in the compression mix. Thus, any rework procedure must be suitably validated so as to ensure that recompressed tablets perform within the specifications of the original product.

A recent publication [54] discussed the use of the Crackulator for recovery of film-coated tablets. Using such equipment, a better separation of tablet and coating fragments was achieved.

IV. COATING EQUIPMENT

An extensive array of equipment is used in modern pharmaceutical coating operations, and includes:

    Coating pans
    Fluid-bed coating columns
    Air-handling equipment (including heat exchangers)
    Coating liquid holding tanks (including mixers)
    Metering/delivery equipment (e.g., pumps)
    Liquid application systems (e.g., spray guns)
    Control systems
    Monitoring systems
    Effluent treatment systems (e.g., dust collectors, solvent recovery
        equipment)

This discussion will focus, for the main part, on coating pans, fluid-bed coating columns, spray equipment, and metering systems.

A. Coating Pans

Coating pans form the basis of any coating process except those that rely on fluid-bed processing equipment. The pan serves as a container for the batch of product being coated, and provides the means for keeping the product (to be coated) in continual motion throughout the process, thus facilitating the uniform distribution of coating fluids.

Over the last 30 years, design of coating pans has undergone some major changes as coating technology has advanced and demands for compliance with GMPs have increased.

Conventional Coating Pans

Originally, pharmaceutical coating pans evolved from designs used for confectionery pan coating. The term conventional coating pan was used to describe spherical, hexagonal, or pear-shaped pans, an example of which is shown in Figure 12.

The simplicity in design made use of such equipment very popular. Drying of the product being coated was typically accomplished by ducting heated air into the opening. An adjacent duct allowed moisture- or solvent-laden air to be exhausted from the pan. Later designs in air-handling equipment involved "fishtailing" of the inlet air duct (to better

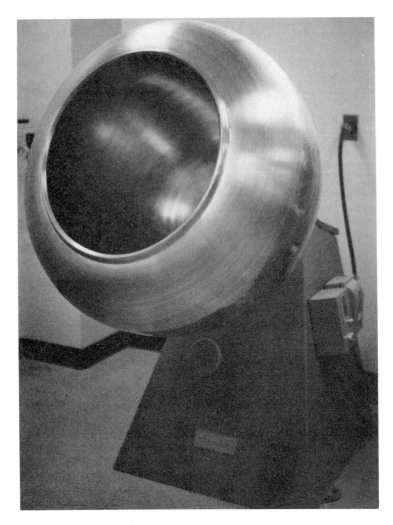

Figure 12   Illustration of conventional coating pan. (Courtesy of Colorcon,
West Point, Pennsylvania.)

distribute the drying air across the bed surface), and placing a hood
(connected to an exhaust plenum to facilitate better extraction of solvent
and dust-laden air from the process) over the pan opening.
  Three major drawbacks of this type of equipment are:

1. Much of the drying takes place on the surface of the bed of mate-
    rial being coated, thus drying efficiency is often low.
2. Mixing efficiency can be poor, and many dead spots (regions of
    low product movement) may exist in the product bed.
3. Improper balance between inlet and exhaust air can, with organic-
    solvent-based film coating, cause solvent vapor to leak into the

general coating area, creating a health hazard and increasing the risk of explosion

While the first of these limitations (i.e., drying efficiency) is not a real problem in sugar coating, it can provide a major constraint in film coating, particularly the aqueous process (where air exchange and, consequently, moisture removal needs to be highly efficient).

Mixing deficiencies can be a major problem, irrespective of the type of process practiced. While mixing can be augmented by addition of baffles (an approach preferred with the film-coating process), improved mixing was usually achieved in sugar coating by the operator "stirring" the tablets by hand.

Since the conventional pan was in common usage at the time film coating was introduced, this type of equipment initially formed the basis for the film-coating process, with lack of drying efficiency being offset by use of highly volatile organic solvents. Unfortunately, significant (and often expensive) modifications in air-handling equipment were required to accommodate the aqueous process.

One modification (the Glatt immersed sword) is shown in Figure 13. This equipment has concentric inlet and exhaust air ducts attached to a perforated "boot" that is immersed in the bed of product being coated. In addition, the opening of the coating pan is closed to isolate the inside of the coating pan from the environment in the coating room, thus further improving air exchange within the pan.

Modified Conventional Coating Pans

An important modification to conventional coating pans is an angular coating pan that rotates on a horizontal axis, with access to the interior of the pan occurring through openings in both the front and back. While several pharmaceutical manufacturers used variants of this style of pan, such equipment was (and still is) available commercially as the Pellegrini coating pan (Fig. 14).

The design of this pan dramatically improves mixing efficiency, which is also aided by the presence of an integral baffle system.

Drying air is introduced into the Pellegrini pan through a duct brought in at the back and connected to a slotted tube that directs air across the tablet surface. Exhausting is accomplished through an air plenum also attached to the back of the pan.

While the standard Pellegrini pan has proven to be an outstanding sugar-coating pan, drying is still somewhat conventional (i.e., restricted mainly to the surface of the bed of product being coated) such that this equipment is limited in capabilities with respect to film coating, especially the aqueous process.

Such limitations in drying capabilities can be offset, however, by installation of the Glatt immersed sword air-handling system.

In addition, the manufacturer of the Pellegrini pan has modified its own equipment to improve drying efficiencies and aid compliance with GMPs. This modification to the Pellegrini pan, known as the Pellegrini-GS coating system, consists of the standard-design Pellegrini pan enclosed inside a stainless-steel, sound-proofing cabinet (Fig. 15). This equipment can be supplied with either of two air-handling systems. The first, called the PLG system, provides drying air (via a slotted tube) across

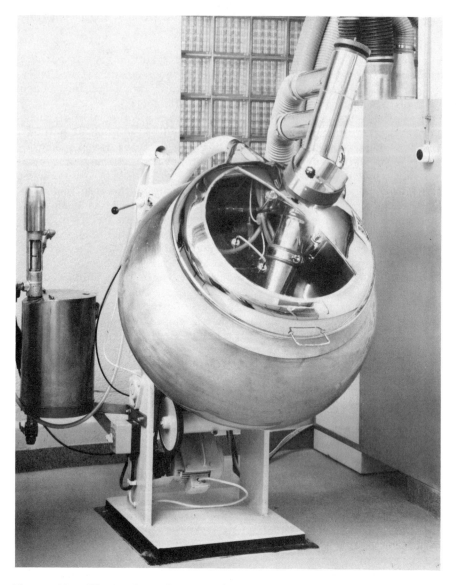

Figure 13   Illustration of conventional coating pan with Glatt "immersion sword" apparatus installed.   (Courtesy of Glatt Air Techniques, Ramsey, New Jersey.)

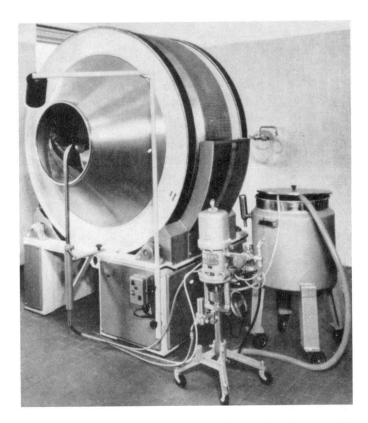

Figure 14   Illustration of Pellegrini coating pan.   (Courtesy of Nicomac, Englewood, New Jersey.)

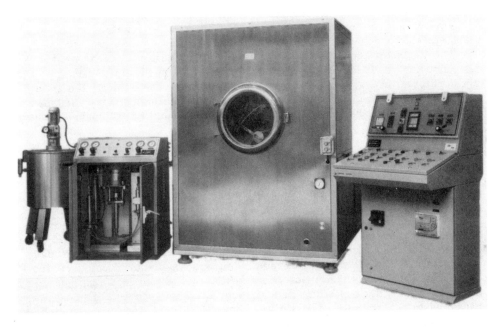

Figure 15   Illustration of Pellegrini-GS coating equipment.   (Courtesy of Nicomac, Englewood, New Jersey.)

the tablet bed and within the tablet bed (by means of two immersed perforated swords), whereas venting is achieved by means of an exhaust
plenum attached to the back of the pan. A second air-handling approach
is achieved with the GS system, which provides drying air via an inlet
plenum attached to the back of the pan, whereas exhaust air is vented via
two perforated swords immersed in the tablet bed. The GS system, which
operates under a negative pressure, is considered to be the more efficient
of the two air-handling systems, and thus is preferred in aqueous film
coating.

As with many of today's pan-coating systems, the Pellegrini-GS equipment is offered as a part of a package that includes liquid delivery
(pumps) and spray and monitoring/control equipment.

Side-Vented Coating Pans

There is no question that aqueous film coating places significant demands
on the drying capabilities of the various types of coating equipment.
Over the last 3 decades, designers of such equipment have sought to increase the interaction between the product being coated and the air responsible for removing solvent (aqueous or otherwise) from the coating
being applied to that product. Some would argue that use of fluid-bed
equipment is the most effective approach for this purpose.

In spite of the advantages of fluid-bed coating equipment, however,
the so-called side-vented pan has surfaced as the design of choice in most
film-coating applications (the major exception being for the film coating of
powders and other particulates).

While a multitude of specific designs of this type of equipment exists,
the basis for them all is one which enables air to be introduced into the
interior of the pan, drawn through the product being coated, and ultimately vented. Typically, such equipment consists of a somewhat angular
pan (fitted with mixing baffles) that rotates on a horizontal axis.

Various approaches to handling airflow in specific types of side-vented
pans are shown schematically in Figure 16.

The penchant today is for most film-coating equipment to be provided
as "turn-key" systems that comprise pan, air-handling, spray-delivery, and
monitoring/control systems. This is certainly the case with all the types
of side-vented pans. In addition, many exhibit clean-in-place (CIP) systems that facilitate cleaning of the pan, cabinets, and appropriate sections
of the air plenums.

ACCELA-COTA. The Accela-Cota equipment (introduced in the 1960s
by Thomas Engineering), based on a design patented by Eli Lilly, was the
pioneer in regard to design of side-vented pans. It has undergone various modifications since first being introduced, and a typical Accela-Cota
pan is illustrated in Figure 17.

Airflow through the pan (and product being coated) is facilitated by
the fully perforated cylindrical portion of the pan. Air is introduced by a
plenum in contact with the top of the pan and is drawn through the pan
and tablets. The air is then exhausted through a plenum located on the
outside of (but in contact with) the exterior of the pan in a position immediately below the cascading bed of tablets. The Accela-Cota pan thus
conforms to the airflow schematic #1, shown in Figure 16.

A modification of the Accela-Cota equipment, based on airflow schematic #2 (see Fig. 16), is used in conjunction with a screen insert to

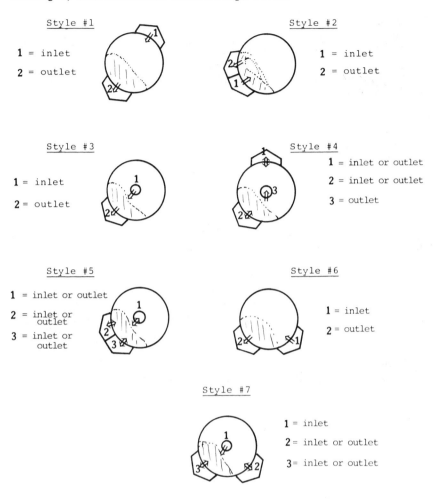

Figure 16 Schematic air flow diagrams for the various types of side-vented coating pans.

facilitate bead/granule coating. This modified design is known as the Multi-Cota coating equipment.

HI-COATER. The Vector-Freund Hi-Coater (Fig. 18) is based on a design that has four perforated segments, each located at 90° to one another in the cylindrical region of the pan. Each of these perforated sections acts as the opening to an exhaust air duct fixed to the outside of the rotating pan, and each duct makes contact with an exhaust plenum as the pan rotates. The exhaust plenum is designed to permit venting through any perforated section that is located approximately between the 6 and 9 o'clock positions as the pan rotates. Drying air is introduced into the pan via an opening located immediately above the door (but inside) of the pan. Thus, the airflow in a Hi-Coater pan conforms to schematic #3 (see Fig. 16).

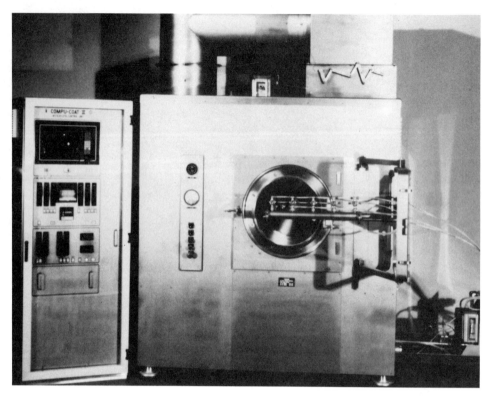

Figure 17 Illustration of Accela-Cota coating equipment. (Courtesy of Thomas Engineering, Hoffman Estates, Illinois.)

DRIACOATER. Unlike the two previously described pans, the Dria-coater pan design is nonagonal rather than cylindrical (Fig. 19). Attached to each of the nine flat sections is a perforated section that is linked via a duct on the exterior of the pan to one of two air-handling systems. Each of these air-handling systems is capable of producing positive or negative airflow (i.e., they can each blow air into or exhaust air from the pan). A third air-handling system, connected to an opening at the back of the pan, provides for exhaust only. This interesting design, which conforms to schematic #4 (see Fig. 16), permits for one of three types of airflow to be achieved:

Direct airflow: air in at the top (through perforated baffles) and
    exhausted through baffles located beneath the tablet bed
Reverse airflow A: air in through baffles located beneath tablet bed
    and exhausted via vaffles at top of pan
Reverse airflow B: air in through baffles located beneath tablet bed,
    and exhausted via plenum connected to opening at back of pan

GLATT PAN-COATING EQUIPMENT. The basis of the Glatt equipment is a fully perforated pan design similar to that of the Accela-Cota. This

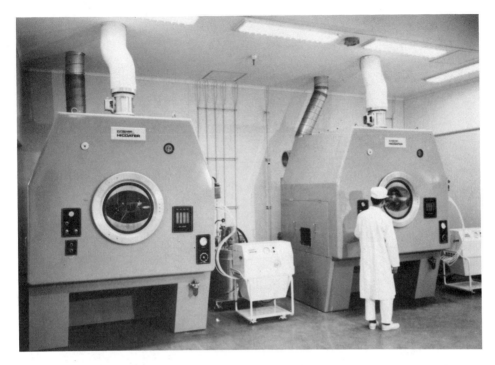

Figure 18 Illustration of hi-coater coating equipment. (Courtesy of Vector Corporation, Marion, Iowa.)

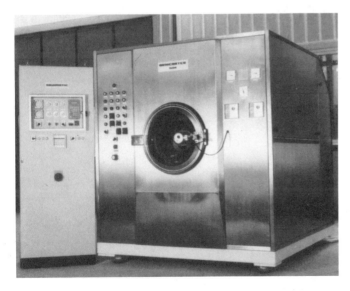

Figure 19 Figure of Driacoater coating equipment. (Courtesy of Driam USA, Spartanburg, South Carolina.)

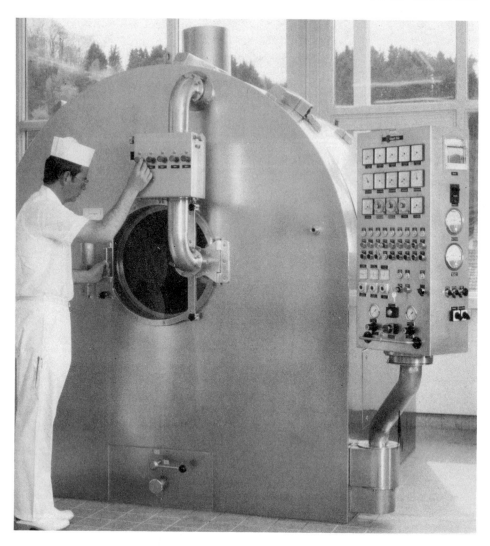

Figure 20   Figure of a Glatt coater.   (Courtesy of Glatt Air Techniques,
Ramsey, New Jersey.)

equipment was initially introduced, as shown in Figure 20, with airflow capabilities conforming to schematic #5 (see Fig. 16). A divided air plenum (located beneath the moving bed of tablets) enables air to be blown into or exhausted from the pan through either or both of the two sections. In addition, another air plenum, connected to an opening above the door (similar to that in a Hi-Coater) also allows air to be blown into or exhausted from the pan.

Consequently, this unusual air-handling system permits either direct or reverse airflow to be accomplished via any one of nine combinations (in direction) of airflow through the three plenums.

This particular design of Glatt pan is recognizable by its "gull wing" doors (that have inflatable seals and permit access to the inside of the cabinet surrounding the pan) and quite comprehensive clean-in-place system.

Unfortunately, owing in part to the flexibility and sophistication built into the design of this equipment, the Glatt coater has proven to be quite expensive. Consequently, a more economical model [called the Pro-Coater (see Fig. 21)] has recently been introduced that features a simpler air-handling system (conforming to schematic #6, Fig. 16). This permits direct airflow while minimizing the impact of airflow on spray patterns.

HÜTTLIN BUTTERFLY PAN. The Hüttlin Butterfly pan (Fig. 22) is rather unique in some aspects of its design. The side-vented pans described so far are often termed perforated pans because air moves in one direction or another through a perforated section of the pan wall. The Butterfly coating equipment, however, has a series of large, angled, slotted openings in the pan wall at the junction of the cylindrical portion with each of the front or back panels. These openings permit air to be exhausted from the pan. They are, however, angled in such a way that during normal rotation (when coating is in progress) the product being coated is prevented from entering the exhaust system. When the coating process is complete reversal of the coating pan allows product to be emptied through those same slotted openings.

Drying air is applied to the surface of the bed of the product being coated by means of a slotted tube (similar to that used in a standard Pellegrini pan) connected to an air plenum introduced through the rear of the pan.

An additional feature of this pan and one from which the name is probably derived, is that the front and back of the pan can be disconnected from the cylindrical, central section and hinged down. This feature allows the cylindrical portion to be removed and replaced with one of a different length. Thus, the capacity of the pan can be changed without resorting to a change in pan diameter (or indeed needing to buy another complete pan).

DUMOULIN IDA.X. The IDA.X (Fig. 23), another pan with a fully perforated cylindrical central section, exhibits airflow capabilities conforming to schematic #7 (see Fig. 16). The two air plenums that function as both inlet or exhaust air systems are located in contact with the outside of the pan, directly adjacent to the perforated cylindrical section of the pan at either the 4/5 o'clock position or the 7/8 o'clock position. In addition, a third plenum, connected to a slotted tube located inside the pan

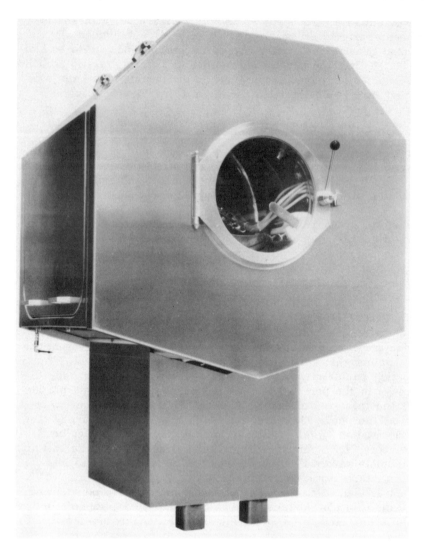

Figure 21   Figure of a Pro-Coater.   (Courtesy of Glatt Air Techniques, Ramsey, New Jersey.)

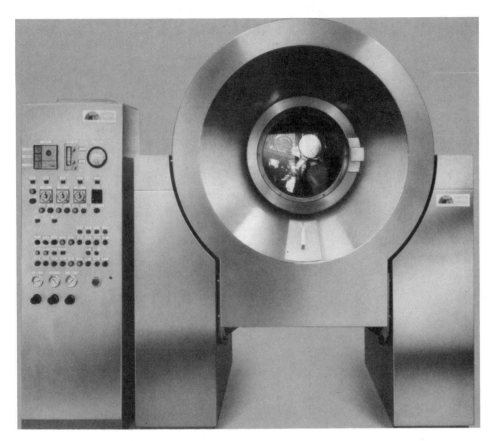

Figure 22 Figure of a Hüttlin Butterfly coating equipment. (Courtesy of Key International, Englishtown, New Jersey.)

and above the cascading product bed allows inlet air only to be directed onto the surface of product being coated.

The various combinations in direction of air flow permit one of four drying approaches to be employed:

1. Single flow: Air is blown onto tablets from above [via plenum (1)] and exhausted through plenum (2) (i.e., the plenum *not* located beneath the tablet bed), thus drying air does not really pass through the bed of product being coated.
2. Reversed single flow: Air is introduced via plenum (3) and exhausted through plenum (2).
3. Double flow: Air is introduced via plenums (1) and (3) and exhausted through plenum (2).
4. Direct double flow: Air is introduced via plenums (1) and (2) and exhausted through plenum (3).

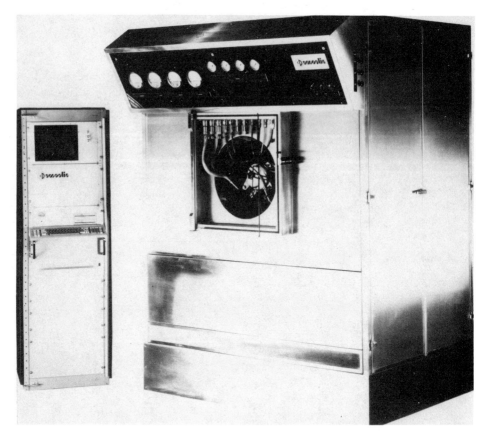

Figure 23 Figure of a Dumoulin IDA.X coating equipment. (Courtesy of Raymond Automation, Norwalk, Connecticut.)

While the unique features of all these types of side-vented pan make them particularly suitable for aqueous film coating, each can also be utilized effectively in the sugar-coating process.

B. Fluid-Bed Coating Equipment

Introduction

Fluid-bed processing technology was first introduced into the pharmaceutical industry over 30 years ago as a means of rapidly drying powdered and granulated materials. Subsequently, in the late 1960s, the addition of spray nozzles allowed fluid-bed drying technology to be extended to cover the granulation process.

The fluid-bed process (or perhaps more appropriately, the air-suspension process) has also been applied to the coating of pharmaceutical solids. Special equipment for this purpose was originally based on a design patented in the 1950s by Wurster [55]. Such a design, commonly called the Wurster process, is shown schematically in Figure 24. The salient features of the Wurster design consist of:

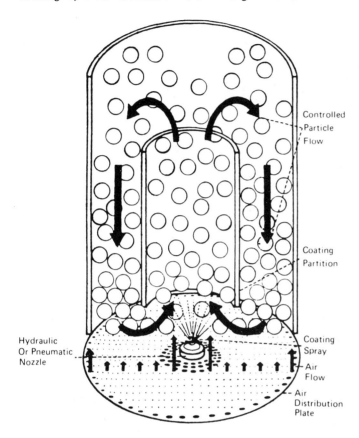

Figure 24 Schematic diagram of Wurster fluid-bed coating process.

Coating chamber

Inner partition, the diameter of which is approximately 50% that of the
   coating chamber

Air-distribution plate drilled with larger diameter holes in the central
   portion than those on the periphery

Spray nozzle located at the center of the air-distribution plate

During normal operation, fluidizing air causes the product being
coated to accelerate rapidly up through the inner partition which defines
the spray zone. Deceleration occurs in the region of the expansion
chamber, causing the product to drop back into the coating chamber into
the region confined by the walls of the chamber and the insert. The
product moves quickly down to the bottom of the coating chamber where
the cycle begins again.

Geometric limitations on the Wurster design normally prevent the diameter of the insert exceeding 9" (which corresponds to a coating-chamber
diameter of 18"). This limitation is imposed by the need to ensure that
all product accelerating through the spray zone is uniformly coated. Consequently, in order to further increase the capacity of the process,
larger-scale Wurster units are based on multiples of the 18" unit. For

example, the 32" unit has a coating chamber diameter of 32", but contains three 9" inserts; similarly, a 46" chamber contains seven 9" inserts.

In the heyday of organic-solvent-based film coating, the Wurster process proved to be very popular for coating tablets. However, most pharmaceutical companies used custom-built equipment, and simply paid appropriate license fees to the Wisconsin Alumni Research Foundation (WARF), to whom the patent rights were assigned.

Commercial manufacturers of fluid-bed processing equipment, initially precluded by patent from adopting the Wurster design, introduced designs of their own for film-coating pharmaceutical products. Such equipment (made available by Glatt, Aeromatic, and Freund) did not really achieve the popularity of the Wurster process. As the Wurster patents have expired, however, these major equipment companies have incorporated the Wurster design as an insert for their own equipment (at the expense of some of their earlier designs).

The product coated in the Wurster process is typically characterized by uniform distribution of coating and high gloss. Additionally, the process itself exhibits excellent drying characteristics. Consequently, it is rather surprising that as the age of aqueous-coating technology dawned, the popularity of the Wurster process waned: surprising when one considers that the aqueous process should benefit from the outstanding drying capabilities of this type of process. Nonetheless, most pharmaceutical manufacturers have preferred to use side-vented coating pans (as described in the previous section) for aqueous film coating of tablets in spite of the benefits of the Wurster process as extolled by Hall and Hinkes [56].

Recent years have witnessed, however, a growing interest in the aqueous film coating of particulates. The rationale for this ranges from a need to apply taste-masking coatings to powders, to that for modifying drug release (with, e.g., enteric- or controlled-release coated products). Since these kinds of film coatings need to be highly functional, the benefits of the fluid-bed process, with its capabilities for applying coatings uniformly and with minimized particle agglomeration, are readily evident, as shown by the data highlighted in Figure 25.

Finally, while the desire to utilize aqueous processes is paramount, some fluid-bed equipment has been specially designed to enable organic-solvent-based coatings to be applied while meeting stringent requirements regarding safety and protection of the environment. An example of such a design has been recently described [57].

Application of Functional Coatings

DIFFERENT APPROACHES IN FLUID-BED COATING. As discussed earlier in this section, the major approach in fluid-bed film coating has been to use the Wurster process. Certainly, this process is the most universally adaptable to most coating situations. However, as coating needs have changed, so has the need to introduce modified designs of coating equipment. For example, the greater demands for coating particulates (compared to coating tablets) has necessitated these changes:

Replacement of coarse filter screens with a filter bag assembly (replete with either a shaking system or blow-back device to dislodge entrained particles)

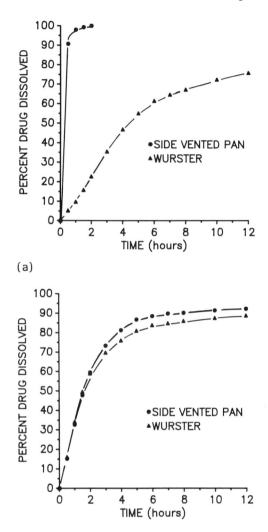

(a)

(b)

Figure 25 Effect of coating process (side-vented pan vs. Wurster) on release of chlorpheniramine from nonpareils coated with ethylcellulose (10% by weight of coating applied). (a) Organic-solvent-based solution of ethylcellulose and (b) aqueous dispersion (Surelease) of ethylcellulose.

Extension of the expansion chamber to permit deceleration of finer
particles and minimize entrainment in the filter system

Additionally, functional coatings are applied for a multiplicity of purposes, including taste masking, enteric coating, and controlled-release
coating. To meet these needs, three basic processing approaches have
evolved:

1. Top spray (essentially similar to that used in the fluid-bed granulation process)
2. Bottom spray (e.g., the Wurster process)
3. Tangential spray (or rotor process), which has developed from
   that used to prepare spheronized granulates and where additional
   particle motion is created by a spinning disc similar to that used
   in traditional spheronizers (such as the Marumerizer)

The schematics of these three processes are shown in Figure 26.
Each approach has its advantages and disadvantages, depending on:

Batch size of product being coated
Functionality of the final coating
Type of coating formulation being applied (e.g., solutions, polymeric
    dispersions, hot melts)
Flexibility with regard to the variety of types of coating that need to
    be applied in one piece of equipment

These advantages and disadvantages have been discussed in detail by
Jones [58] and Mehta [59]. The efficiencies of these types of coating
processes may vary. For example, Olsen and Mehta [60] have described
how the quantities of an organic-solvent-based ethylcellulose formulation

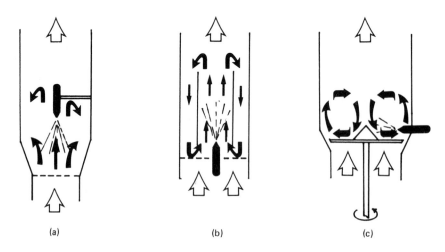

(a)   (b)   (c)

Figure 26   Schematic diagrams for the three basic types of fluid-bed
coating processes. (a) Top spray (granulator), (b) bottom spray
(Wurster), and (c) tangential spray (rotor-processor).

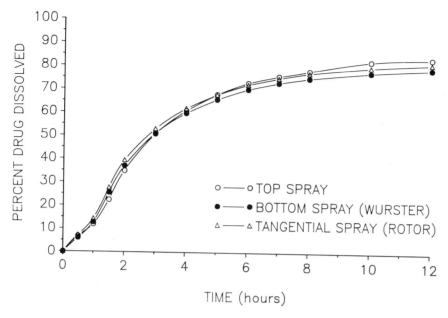

Figure 27 Release of chlorpheniramine from nonpareils coated with an aqueous ethylcellulose dispersion (Surelease 10% by weight of coating applied) in three types of fluid-bed coating processes (based on Glatt GPCG-1 unit).

that needed to be applied to achieve the same end result differed widely when comparing the top spray method with the Wurster process. However, when using aqueous polymeric dispersions, differences in performance between the three types of coating process may not be as significant (Fig. 27).

SCALE-UP CONSIDERATIONS IN FLUID-BED COATING PROCESSES. Scaling up any pharmaceutical process from laboratory to production can often prove difficult. Fluid-bed coating processes need extra special attention because they are associated today with the production of modified-release products (where the applied coating is highly functional).

There are many formulation and processing variables that need to be optimized initially so that ultimately the only variable that has to be dealt with is the change in batch weight as one moves from laboratory scale to full manufacturing scale. In order to facilitate this optimization process, adoption of an appropriate experimental design is essential. Optimization of a fluid-bed process for film coating of multiparticulates, using factorial design, has been described by Johansson et al. [61]. Assuming one particular type of processing equipment has been selected, some of the processing factors that need to be considered in the optimization process are:

Batch size
Fluidizing air volume
Inlet air temperature

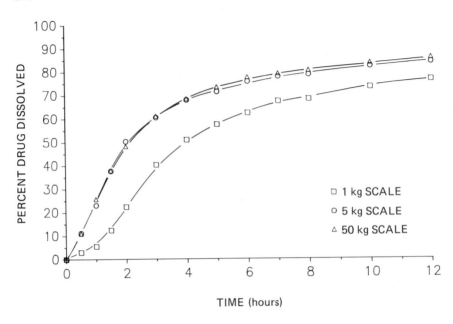

Figure 28   Effect of scale of coating process (Wurster) on release of chlorpheniramine from nonpareils coated with aqueous ethyl cellulose dispersion (Surelease 10% by weight of coating applied).

       Inlet air humidity
       Nozzle location
       Atomizing air pressure/volume
       Spray rate
       Coating liquid solids content

Metha [59] has described in detail the importance of many of these variables and how they relate to the scale-up process. As a word of caution, careful consideration (in the optimization process) should be given to the scale on which the scale-up process is based. Many times, initial studies are conducted on small (0.5–1.0 kg) laboratory scales; unfortunately this may not be an appropriate basis for predicting scale-up factors. By way of example, the data shown in Figure 28 are indicative of how feasibility studies conducted in a 1-kg capacity Wurster may not be entirely predictive of what is likely to happen on scale-up. In this example, a more appropriate starting point is likely to be the 5-kg pilot scale, where results obtained more closely match those obtained on the 50-kg scale.

Commercial Equipment

As discussed earlier, most fluid-bed equipment used for film coating was based on the Wurster design, with many pharmaceutical companies using custom-built equipment under a licensing agreement with WARF. However, in the last 10–15 years, several manufacturers of commercial fluid-bed equipment have adapted their designs to fulfill the needs of the film-coating process. The trend has been to provide equipment designed on the modular concept, where a basic processing unit is intended to accommodate a variety of processing inserts. These inserts can facilitate the use of fluid-bed processes for drying, granulating, spheronizing, and coating.

While many similarities exist for equipment supplied by the various vendors, opportunities for differentiation exists with:

Clamping systems (i.e., the mechanism for clamping the various removable sections together), which are typically either compressed air or hydraulic

Explosion protection, where some manufacturers use 2-bar construction plus explosion-relief venting, whereas others rely on 10-bar construction

Filter-bag assemblies, which can be based on either a split-filter shaking or pulsed-air blow-back systems

Heating units, where typically either conventional steam or electric can be provided, but where there is a growing preference for "face and by-pass" systems that permit more precise control over processing temperatures while facilitating rapid changes (in temperature) to be made when required

The trend is to provide standard equipment with appropriate options so that designs can be more easily customized to meet end-user requirements. Specialized designs, with taller expansion chambers that facilitate appropriate deceleration when coating small particles, are becoming common. As with other types of coating equipment, opportunities for providing completely automated processes now exist.

GLATT FLUID-BED COATING EQUIPMENT. Originally, the Glatt Air Techniques' designs were based on the WSG processing unit, which is capable of accepting a variety of inserts. More recently, however, in order to better address the situation in which the material to be coated is of small particle size (ranging from approximately 100 μm – 2 mm), the emphasis has shifted toward the GPCG processing unit. Inserts can be provided to permit drying, granulating (or top-spray coating), Wurster coating (bottom spray), and rotor granulation/layering/coating (tangential spray).

An example of a 5- to 10-kg pilot GPCG unit is shown in Figure 29. Other common features of the Glatt equipment are:

Filter systems based on the split filter, shaking principle

2-Bar construction with explosion relief (although 10-bar construction, at an added cost, may be available)

Microprocessor-based control panels when non-explosion-proof operating environments are permissible

Hydraulic clamping systems

AEROMATIC FLUID-BED COATING EQUIPMENT. Aeromatic fluid-bed coating equipment is again designed to accommodate a variety of modular inserts. A typical laboratory scale unit, capable of processing up to 3 – 5 kg of material, is shown in Figure 30.

Inserts that can be utilized with this manufacturer's equipment include:

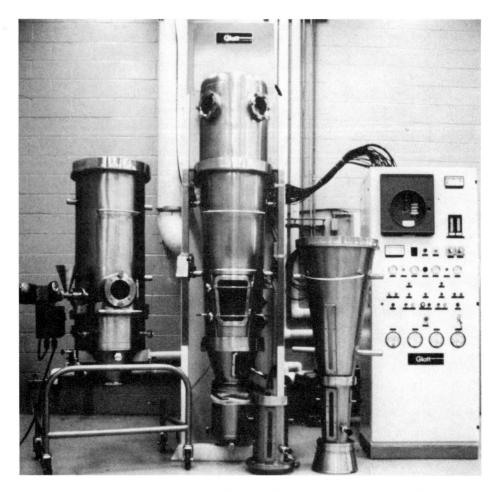

Figure 29   Figure of a Glatt GPCG-5 fluid-bed coating unit. (Courtesy of Glatt Air Techniques, Ramsey, New Jersey.)

Dryer (with options for batch or continuous processing)
Spray granulator (and top-spray coating)
Aero-coater (Wurster, bottom-spray coating)
Ultra coater (bottom/tangential spray for tablet coating)

Some additional features of Aeromatic equipment are:

Sequential blow-back filter system
Clamping system based on compressed air
Standard 10-bar construction

Unlike some of the competitive equipment, the Wurster process (Aero-coater) does not require a completely separate unit, but rather is created by adding the inner Wurster chamber (insert) to the product bowl of the batch granulator unit. This obviously provides some opportunity for economizing on cost.

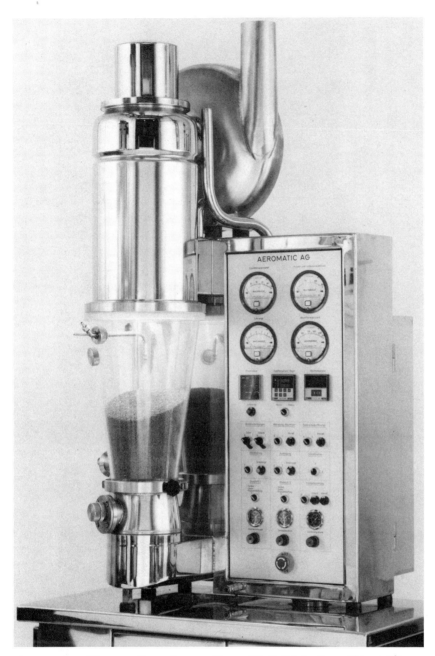

Figure 30 Figure of an Aeromatic multi fluid-bed coating unit.
(Courtesy of Aeromatic, Inc., Columbia, New Jersey.)

VECTOR-FREUND FLUID-BED COATING EQUIPMENT. The design of
the Vector-Freund fluid-bed coating equipment was originally based on
that of the Flowcoater, which features spray nozzles located (and angled
downward) in the sidewalls of the product container. This design permits
the same equipment to be used for fluid-bed drying, coating, and
granulating.

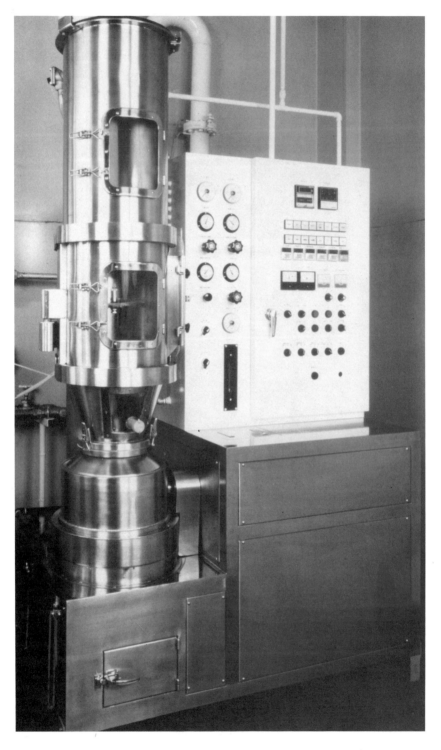

Figure 31 Figure of a Vector-Freund Flowcoater multi fluid-bed coating unit. (Courtesy of Vector Corporation, Marion, Iowa.)

More recently, the Flowcoater multi unit (Fig. 31) has been introduced, which features separate inserts for:

Drying
Granulating (and top-spray coating)
Wurster coating
Spheronizing/layering/coating (a tangential spray, rotor unit that is
     based on the operating principle of the CF granulator)

HÜTTLIN KUGELCOATER. In terms of fluid-bed film coating, the
Kugelcoater is rather unique, both in basic design and for the fact that
it does not consist of a central processor that accepts multiple inserts.

A simplified schematic of the Kugelcoater is represented in Figure 32,
whereas a photograph of the equipment is shown in Figure 33.

The product container of the Kugelcoater is spherical. Inlet fluidizing
air is introduced via a tube that passes down the center of the product
container. The design permits this air to enter the product container at
the bottom. A series of spray nozzles are also located at the bottom of
the product container in such a way that fluidizing air creates a "balloon"
effect to keep the product being coated away from the spray nozzles.

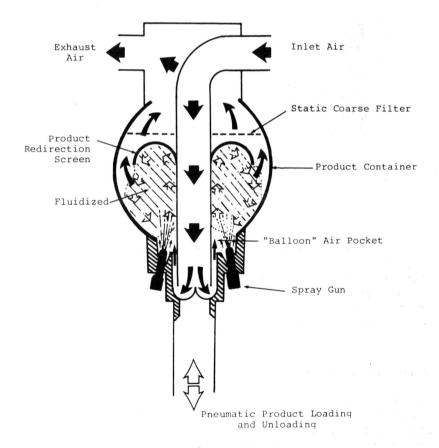

Figure 32   Schematic diagram of a Kugelcoater.

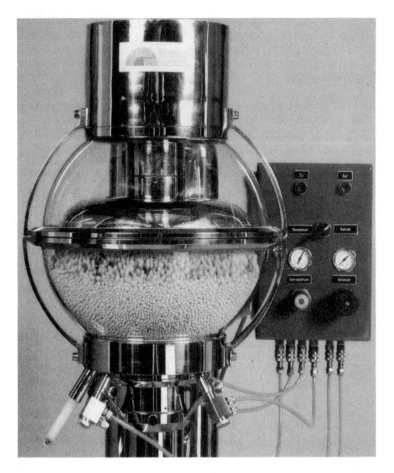

Figure 33   Figure of a Hüttlin Kugelcoater.   (Courtesy of Key International, Englishtown, New Jersey.)

The product fluidization pattern is constrained by a product redirection screen that restricts product entry into the filter system.

This unique design, encompassing the inclusion of multiple spray nozzles intended to maximize uniformity of distribution of the coating, also permits pneumatic loading and unloading of product.

Various sizes of the Kugelcoater are available, ranging from lab models with product container capacities of 2 L to those having capacities of 700 L.

C. Application Equipment

In most modern pan-coating operations, one major emphasis is to provide a means of mechanically applying coating liquids, and thus avoid manual techniques such as ladling.

While there are similarities in requirements (for mechanical application of coating liquids) between the sugar-coating and film-coating processes, certain differences exist that almost certainly influence selection of appropriate equipment.

Sugar-coating liquids typically have solids contents in excess of 70% (w/w), and consequently can be extremely viscous. Contrast this with the fact that film-coating liquids rarely contain greater than 20% non-volatile materials (which typically fall in the range of 5–15%).

Uniform distribution of sugar-coating liquids is achieved by the cascading action (of the product being coated) that takes place within the pan and causes transfer of liquid from one piece to another. This transfer should occur before any substantial drying occurs. Thus, the application equipment needs only to be very simple in design and allow the coating liquid to stream onto the surface of the cascading product.

Conversely, film-coating liquids (almost without exception) need to be applied in a finely atomized state and uniformly distributed across the surface of the product being coated.

In the context of this chapter, mechanical application refers to any method of introducing a coating liquid across the surface in an appropriate manner other than hand ladling.

Application Sparges

Application sparges were discussed earlier in this chapter (and illustrated in Fig. 3) and refer to simple equipment that allow the coating liquid to stream across and onto the surface of the cascading bed of the product being coated.

The simplicity of this type of equipment makes it extremely suitable for use in the sugar-coating process.

Airless Spray Equipment

Airless spray equipment generally consists of a particular design of spray gun that contains a nozzle with an extremely small orifice (typically 200–400 μm or 0.009–0.015"). The coating liquid is delivered under significant pressure (often in the range of 3.5–20.0 MPa or 500–3000 psi) and velocity, and literally explodes into tiny droplets as it emerges from the nozzle. Because of the high shear generated at the nozzle, a nozzle insert or tip made of tungsten carbide is used. Nozzle tips are available in a wide range of configurations that permit cone spray or flat (or ovalized) spray patterns to be generated.

Liquid flow rates through airless spray equipment are typically high. Stearn [62] described how such liquid flow rates, based on examination of fundamental flow theories, are:

Directly proportional to the cross-sectional area of the nozzle orifice
Directly proportional to the square root of hydraulic pressure (of coating liquid)
Inversely proportional to density of the coating liquid

Since a minimum hydraulic pressure is required for optimal atomization of the coating liquid, and there is a practical lower limit on orifice size (before clogging becomes a serious problem), airless spray equipment is mainly restricted to applications where high-volume delivery of coating liquids is required. Such applications include production scale, organic-solvent-based film coating or similar scale sugar coating.

Air-Spray Equipment

Air-spray application equipment is generally less expensive than the corresponding airless equipment, and is capable of delivering coating liquids at
low to relatively high application rates. The functional components of an
air-spray gun are the fluid cap (through which the liquid emerges) and
the air cap (through which compressed air is delivered to create the
driving force for atomization). Typically, the air cap fits over the fluid
cap (or nozzle) and forms an annulus that allows compressed air to impinge
on the stream of coating liquid emerging from the fluid nozzle. This im-
pingement causes the coating liquid to be broken up into tiny droplets.

Droplet size and size distribution are typically controlled by atomizing
air pressure *and* volume. In most pan-coating operations, in order to
allow the coating liquid to be spread out, the air cap also has "wing tips"
that permit compressed air to be directed laterally onto the atomized spray
so that the spray pattern is ovalized. In order to avoid increased risk of
spray drying and turbulence, care should be taken not to try and ovalize
excessively the spray patterns. For this reason, air-spray guns typically
are unable to cover as much of the surface of the product bed as airless
guns, and thus more air-spray guns must be used for a particular application (e.g., in a typical 48" Accela-Cota setup, whereas two airless guns
may provide adequate coverage, three or more air-spray guns may be
required to provide equivalent coverage).

Air-spray equipment is typically suited to small-scale coating operations and all those involving the use of aqueous formulations (where the
atomizing air effectively augments the drying capabilities of the air-
handling system). Air-spray equipment should be used with great care
for organic – solvent-based film coating processes, since the atomizing air
can cause excessive spray drying.

Ultrasonic-Spray Equipment

Recently, attempts have been made to utilize ultrasonic nozzles as a means
of effectively atomizing and applying coating liquids. Such nozzles are
commonly used in oil burners and as part of the lithophotographic process
used in the semiconductor industry, and to apply specialized coatings onto
the surfaces of medical devices.

The major advantages of such nozzles are that they are economical to
operate (although initial capital cost can be high), produce atomized
liquids with uniform size distributions and low velocities, and eliminate
many of the problems associated with overspray and fogging.

While various designs of ultrasonic nozzles are available, those used
for coatings typically have relatively large orifices and conical tips. The
operating principle of an ultrasonic nozzle is similar to that of a speaker
in audio equipment. In this case, ceramic piezoelectric transducers convert electrical energy into mechanical energy, which is transmitted to a
titanium horn that forms the atomizing tip. Coating liquid that is introduced onto the atomizing surface absorbs some of the vibrational energy,
causing a wave motion to be set up in the liquid. If the vibrational
amplitude is carefully controlled, the liquid will break free from the surface of the nozzle as a fine mist (with median droplet sizes in the range
of $20-50$ μm).

So far, the use of ultrasonic nozzles with pharmaceutical coating
liquids has met with very limited success. Most polymeric-coating

solutions appear to present a problem with respect to achieving effective and controllable atomization. This limitation seems to reflect the complex rheological and cohesive properties of these solutions. Such nozzles might be used more effectively where the coating liquid is a dispersion (e.g., many of the formulations used in sugar coating or the aqueous latex systems used in film coating).

Berger [63] has given a more complete description of ultrasonic nozzles, their applications, and limitations.

D. Metering/Delivery Equipment

This discussion of metering/delivery equipment refers to that equipment which enables coating liquid to be delivered from a bulk holding tank to the application equipment described in the previous section (Sec. IV.C).

Pressurized Containers

Pressurized containers (or pressure pots, as they are commonly called) were once commonly used with many organic–solvent-based film-coating systems and have recently been reintroduced as components of some specialized automated delivery systems.

Basically, such a system consists of a special liquid holding tank that can be pressurized by compressed air. Once pressurized, the liquid is forced from the tank through feed lines to the spray nozzle. Fluid delivery rates with such equipment will be dependent on air pressure, liquid viscosity and density, length and internal diameter of the feed lines, and design of the spray nozzles used.

All other things being equal (for a given system and coating liquid), flow rate is controlled via a pressure regulator that determines pressure within the tank.

Precision with such a system may be inadequate when attempting to deliver low-viscosity aqueous-coating liquids (such as latex dispersions).

Peristaltic Pumps

Peristaltic pumps (or "tubing" pumps) are commonly used in many coating operations. The operating principle of these pumps is based on the ability to create liquid flow in a tube by squeezing and stretching that tube. Most common peristaltic pumps have a pump head that allows a piece of tubing to be clamped in a U-shaped fashion against a rotating mechanical device (such as "fingers" or rollers) that squeezes the tube and creates motion of the liquid within the tube. To function effectively, the material from which the tubing is made should have sufficient resiliency that it quickly recovers its original shape after squeezing. For this reason, preferred tubing is made from silicone rubber.

Peristaltic pumps have two major advantages:

1. They are simple and inexpensive (to purchase and operate).
2. They are sanitary (since the liquid being transferred does not come in direct contact with the mechanical pump head), and cleanup is easily accomplished by passing a cleaning liquid through the tubing, and tubing that is difficult to clean can be replaced at little cost.

There are some major drawbacks with such equipment, including:

They are not positive displacement pumps.
Linearity, and often accuracy, decreases as the pump speed is in-
     creased (particularly at the high end of the speed range).
Accuracy decreases as the tubing wears and fatigues.
Their effectiveness is limited by liquid viscosity.

Gear Pumps

Gear pumps are becoming extremely popular in aqueous film coating. They
are positive displacement pumps that rely on two counterrotating gears to
draw liquid into and through the pump housing. Because the gears come
into contact with the coating liquid, they must be made of noncorrodible
materials. Gear pumps can transfer liquids with a wide range of viscosities,
but rely on the inherent "lubricity" of the coating liquid to minimize wear
in the gear mechanism.
    Some limitations of gear pumps are:

Cost
Requirement for more complicated clean-up procedures
Likelihood of excessive wear of mechanism when pumping highly pig-
     mented, low-viscosity coating liquids
Likelihood of inducing coagulation of latex-coating systems as a result
     of shear developed as liquid passes through pump head

While many gear pumps rely on a direct mechanical drive, some recent
models have an indirect magnetic drive.

Piston Pumps

Piston pumps, which are also positive displacement pumps, rely on a re-
ciprocating piston (typically powered by a compressed air motor) to transfer the coating liquid. Such a pump can easily handle very viscous liquids
and so is well suited to sugar-coating and most film-coating operations.
    Those piston pumps driven by air motors usually have a particular
pressure ratio rating (such as 30:1, 10:1, or 5:1). This rating refers to
amount by which pressure supplied by the air operating the pumps is increased when transferred to the liquid being pumped. For example, 10
psi air pressure applied to a 30:1 ratio pump will generate 300 psi of liquid
line pressure. For this reason, such pumps are commonly used as the delivery mechanism in airless spray systems.
    More recently, electrically driven piston pumps, which have variable
speeds and stroke lengths and generate very little line pressure, have
been introduced as components of air-spray systems used in aqueous film
coating. An example of such a pumping system is the volumetric pump
PD 1000/S supplied with the Pellegrini-GS coating system.
    Piston pumps, like gear pumps, are relatively expensive and not as
easy to clean as tubing pumps. In addition, the shearing action as the
pump reciprocates may induce coagulation of latex-coating systems. This
is particularly true when any significant line pressure is generated.

V. AUTOMATED COATING PROCEDURES

A. Introduction

In the early days of tablet coating, the addition of coating liquids, determination of distribution/mixing times, and application of drying and exhaust air were all manual operations. Decisions as to when heated air should be applied, coating liquid should be added, and how long to allow for uniform distribution of the coating liquid were all judgmental factors on the part of the operator.

In order to achieve a high level of reproducibility in the process and simplify the documentation process, it is apparent that the above situation has many limitations.

To effectively automate a process, it is necessary to remove the requirements for direct (and repeated) involvement by the operator. The process must be well developed and precisely defined (when a poorly defined process is automated it will simply produce consistently *unacceptable* results time after time). In particular, it is imperative to avoid using any critical steps that can only be achieved on such a limited basis as to render the whole process impractical.

The benefits to be derived from a well-automated process are:

Independence from operator judgment
Achievement of consistent product quality
Achievement of a fully optimized process with greater potential for
    minimizing processing times
Production of hard-copy documentation

It is critical, however, that an automated process possesses a fail-safe mechanism so that process shutdown takes place in the event of process failure. Such a procedure will reduce the liklihood that a batch of product is ruined.

The automation of a coating process typically involves two basic activities:

1. Timing and sequencing (more appropriate for sugar coating where a sequence of events must occur at specific time intervals)
2. Measuring and controlling appropriate processing parameters

The second of these two activities can be the more difficult, particularly since appropriate precision in measuring devices may be difficult to achieve. Measuring and control devices may be classified as:

Electromechanical
Pneumatic
Electronic

There is no doubt that electronic devices are preferred in order to deal with the complexities of today's coating processes. Electronic devices, however, are subject to drift, and thus must constantly be recalibrated to ensure accuracy and precision.

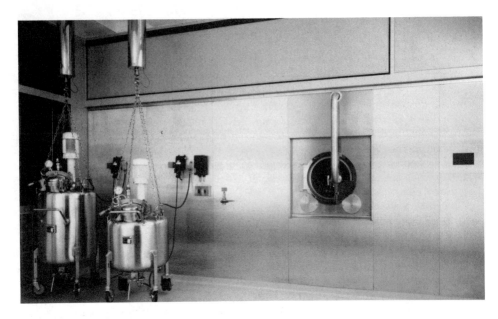

Figure 34   Figure of a totally automated film-coating process. (Courtesy
of Meltech, East Hanover, New Jersey.)

A description of some pan-coating control systems has been given by
Thomas [64], and an example of a modern fully automated tablet coating
process is shown in Figure 34.

B. Automation of Sugar Coating

In basic terms, sugar coating can be considered, from the automation
standpoint, to be a complex, noncritical process. Complexity stems from
the significant number of timing and sequencing functions that are required.
Noncriticality (from a relative standpoint) occurs because many of the coating parameters need not be controlled to extreme accuracies. For example,
accurate control of airflow and temperature is not critical as long as specific objectives (such as achieving a particular state of product dryness
before the next addition of coating liquid occurs) are met.

Early attempts at automation of the sugar-coating process involved
achieving the appropriate sequencing and timing by means of timers.
Such an approach is very simple but has limitations, namely:

  If constant, predictable drying conditions are not achieved (such as
     use of temperature and humidity-controlled drying air), then sea-
     sonal variations in conditions may result in predetermined se-
     quencing and timing to be totally inappropriate for a specific set
     of conditions.
  As coating build-up occurs, there may be a need to adjust the volumes
     of coating liquid applied.

Over the last 25 years, various descriptions of automated procedures have appeared in the pharmaceutical literature [65–67].

An early commercially available system, the Driamat, has been described by Rose [68].

A more recently introduced commercial, fully-automated, sugar-coating process is the Sandomatic system, which was first described by Melliger and Goss [69].

The important independent process variables that need to be monitored and controlled in a typical sugar-coating process are:

Drying air volume (or flow)
Drying air temperature
Drying air humidity
Pan speed
Quantity of coating liquid applied (at each step)

C. Automation of Film Coating

In comparison to sugar coating, film coating is a simpler, but more critical process to automate. Little sequencing is required, but important process conditions must be monitored and controlled to a high degree of accuracy.

Important independent variables that need to be measured and controlled in a film-coating process include:

Drying air volume
Drying air temperature
Drying air humidity
Pan speed
Spray rate (more precisely, the delivery rate from each spray gun in
    a multiple-gun setup)
Atomizing air pressure/volume
Pattern air pressure/volume

In addition, it may be necessary to control various dependent variables, particularly in the aqueous process where the margin for error can be much less than in other types of coating process. Some of the important dependent variables that need to be monitored are:

Tablet bed temperature
Exhaust air temperature
Exhaust air humidity
Tablet bed moisture

Since these variables cannot be controlled directly, it will be necessary to control the interaction between those independent variables that influence a particular dependent variable. For example, exhaust air temperature may be kept under control by maintaining an appropriate balance between:

Inlet air volume
Inlet air temperature
Inlet air humidity
Spray rate

In the aqueous film-coating process, the importance of taking into account the moisture content of the inlet drying air cannot be overemphasized. The simplest way of dealing with this issue is to keep inlet air humidity constant by use of a dehumidificat.on process. Such an approach can, however, prove to be extremely expensive, since the volumes of air that need to be conditioned are typically very large (in an aqueous film-coating process, e.g., a typical 48" Accela-Cota coating a batch of tablets in 90 min will require approximately 5000 m^3 of conditioned air).

An alternative is to compensate for variation in humidity of inlet air by adjusting one or more of:

Air volume
Inlet air temperature
Spray rate

Lachman and Cooper [70] have described an early attempt to automate the film-coating process. More recently, the automation principles of the Sandomatic process have been applied to film coating. Also, virtually every supplier of pan-coating equipment can provide automated equipment, and selection may well depend on the preferences, and individual needs, of the pharmaceutical manufacturer.

REFERENCES

1. Signorino, C. A., U.S. Patent 3,738,952 (1973).
2. Rowe, R. C., *Int. J. Pharm.*, 43:155 (1988).
3. McGinity, J. W., *Aqueous Polymeric Coatings for Pharmaceutical Dosage Forms*. Marcel Dekker, New York, 1988.
4. Skultety, P. F., Rivera, D., Dunleavy, J., and Lin, C. T. *Drug Dev. Ind. Pharm.*, 14(5):617 (1988).
5. Reiland, T. L. and Eber, A. C., *Drug Dev. Ind. Pharm.*, 13(3): 231 (1986).
6. Thoennes, C. J. and McCurdy, V. E., contributed paper at PT Section of 3rd Annual Meeting of AAPS, Orlando, Florida, Oct. 1988.
7. Ebey, G. C., *Pharm. Tech.*, 11(4):40 (1987).
8. Rowe, R. C., *J. Pharm. Pharmacol.*, 29:723 (1977).
9. Fisher, D. G. and Rowe, R. C., *J. Pharm. Pharmacol.*, 28:886 (1976).
10. Rowe, R. C., *J. Pharm. Pharmacol.*, 30:669 (1978).
11. Aulton, M. E., Twitchell, A. M., and Hogan, J. E., Proceedings of AGPI Conference, Paris (1986).
12. Rowe, R. C., *J. Pharm. Pharmacol.*, 32:851 (1980).
13. Rowe, R. C. and Forse, S. F., *Acta Pharm. Tech.*, 28(3):207 (1982).
14. Twitchel, A. M., Hogan, J. E., and Aulton, M. E., *J. Pharm. Pharmacol.*, 39S:128P (1987).
15. Porter, S. C. and Saraceni, K., *Pharm. Tech.*, 12(9):78 (1988).
16. Kara, M. A. K., Leaver, T. M., and Rowe, R. C., *J. Pharm. Pharmacol.*, 34:469 (1982).
17. Rowe, R. C., *Pharm. Int.*, 6(9):225 (1985).

18. Wicks, Z. W., Jr., *Film Formation*. Series on Coatings Technology, Federation of Societies for Coating Technology, Philadelphia (1986).
19. Burrett, H., *Offic. Dig.*, *34*(445):131 (1962).
20. Williams, M. L., Landel, R. F., and Ferry, J. D., *J. Am. Chem. Soc.*, 77:3701 (1955).
21. Wicks, Z. W., Jr., *J. Coatings Technol.*, *58*(743):23 (1986).
22. Entwistle, C. A. and Rowe, R. C., *J. Pharm. Pharmacol.*, *31*:269 (1979).
23. Rowe, R. C., *J. Pharm. Pharmacol.*, *33*:423 (1981).
24. Bindschaedler, C., Gurney, R., and Doelker, E., *Labo-Pharma-Probl. Tech.*, *31*(331):389 (1983).
25. Bradford, E. B. and Vanderhoff, J. W., *J. Macromol. Chem.*, *1*(2): 335 (1966).
26. Gross, H. M. and Endicott, C. J., *D&CI*, *86*(2):170 (1960).
27. Porter, S. C., *Pharm. Tech.*, *4*(3):66 (1980).
28. Crawford, R. R. and Esmerian, O. K., *J. Pharm. Sci.*, *60*(2):312 (1971).
29. Sakellariou, P., Rowe, R. C., and White, E. F. T., *Int. J. Pharm.*, *31*:55 (1986).
30. Woznicki, E. J. and Schoneker, D. R., Coloring agents, In *Encyclopedia of Pharmaceutical Technology*. Marcel Dekker, New York, in press.
31. Porter, S. C., *Int. J. Pharm. Tech. Prod. Mfr.*, *3*(1):21 (1982).
32. Rowe, R. C., *Pharm. Acta. Helv.*, *60*(5/6):157 (1985).
33. Rowe, R. C., *J. Pharm. Pharmacol.*, *33*:51 (1980).
34. Rowe, R. C., *J. Pharm. Pharmacol.*, *36*:569 (1983).
35. Rowe, R. C. and Forse, S. F., *J. Pharm. Pharmacol.*, *35*:205 (1983).
36. Rowe, R. C., *Int. J. Pharm.*, *14*:355 (1983).
37. Banker, G. S., *J. Pharm. Sci.*, 55:81 (1966).
38. Hildebrand, J. and Scott, R., *The Solubility of Non-Electrolytes*, 3rd Ed. Reinhold, New York, 1949.
39. Kent, D. J. and Rowe, R. C., *J. Pharm. Pharmacol.*, *31*(5):269 (1979).
40. Rudin, A. and Wagner, R. A., *J. Appl. Polym. Sc..*, *19*:3361 (1975).
41. Johnson, K., Hathaway, R. D., and Franz, R. M., Presented at the Contributed Paper Session of the 3rd Annual Meeting of AAPS, Orlando, Florida, 1988.
42. Porter, S. C., In *Aqueous Polymeric Coatings for Pharmaceutical Dosage Forms* (J. W. McGinity, ed.), Marcel Dekker, New York, 1988, p. 317.
43. Ozturk, S. S., Palsson, B. O., Donohoe, B., and Dressman, J. B., *Pharm. Res.*, *5*(9):550 (1988).
44. Edgar, B., Bogentoft, C., and Lagerstrom, P. O., *Biopharm Drug Disp.*, 5:251 (1984).
45. Theeuwes, F., *J. Pharm. Sci.*, *64*(12):1987 (1975).
46. Lindholm, T. and Julsin, M., *Pharm. Ind.*, *44*(9):937 (1982).
47. Jambhekar, S. S., Breen, P. J., and Rojanasakul, Y., *Drug Dev. Ind. Pharm.*, *13*(15):2789 (1987).
48. Rowe, R. C., *J. Pharm. Pharmacol.*, *35*:112 (1983).
49. Rowe, R. C., *J. Pharm. Pharmacol.*, *32*:851 (1980).

50. Breech, J. A., Lucisano, L. J., and Franz, R. M., *J. Pharm. Pharmacol.*, *40*:282 (1988).
51. Rowe, R. C. and Forse, S. F., *Acta. Pharm. Technol.*, *28*(3):207 (1982).
52. Kim, S., Mankad, A., and Sheen, P. *Drug Dev. Ind. Pharm.*, *12*(6): 801 (1986).
53. Down, G. R. B., *J. Pharm. Pharmacol.*, *34*(4):281 (1982).
54. Shah, B. B., Contractor, A. M., and Auslander, D. E., *Pharm. Res.*, *5*(10):S-253 (1988).
55. Wurster, D. E., U.S. Patent 2,648,609 (1953).
56. Hall, H. S. and Hinkes, T. M., Presented at the Symposium on Microencapsulation: Processes and Applications, American Chemical Society, Chicago, Aug. 27–31, 1973.
57. Glatt Technically Speaking, *2*(1):1 (1989).
58. Jones, D. M., *Pharm. Technol.*, *9*(4):50 (1985).
59. Mehta, A. M., *Pharm. Technol.*, *12*(2):46 (1988).
60. Olsen, K. W. and Mehta, A. M., *Int. J. Pharm. Tech. Prod. Mfr.*, *6*(4):18 (1985).
61. Johansson, M. E., Ringberg, A., and Nicklasson, M., *J. Microencapsul.*, *4*(3):217 (1987).
62. Stern, P. W., *J. Pharm. Sci.*, *63*(7):1171 (1974).
63. Berger, H. L., *Machine Design*, July 1988.
64. Thomas, R., *Pharmaceut. Eng.*, *16*:Aug.–Oct. (1981).
65. Rieckmann, P., *Drugs Made in Germany*, *6*:162 (1963).
66. Heyd, A. and Kanig, J. L., *J. Pharm. Sci.*, *59*(8):1171 (1970).
67. Fox, D. C., Buckpitt, A. E., Laramie, M. V., and Miserany, M. E., Presented at A.I.Ch.E. Meeting, New York, Nov. 17, 1977.
68. Rose, F., *D&C.I.*, *44*:Nov. (1971).
69. Melliger, G. and Goss, L., Presented at A.Ph.A. Annual Meeting, New York, April 1977.
70. Lachman, L. and Cooper, J., *J. Pharm. Sci.*, *52*(5):490 (1963).

3
Particle-Coating Methods

Dale E. Wurster

University of Iowa, Iowa City, Iowa

I. INTRODUCTION

There are many important pharmaceutical reasons for applying coatings to both pure chemicals used as medicinal agents and to physical–chemical systems employed as dosage forms [1–4]. Similar coatings are also widely used in other industries to coat particulate solids. One of the most widespread pharmaceutical uses today is for the control of drug release from various types of oral or parenteral dosage forms designed to have either an enteric, a timed, or a sustained-release effect. Thus, particle coatings can be formulated so that the escape of the drug from the dosage form occurs primarily via a diffusional process. The various physical parameters influencing diffusion can then be modified in order to control the rate of drug release. In other systems, the dissolution kinetics of the applied coat serve to control the availability of the contained drug. In still other cases, drug release can be controlled by chemical reactions involving the coating material or by simple attritional effects on the coat. No matter what mechanism of controlled drug release one wishes to use, it is apparent that this can usually be achieved by the proper formulation of coating materials and the manner in which they are applied.

A second type of effect achieved by coating procedures is the enhancement of the chemical stability of drugs. It is possible to formulate coating materials to guard against the penetration of substances which will cause specific degradation reactions. Thus, coatings can be designed to resist the penetration of water vapor when the product contains drugs which are susceptible to hydrolytic decomposition. For those drugs which degrade by oxidative reactions, coatings can be used which inhibit the transport of oxygen to the labile compound. In cases where detrimental

interactions result from materials contained within the physical system rather than from external influences, the incompatible materials can be separated by suitable coatings.

Of course, coating procedures have long been used to occlude drugs
with an unpleasant taste from the taste receptors, or to impart pleasing
colors to a product to make it more attractive visually. Certain other
physical parameters, such as particle density, surface characteristics, or
geometry, can also be altered by the use of coatings to obtain processing
advantages. For example, coatings can sufficiently change the geometry
and surface of small particles so that the flow properties of a powder are
enhanced.

It is the primary intent of this chapter to present a discussion of
those processes which are useful in particle coating to meet the above
needs. While the theoretical mechanisms involved in controlling such factors as drug release and chemical stability are of great interest to all who
work with these systems, a discussion of these mechanisms is not within
the scope of this chapter. Primary emphasis is, therefore, directed toward
the processes which are useful for the coating of solid particles. However,
methods which are mainly useful for the microencapsulation of liquids are
also briefly discussed. This is because these processes can usually be
modified so that, in some manner, particulate solids can also be coated.

II. WURSTER PROCESS

A. Introduction

The commonly called air-suspension particle-coating method, also known as
the Wurster process,* has been utilized for many years by the pharmaceutical, chemical, food, agricultural, and other industries. The rapidity
of the operation, the ability to control variables, the uniformity of the coat
produced, and the fact that it can be used to coat particles varying greatly in size, shape, and density are some of the main advantages of the
process. Further, the process does not restrict either the kind of coating
materials used or the solvents employed in the coating fluids. Even chemical reactions designed to produce polymer coatings from applied monomer
solutions can be easily conducted in the column.

Because it is possible to control the variables of the process the method is sufficiently flexible to make it extremely versatile. Thus, the
process can be utilized to coat medicinal tablets [5–13] or other large particles, to microencapsulate fine particles [14], to control drug release from
coated particles [15,16], and to prepare compressed tablet granulations
[17,18] or the like. By the proper adjustment of process conditions, it is
possible to either coat solid particles or to cause particles to aggregate.
It is also possible to control the density, geometry, friability, and other
physical parameters, of the treated particles.

There is little doubt that the Wurster process provides the most rapid,
efficient, and cost-effective method of producing film-coated compressed

---

*Wisconsin Alumni Research Foundation, Madison, Wisconsin.

tablets. Similar advantages are gained in microencapsulation and compressed-tablet granulation procedures.

B. General Description

The Wurster process* can be appropriately be described as an upward-moving, highly-expanded pneumatically transported bed of particles coupled with a downward-moving, more condensed, fluidized bed of particles on the periphery of a vertical column. The two beds are separated by the tubular central partition. Figure 1 is a schematic drawing of the equipment. As indicated above, the particles to be coated are pneumatically conveyed upwardly through the central tube, (b), of the coating chamber. As the particles pass the atomizer, (d), they are wetted by the coating fluid and then immediately subjected to drying conditions created by the heated conveying air moving upwardly in the column. The partially coated solid particles move downwardly in a near-weightless condition along the periphery of the column, (c), where further drying occurs. When the solid particles reach the lower end of the column they are directed back into the upwardly-moving bed and the entire process is repeated. The air pump, (g), and heater (f), provide the heated support air for the process, and the distribution plate (e) directs the proper volume of air to the central and peripheral regions of the column.

The proper adjustment of the airflow, the temperature, and the fluid application rate are all critical to the successful operation of the process. Obviously, the drying kinetics are influenced by the airflow rate and the temperature of the air. These kinetics in turn dictate the fluid application rate. Since drying is a cooling process, the temperature of the particle surface is lower than either the inlet or exhaust air temperatures. This permits the coating of heat-sensitive materials, since process conditions can be adjusted so that the exhaust temperature will not exceed the temperature which the product can tolerate. Thus, it is readily apparent that the drying kinetics can be enhanced by increasing either the airflow rate or the air temperature while maintaining the fluid application rate constant.

C. Control of Airflow

The proper airflow rate is most important for the successful operation of the Wurster process. It is apparent from the general description of the process that the two-component fluidized bed employed in this process

---

*Before using this or other fluidized bed processes, it is important to become familiar with the basic principles that govern fluid-bed systems. The following textbooks are included in a long list of textbooks that are very useful for this purpose. (1) Cheremisinoff, N. P., *Hydrodynamics of Gas—Solids Fluidization*, Gulf Publishing Co., Houston, 1984; (2) Davidson, J. F., *Fluidization*, Academic Press, New York, 1971; and (3) Howard, J. R., *Fluidized Beds*, Applied Science Publishers Ltd., London, 1983.

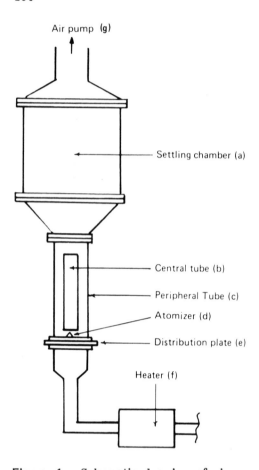

Figure 1   Schematic drawing of air-suspension coating apparatus.

differs considerably from a conventional fluidized bed. Since the solid particles undergo pneumatic transport up the central portion of the column
and descend in the peripheral region, different air velocities are required
in the two regions. Although an air distribution plate is positioned at the
base of the column (see Fig. 1), an air distribution zone also exists just
above the plate. It is in this zone in the loaded column that the air undergoes further distribution to the directional flow and velocity conditions
which prevail above the plate and which differ markedly from the conditions imposed by the plate alone [19]. Nevertheless, it is extremely important that the plate is properly designed for the particular production
process for which the method is being used.

Minimum Fluidization Velocity

When particulate solids are placed on a perforated plate in a vertical column and a gas, usually air, is passed upwardly through the bed of particles the bed at lower air velocities will initially remain fixed. However,
as the air velocity is increased the particulate bed expands, the individual

particles begin to move in the air stream, and an increase in the void space of the bed is observed. The transition of the bed from the fixed to the fluidized state occurs at the point where the pressure drop across the bed is equal to the weight of the bed per unit of cross-sectional area. This is often referred to as incipient fluidization, and the air velocity required to produce this state is known as the minimum fluidizing velocity. Thus, the pressure drop across the bed at incipient fluidization is given by [20,21]

$$\Delta P_b = (1 - \varepsilon_{mf})(\rho_s - \rho_g)H_{mf}\, g \tag{1}$$

where ΔP_b = pressure drop across bed

ε_{mf} = bed voidage at condition of minimum fluidization

ρ_s = density of solid particles

ρ_g = density of fluidizing gas

H_{mf} = height of bed at minimum fluidization

g = gravitational constant

For uniform, small spherical particles in the approximate range of 20–100 μm and densities up to 1.4, the equation derived by Kozeny [20–23] and tested by Carman over the range of bed voidages of 0.26–0.89 [24,25] shows that the relationship between the pressure drop and the minimum fluidizing velocity at incipient fluidization can be written in the following manner

$$V_{mf} = \frac{\varepsilon_{mf}^3}{5(1 - \varepsilon_{mf})^2}\, \frac{\Delta P_b}{S^2 \mu H_{mf}} \tag{2}$$

Here V_{mf} = gas velocity at minimum fluidization

S = specific surface area of solid particles

μ = the viscosity of the gas

From equations (1) and (2), it follows that

$$V_{mf} = \frac{\varepsilon_{mf}^3}{5(1 - \varepsilon_{mf})}\, \frac{(\rho_s - \rho_g)\, g}{S^2 \mu} \tag{3}$$

If it is assumed that the bed is composed of uniform spherical particles, $S = 6/d$, where d is the particle diameter and correspondingly, the bed voidage, ε_{mf}, is considered to be 0.4 then [20]

$$V_{mf} = \frac{0.4^3}{5(1 - 0.4)}\, \frac{d^2(\rho_s - \rho_g)\, g}{6^2 \mu} \tag{4}$$

Another simple and convenient method for predicting the approximate minimum fluidization velocity for solid particles in the 50- to 500-μm size range takes advantage of the mathematical expression recommended by Woodcock [21, 26]

$$V_{mf} = 420 \; \rho_p \; d_v^{\,2} \tag{5}$$

Here V_{mf} = minimum fluidization velocity in m/s

ρ_p = the solid particle density in kg/m^3

d_v = mean particle diameter in meters

When the bed is composed of larger particles it has been suggested by some [20] that more general type equations such as those given by Ergun [27] and Black [28] be employed to arrive at the pressure drop across the bed.

Effects of Increasing Air Velocity

The influences on the bed created by increasing air velocities are shown in the idealized graph [29] presented in Figure 2. As stated previously, the pressure drop across the bed increases with an increase in the velocity of the air directed through the bed. Initially, the bed remains fixed, but as the air velocity is further increased the bed expands somewhat and the

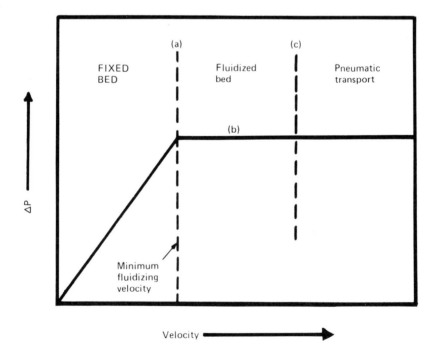

Figure 2   Pressure drop versus air velocity.

point of incipient particle fluidization and the minimum fluidizing air velocity is reached at point (a). A further increase in the air velocity to
point (b) does not yield a concomitant increase in the pressure drop; however, the bed does further expand, bed voidage changes, and the nature
of the bed changes drastically as it passes from smooth fluidization through
bubbling fluidization, slugging, and fast fluidization phases. Ultimately,
as the air velocity is further increased pneumatic transport of the solid
particles begins at point (c).

A graph of the type shown in Figure 2 can also be readily prepared
from the experimental data obtained on a particular type of bed. Of
course, in this case, the particle size, shape, and density will remain constant. This type of experimental graph is particularly useful to show the
pressure drop across the bed and the air velocity required to produce the
various phases of bed fluidization. Since the Wurster process employs a
two-component fluidized bed, it is most important to know the minimum
fluidization and pneumatic transport velocities. Other types of experimentally derived graphs will also be found to be most useful for a coating
column of a given diameter. For example, the manner in which a change
in the size of the solid particles in the bed, but which have the same shape
and density, influence the required velocities can be shown by plotting the
air velocity in cubic feet per minute (cfm) or the pitot tube reading in
inches of water versus the particle size of the mesh size [30].

When there is a tendency for the solid particles in the bed to inter-
lock with one another the pressure drop across the bed actually increases
and departs from theoretical, as is shown in curve (a) of Figure 3. If the
bed is composed of large and unevenly sized particles, the departure from
the theoretical pressure drop is manifested by a pressure decrease owing
to uneven support of parts of the bed and uneven bed fluidization, as is
shown in curve (b) of Figure 3.

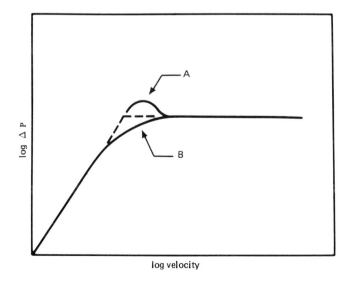

Figure 3   Pressure drop versus air velocity.   A = Interlocking particles,
B = large particles.

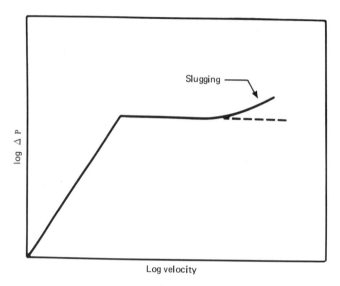

Figure 4   Pressure drop versus air velocity in a slugging bed.

Changes in the pressure drop as the bed response changes from ideal to a vigorous bubbling or a slugging bed also occur. The pressure drop change in a slugging bed is shown in Figure 4.

Following the fixed bed and smooth fluidization phases, the various bed phases which occur as the air velocity is further increased are shown in Figure 5.

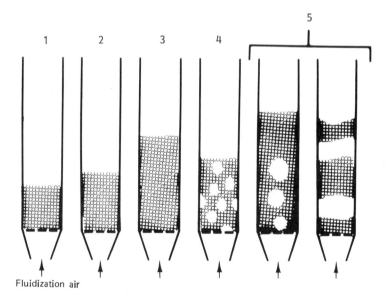

Figure 5   Various bed phases. 1, fixed bed; 2, incipient fluidization; 3, smooth fluidization; 4, bubbling fluidization; and 5, slugging beds.

Particulate and Aggregative Fluidization

There are two main types of fluidization commonly referred to in fluidized
bed utilization. When the solid particles are small in size, of relatively low
density, and the air velocity is also low the bed will often fluidize in a
smooth and even manner. The solid particles will then move freely and individually through a relatively mean free pathway. The dense phase of
the bed will appear to flow quite similarly in appearance to a viscous liquid.
This is referred to as particulate fluidization. If the solid particles are
large in diameter and higher in density, a higher air velocity is required
for fluidization. Under these conditions, the bed fluidizes unevenly and
the air passes through the bed in the form of bubbles. As the bubbles
rise in the bed, they increase in size primarily by the process of coalescence. Such bubbling bed-type fluidization is often referred to as aggregative fluidization.

As the large air bubbles pass through the bed, a bubble wake is
formed. Other smaller bubbles as well as solid particles are aspirated into
the wake to not only produce larger bubbles, but to create a very turbulent bed condition. All of these factors combine to produce good mixing
of the solid components. A fluidized bed is, in fact, one of the very best
methods of mixing solids.

Minimum Bubbling Velocity

The velocity at which air bubbles first appear and pass through the bed is
known as the minimum bubbling velocity. This occurs at velocities only
slightly greater than minimum fluidization velocities. The Froude number
has been employed by some to differentiate between particulate and bubbling
fluidization [21]. Here the critical Froude number is assumed to be 0.1
based on the superficial air velocity and the particle diameter [31].

$$Fr = \frac{V_f^2}{d_p g} \tag{6}$$

where Fr = the Froude number

V_f = the superficial air velocity

d_p = the solid particle diameter

g = the gravitational constant

Smooth bed fluidization will usually remain when the air velocity is increased
up to and beyond a twofold increase in the minimum fluidization velocity.
When the Froude number is at unity or greater only the aggregative type
of fluidization can be expected to exist in the bed [21].

Problems and Solutions of Bubbling and
Slugging Beds

The more turbulent bubbling and slugging bed phases create conditions
which give rise to many problems when fluidized bed processes are employed for particle coating, granulation, and microencapsulation procedures.
Two of the more troublesome problems which occur are the attrition of solid

particles and the aggregation of solid particles. The Wurster process is very carefully designed to delete these type problems from the process. As previously stated, particles are pneumatically transported upward in the center column. Under these conditions, the interparticle distance is very large so that particle attrition is minimized, and the drying kinetics of applied fluids are enhanced. The combination of interparticle distance and rapid drying conditions greatly inhibit the aggregation of the solid particles. In the peripheral, downward-moving, smooth-flowing, fluidized bed the air flow approximates the minimum fluidizing air velocity and contributes to the terminal drying of the particles. Thus, only the uniform smooth fluidization phase and the pneumatic transport phase are permitted to exist in this process, and the troublesome turbulent bubbling and slugging phases are not allowed to occur because of the type of two-component bed employed.

D. Fluid Application Rate

It is possible to calculate a fluid application rate which will conform to the desired column conditions [30]. By knowing the water vapor content of the incoming air, the air flow rate, and the desired inlet and outlet air temperatures, the amount of water which can be introduced into the system in the coating fluid can be determined. A humidity chart can be used here as a matter of convenience and the following will serve as an example of this simple method. On the humidity chart shown in Figure 6, point 1 shows that the inlet air has a dry bulb temperature of 80°F and a wet bulb temperature of 65°F. Thus, the inlet air has a humidity of about 45%. If the inlet air is then heated to 124°F, point 2, and water is sprayed into the system so that the exhaust air is cooled to 80°F and has a 90% humidity condition, point 3, then the drying capacity is the vertical difference between points 1 and 3 or $0.02 - 0.01 = 0.01$ lb water/lb of air on the left scale or $0.64 - 0.32 = 0.32$ ml water/ft^3 of air on the right scale. Now if the particles to be coated require 100 cfm of support air, the drying rate would be $100 \times 0.32 = 32$ ml of water/min. The fluid application rate for a given coating fluid can now be calculated if the water concentration is known. For example, if the coating solution contains 30% water, it is obvious that a fluid application rate of 106.67 ml min^{-1} can be used.

If, in the above example, the material to be coated could readily tolerate a higher temperature, then it is apparent that the fluid application rate can be increased. Thus, at an inlet air temperature of 177°F and an exhaust temperature of 92°F, the fluid application rate could actually be doubled, which, of course, permits a much faster coating process.

The presence of certain chemical components in the coating fluid may significantly decrease the solvent vapor pressure, which in turn reduces the drying capacity normally observed for a given set of conditions. When this is the case it is necessary to operate at either a slower fluid application rate or a higher inlet and exhaust temperature to compensate for this effect and to inhibit particle aggregation.

It is evident that when the coating materials are tacky in the partially dried state particle aggregation will occur if residual solvent remains in the applied coat. The residual moisture or solvent concentration in the coated product is, of course, a function of the operating conditions. If the process is operated under such conditions that the humidity approaches the dew point, then particle aggregation occurs. If a very dry condition

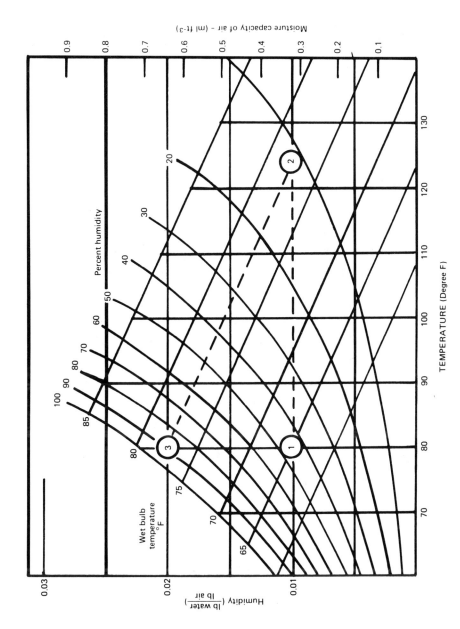

Figure 6. Humidity chart.

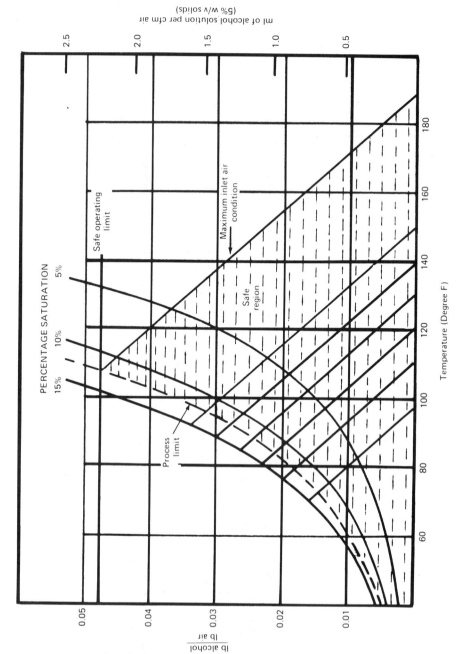

Figure 7   Alcohol-drying chart for coating solution.

is maintained, then attrition of the particles may occur. In actual practice, then, a humidity condition above 85% for some materials can lead to aggregation, whereas below 45% attrition may occur.

Drying charts can be constructed and used for organic solvents or solvent mixtures in a manner similar to the above use of the humidity chart. In Figure 7, a drying chart for ethyl alcohol solutions of coating materials is shown. The required calculations for chart construction are conventional and need not be treated here.* As in the case of humidity charts, these charts ignore the influence of dissolved substances on the solvent removal rate.

The determination of the fluid application rates using solvent-drying charts such as shown in Figure 4 differs slightly from that of a humidity chart. This, of course, is because the atmosphere employed as the support air does not normally contain a significant amount of the organic solvent. From the alcohol-drying chart shown in Figure 5, it can be observed that if the air is 140°F and if an outlet temperature of 98°F is desired, then 0.024 lb of alcohol/lb of dry air can be used. From the right-hand scale it can be observed that under the above conditions, 1.13 ml of the coating solution per cubic foot per minute of air can be employed. Then if the support air is 100 cfm, the fluid application rate for the coating solution is 113 ml min^{-1}.

Since alcohol is an inflammable solvent, the process conditions can be set so that a wide margin of safety exists. The lower inflammability limit for alcohol is 0.0716 lb of alcohol vapor/lb of dry air. In Figure 4, the safe operating limit is set at two-thirds of this value or 0.0477 lb of alcohol/lb of dry air. The maximum inlet temperature is also indicated as is the process limit. By setting operating conditions within these parameters, a wide margin of safety is achieved [30].

E. Drying Properties of the Process

When particles are wetted by a solvent it can be assumed that normally the solvent penetrates into the particle and also that a pool of solvent resides on the surface. When the wetted particle is subjected to a drying process, the solvent on the surface is readily removed at a constant rate or a steady state exists. The solvent which has penetrated the particle subsequently returns to the surface by diffusion and capillarity, and thus a nonsteady state exists for the removal of the solvent residing within the particle. Figure 8 shows a typical drying curve for the solvent loss from a particle as a function of time.

In the Wurster process, a thin layer of the coating fluid is atomized onto the surface of the solid particles. Because of the elevated temperatures and the large volume of air passing over the particles, the solvent is rapidly removed and drying occurs primarily under the steady-state condition.

---

*The interested reader is referred to Perry, R. H. and Chilton, C. H., *Chemical Engineers' Handbook*, 5th Ed., McGraw-Hill Book Company, New York, 1973, Chap. 20; and *Pilot Plant Operation, Wurster Coating and Granulating Process*, Wisconsin Alumni Research Foundation, Madison, Wisconsin, Sec. VI.

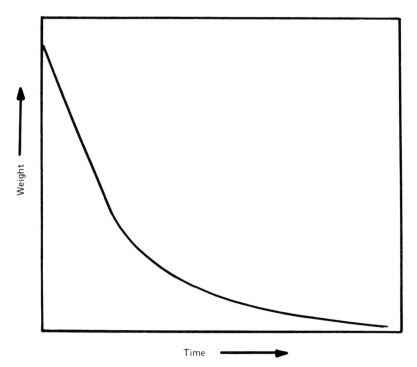

Figure 8   Water loss as a function of time.

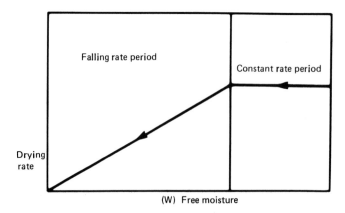

Figure 9   Drying rate versus free moisture.

In drying processes, the nonsteady state or falling rate and the steady state or constant rate of solvent removal is often depicted as shown in Figure 9, in which the drying rate is plotted against the free solvent content. The following relationship is also often employed to determine the constant drying rate in conventional drying processes [32].

$$\frac{dw}{dt} = \frac{h_t \, A \, (t_a - t_s)}{\lambda} = k_g A \, (P_s - P_a) \tag{7}$$

where $\dfrac{dw}{dt}$ = drying rate in lbs. H_2O/h

$\quad h_t$ = total heat transfer coefficient in $BtU/(hr)(ft^2)(°F)$

$\quad A$ = area in ft^2

$\quad \lambda$ = latent heat of evaporation at t_s

$\quad t_a$ = air temperature

$\quad t_s$ = wet surface temperature

$\quad k_g$ = mass transfer coefficient in $lb/(hr)(ft^2)(atm)$

$\quad P_s$ = vapor pressure of H_2O at t_s

$\quad P_a$ = the partial pressure of H_2O in air

To obtain the falling rate in drying processes, we can use [32]

$$\left(\frac{dw}{dt}\right)_F = K \, (W - W_e) \tag{8}$$

Here $\quad W$ = average moisture content at time, t (dry basis)

$\quad W_e$ = average moisture content (in equilibrium with external conditions)

$$\left(\frac{dw}{dt}\right)_{C, W=W_c} = \left(\frac{dw}{dt}\right)_{F, W-W_c} = K \, (W_c - W_e) \tag{9}$$

where W_c = critical moisture content, and F = falling rate and C = the constant rate, or

$$K = \frac{(dw)/(dt)_c}{W_c - W_e} \tag{10}$$

$$\left(\frac{dw}{dt}\right)_F = \frac{W - W_e}{W_c - W_e} \left(\frac{dw}{dt}\right)_c \tag{11}$$

Figure 10 shows the difference in the rate at which water is removed from a product in the air-suspension method as compared to more traditional drying methods. As indicated previously, the process can be monitored by following the exhaust temperature. Also, as shown in Figure 11,

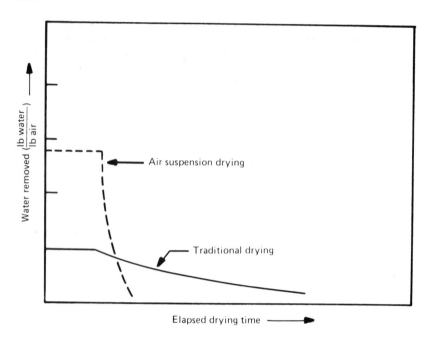

Figure 10   Comparison of air-suspension drying with traditional drying methods.

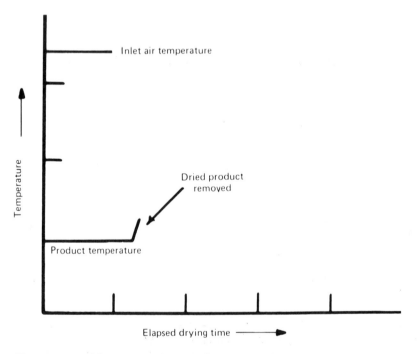

Figure 11   Air-suspension drying.

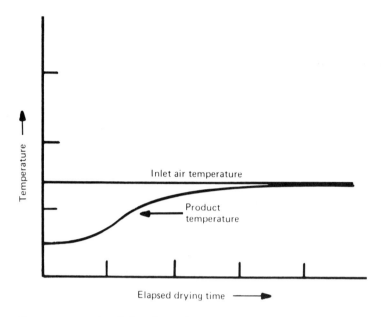

Figure 12   Traditional drying process.

the exhaust temperature remains relatively constant during the steady-state drying which occurs during the coating process. When atomization is stopped, the temperature rapidly rises and the dried product can be immediately removed without exposing it unnecessarily to a high temperature for a long time. If during the actual coating process the exhaust temperature falls below that set for the process, this suggests that the fluid application rate is too great; the particles may become too wet, and aggregation will occur. Conversely, if the exhaust temperature rises, then the column condition is drier than desired and particle attrition may occur. The equipment can be instrumented to monitor such changes and to make corrective changes. Figure 12 shows the drying curve of a wetted product by more traditional methods. In the case of substances which form hydrates, the slight temperature changes can actually be utilized to follow the conversion of one hydrate form to another (Fig. 13).

F. Uniformity of Coat

One of the main advantages of the air-suspension coating process is the uniformity of coat that can be achieved on both small and large particles. If the coating fluid is applied at a constant rate, both the weight of the particles and the cube of the radius for spherical particles should increase linearly with time. Figures 14 and 15 show this to be the case [5]. Even a very thin, 1-μm thick coat applied to a small crystal is extremely uniform, as is shown in Figure 16.

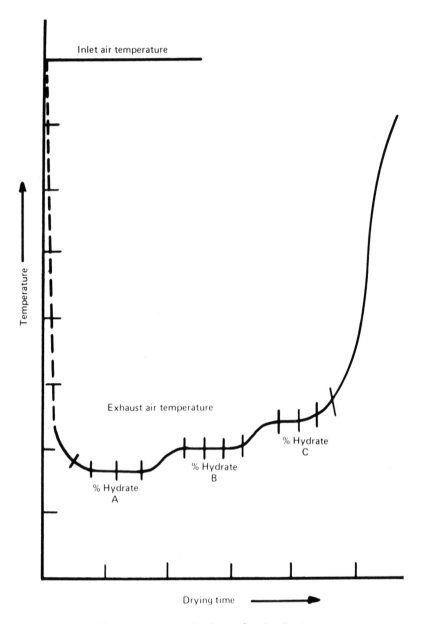

Figure 13   Air-suspension drying of a hydrate.

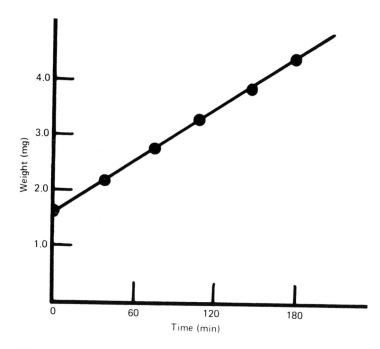

Figure 14 Weight of particles as a function of process time (constant atomization rate).

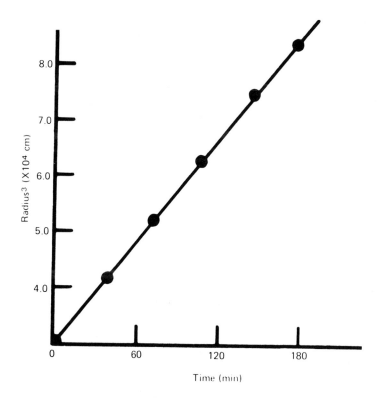

Figure 15 Particle size of spheres as a function of process time (constant atomization rate).

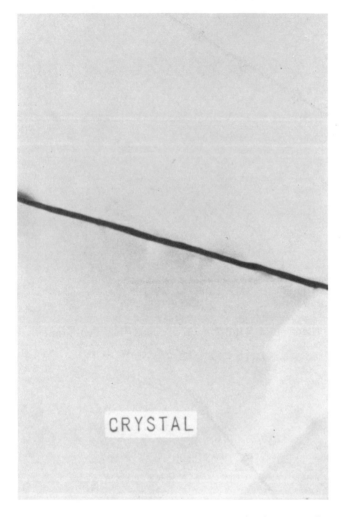

Figure 16   A 1-μm thick coat on a single crystal.

G. Particle Aggregates, Granulations, and Particle Build-Up

As previously stated, it is possible to prepare particle aggregates of different densities and geometries depending upon column conditions. For example, one can prepare aggregates which are comparable to those made for a compressed tablet granulation by the wet method. By utilizing materials which are tacky when wet, a column condition approaching saturation of the support air can be employed. In the case of water solutions containing such materials as sugars and gums, a humidity condition in the column exceeding 85% relative humidity (RH) will usually result in particle aggregation. Irregular particles prepared by this process are shown in Figure 17. If a friable, low-density spherical particle is desired, this

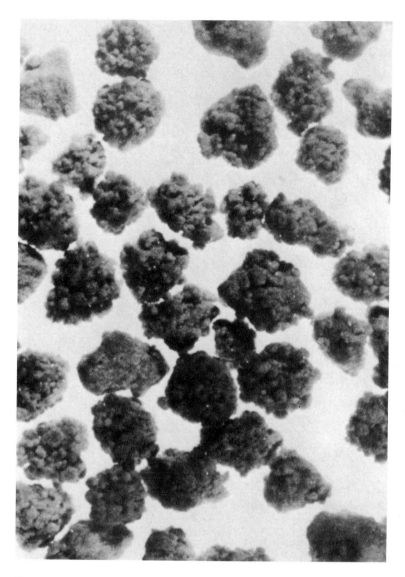

Figure 17 Irregular aggregate of particles (1500 µm).

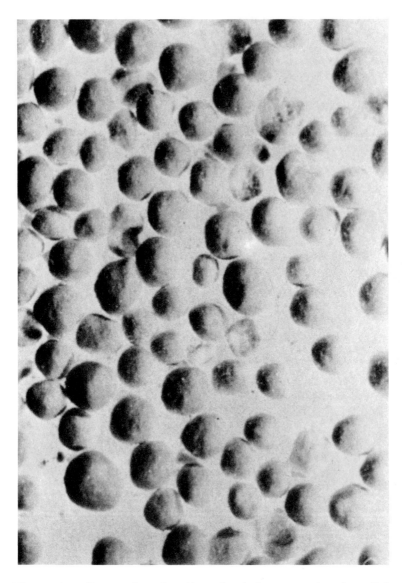

Figure 18   Porous low-density spherical aggregate of particles (1000 μm).

can also be accomplished. In this case a high-humidity column condition together with the atomization of the binder solution as large liquid particles is required. By utilizing a very small particle size of the solid material (less than 15 μm) and a large droplet size of the atomized solution, the small solid particles are allowed to impinge upon and be entrapped by the large liquid particles. Upon the subsequent removal of the solvent, a porous, low-density particle results. This type of particle is shown in Figure 18. The fragility of this type particle is evident by the presence of the fractured spheres in the figure.

Spherical particles of near-theoretical density can be prepared by coating particles with a slurry which contains both suspended solids and a binder. In this case, column conditions are adjusted so that a coating process rather than an aggregation process results (Fig. 19). If water is

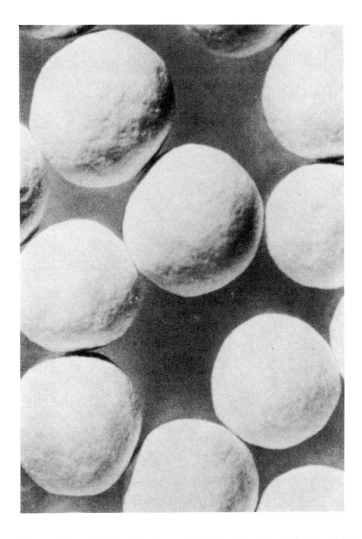

Figure 19   High-density, slurry-coated particles (2000 μm).

the solvent, a 65% humidity condition in the column can be used as a starting point.

Granulations of effervescent materials are normally quite difficult to prepare by conventional methods because of the close control which is required over the reaction rate, the drying rate, and the residual water. The air-suspension process is well suited for the preparation of these granulations [33] because of the ease with which the process conditions can be controlled and monitored.

In air-suspension coating procedures, the lower particle size limit is approximately 50 μm, but smaller particles have been coated. There is no practical upper limit for larger particles. In fact, very large particles are efficiently coated with great ease. When particle aggregates (tablet granulations, etc.) are prepared, very fine particles of only a few micrometers can be aggregated into larger particles without difficulty. Of course, the particle aggregates can subsequently be coated, if desired, without removing them from the column.

Lastly, because the air-suspension process operates as a closed system with respect to the working area, people are protected from exposure to dangerous chemicals and solvents. Similarly, the loss of solids can be prevented and solvents can be reclaimed from the exhaust so that contamination of the environment does not occur.

III. CENTRIFUGATION

The centrifugation method* is a unique modification of the simple extrusion technique of producing microcapsules [34−40]. As shown in Figure 20, the simple extrusion method utilizes a device consisting of two concentric tubes containing aligned fluid nozzles. The liquid material to be coated is extruded through the nozzle of the inner tube into the coating fluid contained in the outer tube. Initially, the fluid extrudes as a rod surrounded by the coating fluid, but the rod ultimately breaks up into droplets which are then immersed in the coating fluid. As the extruded droplets pass through the nozzle orifice of the outer tube, the coating fluid forms a surface coat which encases the extruded particle. Spherically shaped particles are formed by the surface tension of the liquid. By suitable means the formed coat is converted to a more rigid structure. Hardening baths are usually employed for this purpose. These baths are designed according to the coating material used. Thus, in some cases the bath contains a chemical agent which will react with the coating material to yield an insoluble compound. A common example of this is the use of calcium chloride in the bath to convert sodium alginate in the coat to the insoluble calcium alginate [39]. In other cases, the bath may simply be a nonsolvent for the coating material, whereas in still other cases only a decrease in temperature is needed to harden the coat.

This process is primarily employed to prepare microcapsules of liquids. Thus, the coating fluid is immiscible with the liquid to be encapsulated. As previously stated, however, the main concern of this chapter is a discussion of methods by which discrete solids can be coated. When this

*Southwest Research Institute, San Antonio, Texas.

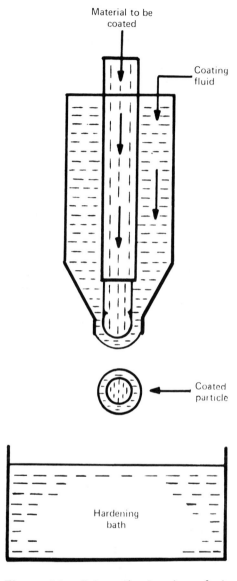

Material to be
coated

Coating
fluid

Coated
particle

Hardening
bath

Figure 20   Schematic drawing of simple extrusion.

method is used to coat solid drugs it is convenient to prepare a slurry of the solid material. The slurry is then encapsulated in the same manner as described above for a liquid. Also, in some cases solids, such as fats, resins, waxes, or like materials, can be extruded and coated while in the molten state [37]. Obviously, other particulate solids can also be included in the molten solid. Substances in the molten state can also be used as coating materials.

The initially employed gravity flow and simple extrusion devices were found to have some general processing problems. Thus, in gravity flow systems it is apparent that certain limitations are imposed upon the size of the capsule produced. Also, with simple extrusion devices capsule uniformity is a problem. To overcome such problems and yet maintain a high output of product, devices utilizing centrifugal force and having multiorifice extrusion heads, as shown in Figure 21, were designed. It is important to note here that the capsule size can be controlled by varying such factors as the orifice size, the rotational speed, and the flow rate of the fluid to be encapsulated. As would be expected, with a uniform orifice size and a constant rotational speed, an increase in the fluid flow rate results in an increase in the capsule size. Conversely, with a uniform orifice size and a constant fluid flow rate, an increase in the rotational speed yields smaller

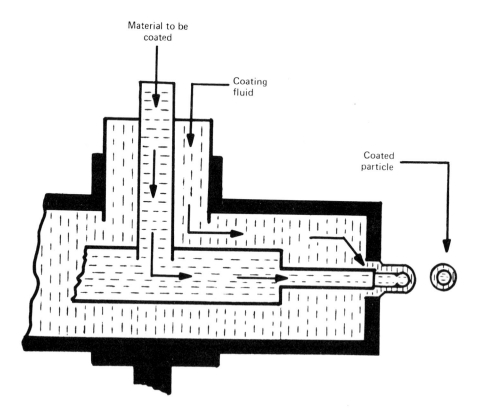

Figure 21 Schematic drawing showing one nozzle unit of a multiorifice centrifugal extrusion head.

capsules. The centrifugation method is capable of producing microcapsules in the 100–200 μm range.

A still further modification [39] of this method, the so-called submerged nozzle, utilizes three concentric tubes in which the outermost tube contains a carrier fluid. As the fluid to be encapsulated is extruded from the innermost tube, it is surrounded by the coating fluid in the center tube and encapsulation is effected in a manner similar to that described above. However, in this case the carrier fluid in the outermost tube carries the microcapsules away from the nozzle. Naturally, the carrier fluid must not be miscible with the coating fluid. This modification of the process is stated to be most useful when the fluid coat is fragile and ruptures upon impact with the hardening bath used with the centifugal devices. The size of the microcapsules produced in this system is again a function of the nozzle size and fluid flow rate; however, the carrier fluid flow rate is also important in this regard. Thus, an increase in the carrier fluid flow rate, other factors remaining constant, results in a decrease in the capsule size.

IV. SPRAY DRYING

The application of the spray-drying process to the production of microcapsules has been found to be useful for a variety of materials and can be

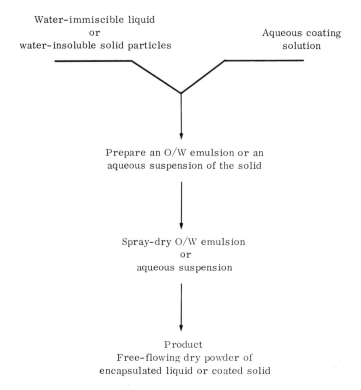

Water-immiscible liquid
or
water-insoluble solid particles

Aqueous coating
solution

Prepare an O/W emulsion or an
aqueous suspension of the solid

Spray-dry O/W emulsion
or
aqueous suspension

Product
Free-flowing dry powder of
encapsulated liquid or coated solid

Figure 22 Flow chart for spray-dry process of coating liquid or solid particles.

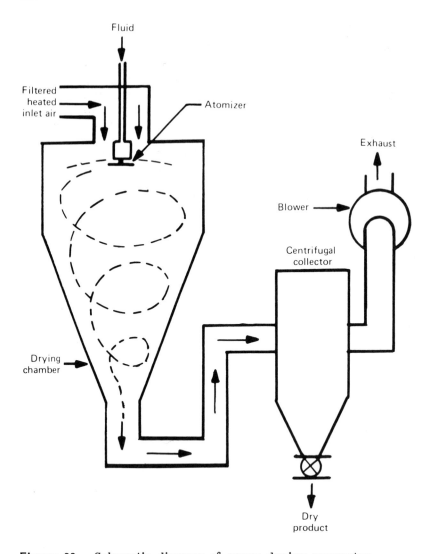

Figure 23   Schematic diagram of spray-drying apparatus.

employed to encapsulate both liquids and solids [1,41–46]. In the case of liquids, the fluid to be coated is first emulsified. The film-forming coating material is contained in the continuous phase of the emulsion and the fluid to be coated becomes the dispersed phase. The emulsion is subjected to the spray-drying process and the solvent constituting the continuous phase is removed. The film former is thus deposited upon the surface of the dispersed particles. The resulting product is a free-flowing powder-like material containing the encapsulated liquid. Essentially, the same procedure is followed when this method is used to produce coated solids. Here, however, a suspension of the solid particles in a solution containing material is first prepared. Solvent removal during the spray-drying process deposits the coating material on the surface of the solid particles.

The spray-dry process usually produces coated aggregates rather than coated single particles. A simplified flow chart for the overall process is shown in Figure 22, and a schematic drawing of the spray-drying equipment is presented in Figure 23. Since emulsion systems are employed in the interfacial polymerization microencapsulation method (see page 194), the spray-drying process may also be utilized to recover the microcapsules prepared by this technique. The principles governing the spray-drying process are well known and need not be treated here.

V. AQUEOUS-PHASE SEPARATION, COACERVATION

In the coacervation coating method* [1,47−61], an aqueous colloidal solution of a hydrophilic polymer having film-forming properties is employed. The material to be coated may be either a liquid or a solid. When liquids are microencapsulated an oil-in-water−type emulsion is prepared, with the liquid to be coated occupying the dispersed phase and the aqueous colloidal solution the continuous phase. When solids are coated, a suspension of the particulate solid in the aqueous colloidal solution is prepared. In either case, by suitable means, phase separation is produced with a layer of the coacervate derived from the hydrophilic colloid forming around the dispersed particles. Finally, the coacervate layer is treated to cause it to become more firm. The process can be one of simple coacervation involving only a single colloidal solute, or complex coacervation utilizing two or more colloidal solutes can be employed.

The steps involved in the coating process are presented in a general manner in Figure 24.

In simple coacervation, the single colloid contained in the continuous phase can be caused to deposit on the surface of the dispersed particles as a result of such physical influences as salting-out effects or the addition of another solvent. Such influences, of course, result in the dehydration of the hydrophilic colloid. Gelatin is commonly employed as the hydrophilic colloid here, since the above effects are readily observed by the addition of a highly soluble salt such as sodium sulfate or ammonium sulfate, or by the addition of alcohol. A flow chart of the simple coacervation process is shown in Figure 25. The process allows the use of other hydrophilic film-forming colloids as well as other dehydrating and film-hardening agents.

A. Particle-Coating Methods

Complex coacervation, in contrast to simple coacervation, requires at least two hydrophilic colloids in the continuous phase of the fluid system. This type of procedure allows the application of the well-known phenomenon whereby two oppositely charged colloids discharge with each other to produce a coacervate, as is shown in the following general-type reaction:

$$[\text{Colloid } 1]^+ + [\text{colloid } 2]^- \longrightarrow [\text{colloid } 1]^+[\text{colloid } 2]^- \downarrow$$

---

*National Cash Register Company, Dayton, Ohio.

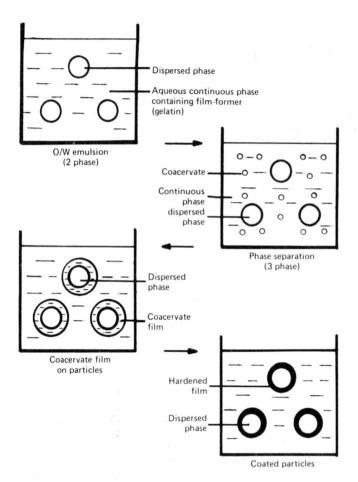

Figure 24   Schematic diagram of steps involved in coacervation coating.

Unless the coacervate remains highly hydrated it will separate from solution.   Thus, when such a weak union between the charged colloids occurs fine droplets initially appear which subsequently coalesce to produce a continuous phase.   Figure 26 is a flow chart for the complex coacervation process.

The process is a batch method and can be conducted on an experimental basis with ordinary laboratory equipment.   Pilot plant and production-scale operations require only such simple equipment as suitable tanks, filtration, or other separation equipment and means to control such process conditions as pH and temperature.

The particle size of the dispersed phase (i.e., the solid particles or liquid droplets to be coated) will govern to a large degree the size of the coated particles produced.   From this it is evident that coated particles, varying widely in size, can be prepared.   The literature indicates this size range to be 5–5000 μm in diameter [2].   The thickness of the coat is, of course, a function of the amount of coating material on the surface of the particle.   In normal commercial coating procedures the weight of the

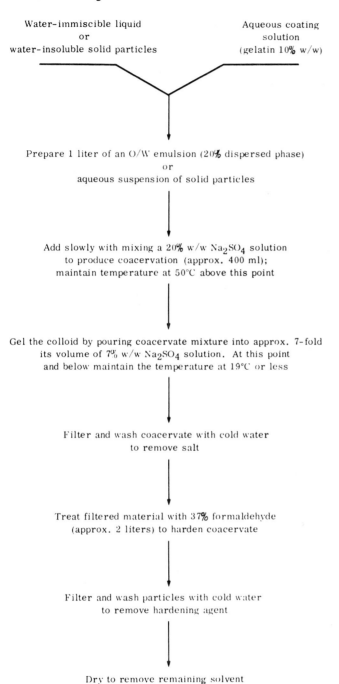

Figure 25 Flow chart for simple coacervation process.

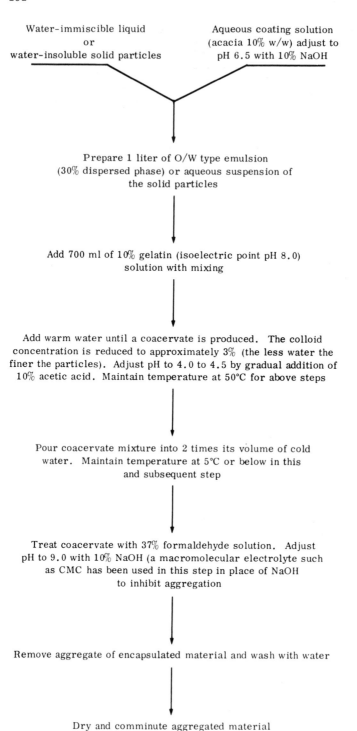

Figure 26   Flow chart for complex coacervation process.

coat varies between 3 and 30% of the particle weight, but coatings of 1-70% have been applied.

The flexibility of this coating process is further emphasized by the wide variety of coating materials that can be utilized. A partial list of suitable coating materials which can be employed, depending on whether the aqueous-phase separation or nonaqueous-phase separation method is used, follows:

Gelatin
Gelatin/acacia
Gelatin/acacia/vinylmethylether maleic anhydride
Gelatin/acacia/ethylenemaleic anhydride
Carboxymethylcellulose
Propylhydroxycellulose
Polyvinylalcohol
Cellulose acetate phthalate
Ethylcellulose
Ethylenevinylacetate
Nitrocellulose
Shellac
Wax

While the coacervation method is capable of coating a large number of materials, it is readily apparent that the material to be coated must be stable to the process conditions. Particular consideration must therefore be given to the influence of temperature, pH, solvent system, etc., on product stability.

VI. NONAQUEOUS-PHASE SEPARATION

Phase separation [2,62,63] can be induced in organic solvent systems as well as aqueous systems. Again, the suspended particle may be either a solid or an immiscible liquid. Thus, for dispersed liquids, emulsions of the W/O type are employed in contrast to the more conventional coacervation method in which O/W-type emulsions are used. Obviously, water-soluble solids can also be included either by suspending them in the organic solvent or by dissolving them in the internal phase of the W/O-type emulsion.

The polymeric coating material is dissolved in the continuous organic solvent phase. Phase separation and the coating of the solid or liquid dispersed particles is accomplished by adding a solvent which is miscible with the continuous organic solvent phase but which is a nonsolvent for the polymeric coating material. Triangular phase diagrams are a most useful tool when dealing with phase separation in either nonaqueous [62] or aqueous [64] systems.

Hardening of the polymer coat on the particles is usually accomplished either by the addition of more of the nonsolvent or by separating the coated particles from the system, washing them with a nonsolvent liquid, and drying.

VII. INTERFACIAL POLYMERIZATION

The interfacial polycondensation or polymerization technique [63-65] has been applied to the microencapsulation of various liquids. However, as with the other processes discussed in this chapter, particulate solids can be suspended in the liquid so that the microencapsulated particle contains both the solid and the liquid.

The process consists of bringing two reactants together at the interface of the dispersed and continuous phases in emulsion systems [66]. This is usually accomplished by emulsifying the liquid containing the first reactant (dispersed phase) into the continuous phase, which is initially devoid of the second reactant. Additional continuous phase containing the second reactant is then added. This interfacial polymerization reaction produces a continuous film of the formed polymer around the dispersed phase. A diagram of the interfacial process is shown in Figure 27. The recovery of the microcapsules from the continuous phase can be accomplished by spray drying, flash evaporation, filtration, or other separation techniques [67]. A flow chart of the process is shown in Figure 28.

The various polymer-coating materials which have been utilized to prepare microcapsules by the described process include polyamides (nylon), polyurethanes, polysulfonamides, polyesters, polycarbonates, and polysulfonates. The particle size of the product created by this method varies in accordance with the particle diameter of the dispersed phase. Therefore, particles varying greatly in size, from approximately 3 to 2000 μm in diameter, can be prepared.

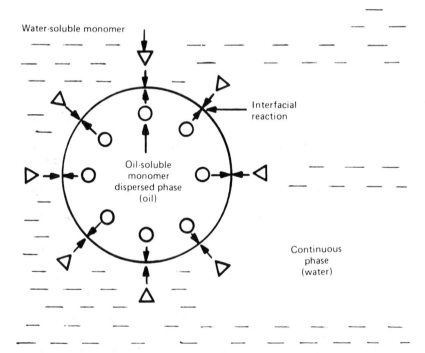

Figure 27   Schematic diagram of interfacial polymerization coating process in an O/W emulsion system.

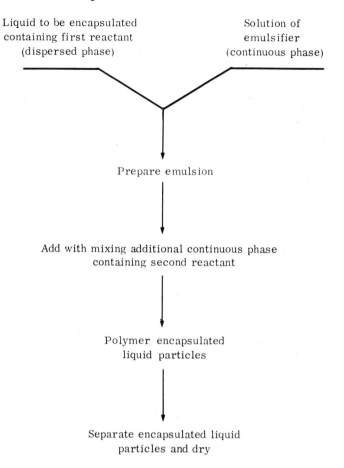

Liquid to be encapsulated
containing first reactant
(dispersed phase)

Solution of
emulsifier
(continuous phase)

Prepare emulsion

Add with mixing additional continuous phase
containing second reactant

Polymer encapsulated
liquid particles

Separate encapsulated liquid
particles and dry

Figure 28 Flow chart of interfacial polymerization coating process.

Because the interfacial polymerization method is best suited for the encapsulation of liquids, other methods may be found to be more useful for solids. The reader is therefore referred to those methods specifically designed to handle solids. For example, in the air-suspension method, polymers soluble in solvents can be directly applied to the solid surface. Surface reactions similar to interfacial reactions can also be accomplished by coating the reactants onto the solid surface and adjusting the column temperature to accommodate the polymerization process.

REFERENCES

1. Bakan, J. A. and Anderson, J. L., Microencapsulation: The theory and practice of industrial pharmacy (L. Lachman, H. A. Lieberman, and J. L. Kanig, eds.), Lea & Febiger, Philadelphia, 1976, pp. 420–438.

2.   *Microencapsulation of Pharmaceuticals*, Capsular Products Division, The National Cash Register Company, Dayton, Ohio, 1971.

3.   Luzzi, L. A., Encapsulation techniques for pharmaceuticals: Considerations for the microencapsulation of drugs. In *Microencapsulation* (J. R. Nixon, ed.), Marcel Dekker, New York, 1976, pp. 193–206.

4.   Bakan, J. A. and Sloan, F. D., *Drug Cosmet. Ind.*, *110*:34 (1972).

5.   Wurster, D. E., *J. Am. Pharm. Assoc. (Sci. Ed.)*, *48*:451 (1959).

6.   Brudney, N. and Toupin, P. Y., *Can. Pharm. J.* (July 1961).

7.   Chilson, F., *Drug Cosmet. Ind.*, *84*:217 (1959).

8.   Wurster, D. E., U.S. Patent 2,648,609 (1953).

9.   Wurster, D. E., U.S. Patent 2,799,241 (1957).

10. Wurster, D. E., U.S. Patent 3,196,827 (1965).

11. Wurster, D. E., U.S. Patent 3,207,834 (1965).

12. Wurster, D. E., U.S. Patent 2,253,944 (1966).

13. Wurster, D. E., U.S. Patent 3,241,520 (1966).

14. Lindolf, J. A. and Wurster, D.E., U.S. Patent 3,117,027 (1964).

15. Coletta, V. and Rubin, H., *J. Pharm. Sci.*, *53*:953 (1964).

16. Wood, J. and Syarto, J., *J. Pharm. Sci.*, *53*:877 (1964).

17. Wurster, D. E., *J. Am. Pharm. Assoc. (Sci. Ed.)*, *49*:82 (1960).

18. Wurster, D. E., U.S. Patent 3,089,824 (1959).

19. Royce, F., *Momentum Transfer in Wurster Air-Suspension Coating Equipment*. Wisconsin Alumni Research Foundation, Madison, Wisconsin, 1963.

20. Richardson, J. F., Incident fluidization and particulate systems: Fluidization (J. F. Davidson and D. Harrison, eds.), Academic Press, New York, 1971, pp. 25–64.

21. Cheremisinoff, N. P. and Cheremisinoff, P. N., *Hydrodynamics of Gas–Solids Fluidization*, Gulf Publishing Company, Houston, 1984, pp. 137–206.

22. Botterill, J. S. M., Fluidization bed behavior: Fluidized beds (J. R. Howard, ed.), Applied Science Publishers, London and New York, 1983, pp. 1–36.

23. Kozeny, J., *Sitzber, Akad. Wiss. Wien, Math-naturw. kl (Abt. IIa)*, *136*:271 (1927).

24. Carman, P. C., *Trans. Inst. Chem. Engrs. (Lond)*, *15*:150 (1937).

25. Carman, P. C., *J. Soc. Chem. Ind. (Lond)*, *57*:225 (1938).

26. Woodcock, C. R., *Economical Transport of Bulk Particulate in Air-Assisted Gravity Conveyors and an Approach to Their Design*, International Conference on Pneumatic Conveying, Cafe Royal, London, January 1979.

28. Blake, C. F., *Trans. Amer. Inst. Chem. Engrs.*, *14*:415 (1922).

29. Kunii, D. and Levenspiel, O., *Fluidization Engineering*. Wiley, New York, 1959, Chap. 3.

30. *Pilot Plant Operation, Wurster Coating and Granulating Process*, Wisconsin Alumni Research Foundation, Madison, Wisconsin.

31. Wilhelm, R. H. and Kwauk, M., *Chem. Eng. Prog.*, *44*:201 (1948).

32. Perry, R. H., Chilton, C. H., and Kirkpatrick, S. D., *Chemical Engineers' Handbook*, 4th Ed., McGraw-Hill, New York, 1963, Chap. 15, pp. 38–40.

33. Coletta, V. and Kennon, L., *J. Pharm. Sci.*, *53*:1524 (1964).

34. Raley, C. F., Jr., Burkett, W. J., and Searingen, J. S., U.S. Patent 2,766,478 (1956).

35. Somerville, G. R., U.S. Patent 3,015,128 (1962).
36. Somerville, G. R., U.S. Patent 3,310,612 (1967).
37. Somerville, G. R., U.S. Patent 3,389,194 (1968).
38. Schultz, E., U.S. Patent 2,857,281 (1958).
39. Goodwin, J. T. and Somerville, G. R., Physical methods for preparing microcapsules. In *Microencapsulation: Process and Application* (J. E. Vandegaer, ed.), Plenum, New York, 1974, pp. 155–163.
40. Luzzi, L. A., *J. Pharm. Sci.*, *59*:1367 (1970).
41. Miles, J. M., Mitzer, B., Brenner, J., and Polak, E., *J. Soc. Cosmet. Chem.*, *22*:655 (1971).
42. Wurzburg, O. and Herbst, W., U.S. Patent 3,091,567 (1961).
43. Evans, R. and Herbst, W., U.S. Patent 3,159,585 (1961).
44. Macaulay, N., U.S. Patent 3,016,308 (1962).
45. Grevenstuk, A. B. and Hougesteger, F., U.S. Patent 3,202,731 (1965).
46. Marotta, N. G., Boettger, R. M., Nappen, B. H., and Szymanski, C. D., U.S. Patent 3,455,838 (1969).
47. *Microencapsulation the Process and Its Capabilities*. Capsular Products Divison, National Cash Register Company, Dayton, Ohio, 1971.
48. Green, B. B., U.S. Patent 2,712,507 (1955).
49. Green, B. K. and Schleicher, L., U.S. Patent 2,730,456 (1956).
50. Green, B. K. and Schleicher, L., U.S. Patent 2,730,457 (1956).
51. Green, B. K. and Schleicher, L., U.S. Patent 2,800,457 (1957).
52. Green, B. K., U.S. Patent 2,800,458 (1957).
53. Luzzi, L. A. and Cerraughty, R. J., *J. Pharm. Sci.*, *53*:429 (1964).
54. Phares, R. E., Jr. and Sperandio, G. J., *J. Pharm. Sci.*, *53*:515 (1964).
55. Luzzi, L. A. and Gerraughty, R. J., *J. Pharm. Sci.*, *56*:364 (1967).
56. Luzzi, L. A. and Gerraughty, R. J., *J. Pharm. Sci.*, *56*:1174 (1967).
57. Paradissis, G. N. and Parrott, E. L., *J. Clin. Pharmacol.*, *8*:54 (1968).
58. Madan, P. L., Luzzi, L. A., and Price, J. C., *J. Pharm. Sci.*, *61*: 1586 (1972).
59. Brynko, C. and Scarpelli, J. A., U.S. Patent 3,190,837 (1965).
60. Brynko, C., Bakan, J. A., Miller, R. E., and Scarpelli, J. A. U.S. Patent 3,341,466 (1967).
61. Bakan, J. A., U.S. Patent 3,436,355 (1969).
62. Dobry, A. and Boyer-Kawenoki, F., *J. Poly. Sci.*, *2*:90 (1947).
63. Powell, T. C., Steinle, M. E., and Yoncoskie, R. A., U.S. Patent 3,415,758 (1965).
64. Phares, R. E., Jr. and Sperandio, G. J., *J. Pharm. Sci.*, *53*:518 (1964).
65. Nack, H., *J. Soc. Cosmet. Chem.*, *21*:85 (1970).
66. Watanabe, A. and Hayashi, T., Microencapsulation techniques of Fuji Photo Film Co. Ltd., and their applications. In *Microencapsulation* (J. R. Nixon, ed.), Marcel Dekker, New York, 1976, pp. 13–38).
67. Baxter, G., Microencapsulation processes in modern business forms. In *Microencapsulation: Processes and Applications* (J. E. Vandegaer, ed.), Plenum, New York, 1974, pp. 127–143.

4

Sustained Drug Release from Tablets and Particles Through Coating

Rong-Kun Chang

Schering Research, Miami, Florida

Joseph R. Robinson

University of Wisconsin, Madison, Wisconsin

I. INTRODUCTION

Probably the earliest work in the area of sustained drug delivery dosage forms can be traced to the 1938 patent of Israel Lipowski [1]. This work involved coated pellets for prolonged release of a drug, and was presumably the forerunner to the development of the coated-particle approach to sustained drug delivery that was introduced in the early 1950s. There has been 40 years of research and development experience in the sustained drug release area since that patent, and a number of strategies have been developed to prolong drug levels in the body. These range from the very simple slowly dissolving pellets or tablets to the more technologically sophisticated controlled drug-release systems which have recently started to appear on the market and in the pharmaceutical literature [2–13]. The endpoint in all of these systems is the same in that extended durations of drug levels are sought, but the method of achieving this endpoint and the clinical performance of these products can vary considerably. Successful fabrication of sustained-release products is usually difficult and involves consideration of the physical–chemical properties of the drug, pharmacokinetic behavior of the drug, route of administration, disease state to be treated and, most importantly, placement of the drug in a dosage form that will provide the desired temporal and spatial delivery pattern for the drug. This chapter is devoted to an examination of one method of sustained-release drug delivery; namely, coating.

The approach in this chapter is to present the requirements for a sustained-release product in terms of the appropriate release rate of drug from the dosage form, a brief review of those factors influencing the design and performance of a sustained-release product, such as the physical–

Table 1   Some Therapeutic Advantages of Sustained-Release Systems

1. Avoid patient compliance problems	
2. Employ less total drug	Minimize or eliminate local side effects
	Minimize or eliminate systemic side effects
	Less potentiation or reduction in drug activity with chronic use
	Minimize drug accumulation with chronic dosing
3. Improved efficiency in treatment	Cure or control of condition more promptly
	Improved control of condition; i.e., less fluctuations in drug level
	Special effects, e.g., sustained-release aspirin provides sufficient drug so that on awakening the arthritic patient has symptomatic relief

Source: From Ref. 21.

chemical properties of the drug and the type of delivery system employed, and lastly, a reasonably critical review of coating as an approach to sustained-drug delivery. Numerous chapters and articles have been written about the technology of specialized coatings, the theoretical foundation for these products, and the resulting clinical and pharmacokinetic assessment. We have no intention of duplicating this effort and, for the sake of brevity, our approach will be to touch on each of these areas without attempting to be comprehensive. Thus, this chapter should serve as a starting point for the pharmaceutical scientist wishing to prepare a coated sustained-release product.

At the outset it may seem unnecessary to justify sustained-release products, but there are some who still view these products as convenience items that offer little clinical benefit to the patient. Indeed the therapeutic advantages of sustained-release products over their nonsustained counterparts are well documented in the literature. Some of these advantages are shown in Table 1. Aside from the enormous advantage of overcoming patient compliance problems, well-designed sustained-release dosage forms offer considerable potential in terms of the temporal and spatial delivery of drug and the resulting maintenance of drug levels in tissues of the body. This suggests that all drugs ought to be placed in a sustained-release form, but this is often not feasible and/or practical.

There are many different definitions of sustained release, but we will adopt the brief, simple definition of sustained-release drug systems as *any drug or dosage form modification that prolongs the therapeutic activity of the drug.* Further, in the absence of suitable clinical evidence of this sustaining effect, we shall accept prolongation of drug levels in the blood. Accordingly, a prodrug or analog modification of the drug that sustains drug activity, or blood drug levels, is viewed as a sustained-release system in the same sense as an alteration in the dosage form.

There are literally dozens of names associated with sustained-release products, such as timed release, prolonged release, controlled release, etc., and this has led to a great deal of confusion. We shall adopt the term *sustained release* to indicate a prolonged release of drug from the dosage form, irrespective of the mechanism or duration of this sustaining effect. Thus, a repeat-action dosage form will be referred to as a sustained-release product, as will the more common prolonged-release type. Moreover, we will use the terms prolonged release and sustained release interchangeably.

Sustained-release products have received a substantial amount of attention in recent years, and several good reviews are available for the interested reader [3-7, 14-20]. These reviews provide not only a description of the available mechanisms and technology for production of these dosage forms, but also information on clinical evaluation and performance. Information on coating technology for sustained-release products, although extensive in the pharmaceutical industry is, unfortunately, rather sparse in available published form. Fields outside of pharmacy making use of sustained-release principles do contain a relatively rich supply of information, specially about polymer properties [22-25], that can sometimes be used for pharmaceutical application. However, this information usually cannot be directly translated into pharmaceutical practice because of the uniqueness of the pharmaceutical dosage form.

II. REQUIREMENTS FOR SUSTAINED DRUG RELEASE

Design of a sustained-release product is normally a very difficult task because of the interplay of the physical-chemical-biological properties of the drug, the patient-disease state, and technological limitations in fabrication of the final dosage form. Depending on the drug, disease state, route of administration, and the like, some of these points will be less important than others, but before a final decision is made to proceed with the dosage form, all of these factors must be considered. To give some perspective on the deliberations that are required as well as establish some guidelines for design of sustained-release products it is worthwhile to briefly review those factors playing a substantial role in the design of sustained-release products.

A. Release Rate and Dose Concentrations

An ideal type of sustained-release product would be one in which the rate of drug delivery is phased to the needs of the condition at hand. Thus, such factors as moment-to-moment variations in drug needs of the condition could be incorporated into the drug-release pattern [26, 27]. However, we generally lack the technological sophistication to prepare a

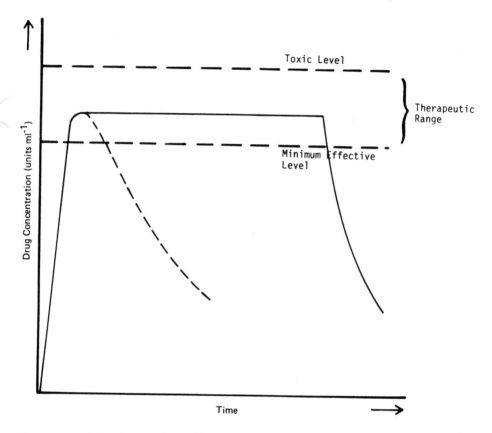

Figure 1 "Ideal" sustained blood or tissue drug level versus time profile. The corresponding level from a nonsustained unit is shown as the dashed line.

product with such a variable release rate, and indeed we frequently do not understand the drug needs of the condition sufficiently to incorporate this into the design of the product. In fact, we can think of only one sustained-release system that meets the criteria of an ideal product, and that is the so-called artificial pancreas. In this system, an implantable electrode monitors the level of circulating glucose and releases an amount of insulin based on the needs of the condition [28].

What is more commonly done with a sustained-release product is to generate a tissue or blood drug concentration versus time profile whereby the level of drug is maintained constant throughout therapy, as is depicted in Figure 1. In this approach, it is assumed that the biological activity of drug instantaneously mirrors blood or tissue drug levels. This is a reasonable assumption that is borne out with many drugs.

For the sake of discussion, the model for oral drugs shown in Scheme 1 will be used to describe drug movement in the body, where k_r, k_a, and k_{el} represent the rate constants for drug release, absorption, and elimination, respectively. For a sustained-release dosage form k_r is much

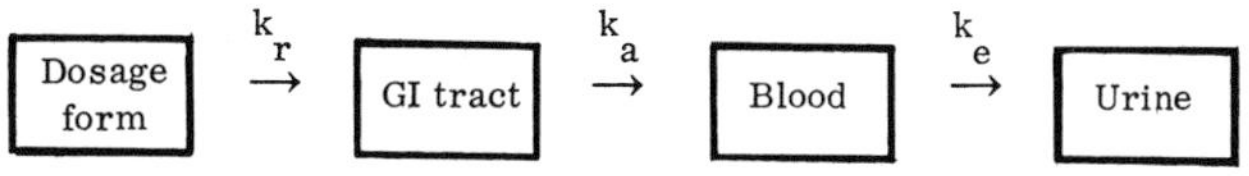

Scheme 1

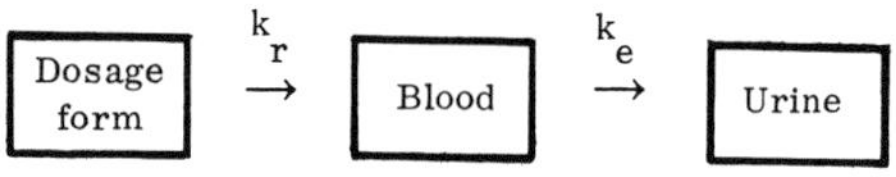

Scheme 2

smaller than k_a, thus becoming rate limiting in the above catenary scheme and reducing the model to that shown in Scheme 2.

If indeed we wish to maintain a constant level of drug in some desired target tissue, the next logical question is what release pattern from the dosage form (drug input) is needed to produce such a profile. It can easily be shown that a zero-order release of drug from the dosage form or, conversely, availability to the body is the most appropriate release pattern [3,29]. The following discussion is pertinent to the question of the desired release rate. For a drug whose disposition in the body can be described by a simple, one-compartment open model, the rate of drug loss at any point in time can be described as

$$\text{rate out} = k_r^0 = C_t k_{el} V_d \tag{1}$$

where C_t is the concentration of drug in the blood (or tissue) at a particular point in time, k_{el} is the total elimination rate constant, and V_d is incorporated into the equation to convert from concentration to an amount basis and is the apparent volume of distribution for the drug. For illustration purposes refer to Figure 1; the desired concentration of a drug is shown as the plateau concentration or maximum in the nonsustained blood drug level profile, which presumably would be the midpoint of the therapeutic range. If we wish to maintain this drug level indefinitely, it is only necessary to put the drug back in at the same rate it is being removed, or

$$\text{rate in} = \text{rate out} = k_r^0 = C_t k_{el} V_d \tag{2}$$

Note that the units resulting from equation 2 are weight (dose) per unit time or that to maintain a constant level of drug it is necessary to provide drug at a constant rate to replace that which is lost. One can envision the simplest sustained drug product as an intravenous drip whereby the rate of drug supply matches that which is lost and is constant (zero-order). For oral and other routes of drug administration, we therefore wish to provide drug via a zero-order pattern whose rate constant describing delivery is determined by the terms shown in equations 1 and 2. For drugs showing more complex disposition patterns than a simple one-compartment model, suitable mathematics can be generated to produce the appropriate rate constant for release of drug from a sustained-release unit [26,27].

To determine the total amount of drug for the dosage form one merely adds the amount of drug needed to achieve the desired blood level quickly (the immediately available portion) to the sustaining portion. The sustaining portion is determined by multiplying the zero-order rate constant for sustained drug delivery, k_r^0, by the desired sustaining time, h [29]:

$$W = D_i + k_r^0 h \tag{3}$$

where W is the total dose and D_i is the initial dose. If drug is released via a first-order process, the appropriate equation [29] is

$$W = D_i + \frac{k_{el} C_t V_d}{k_r^1} \tag{4}$$

where k_{el} is the total elimination constant for the drug, C_t is the desired blood concentration, V_d is the volume of distribution for the drug, and k_r^1 is the first-order drug-release rate constant. The last term in equation 4 results from the approximation $D_m = k_{el} C_t V_d / k_r^1$, where D_m is the maintenance dose [29]. For those drug-delivery systems where drug from the sustaining dose is provided to that from the immediate dose at early times, that is, both release drug from time zero, an appropriate correction to the immediately available dose needs to be made [29].

The following example of how the previously described equations can be used will help clarify the discussion.

Sample Calculation for a Sustained-Release Tablet

From a single 500-mg nonsaturated dose of a tablet, the following pharmacokinetic parameters were determined from the blood drug concentration versus time profile:

k_a (absorption) = 2.0 h^{-1}

k_{el} (elimination) = 0.2 h^{-1}

C_t = desired blood level = 10 $\mu g \ ml^{-1}$

V_d = volume of distribution = 42 L

D_i = initial dose = 500 mg or 5,000,000 μg

It is desired to formulate this drug into a sustained-release product releasing drug over a 12-h period such that the serum level is maintained at 10 $\mu g \ ml^{-1}$. Step 1: Using equation 2 from the text

$$\text{Rate in} = \text{rate out} = k_r^0 = C_t k_{el} V_d$$

$$= 10 \ \mu g \ ml^{-1} \times 0.2 \ h^{-1} \times 42,000 \ ml$$

$$= 84,000 \ \mu g \ h^{-1}$$

Step 2: After calculating the zero-order release rate constant, k_r^0, calculate the total dose per tablet. Using equation 3 from the text

$$W = D_i + k_r^0 h$$

$$= 500,000 \ \mu g + (84,000 \ g \ h^{-1} \times 12 \ h)$$

$$= 1,508,000 \ \mu g$$

$$= 1.5 \ g \ per \ tablet$$

Since a large tablet will be generated, the formulator may wish to prepare 0.75-gm tablets so that the patient takes two tablets every 12 h. Conversely, it is possible to reduce the size of the tablet by recalculating for a shorter sustaining time. For example, suppose 6 rather than 12 h of sustaining time is used.

$$W = 500,000 \ \mu g + (84,000 \ g \ h^{-1} \times 6 \ h)$$

$$= 1,004,000 \ \mu g$$

$$= 1.0 \ gm \ per \ tablet$$

Suppose the formulator finds that the particular sustaining mechanism is better approximated by first-order rather than zero-order release. From the earlier calculations, the formulator knows that for 12 h of release the tablet should contain about 1.5 gm and the zero-order release rate is 84,000 $\mu g \ h^{-1}$. From these data it is possible to approximate the first-order rate constant k_r using equation 4

$$W = D_i + \frac{k_{el} C_t V_d}{k_r^1}$$

$$k_r^1 = \frac{k_{el} C_t V_d}{W - D_i}$$

$$= \frac{0.2 \ h^{-1} \times 10 \ \mu g \ ml^{-1} \times 42,000 \ ml}{1,508,000 - 500,000 \ \mu g}$$

$$= 8.33 \times 10^{-2} \ h^{-1}$$

B. Drug Properties Considerations

There are a number of physical–chemical and derived biological properties of the drug that either preclude placement of the drug in a sustained-release system or have an adverse influence on product design and performance. Some of these considerations are listed in Table 2. With almost all of these properties we refer to them as restrictive factors, making formulation of a sustained-release system difficult, but not impossible. Thus, by changing the type of sustaining mechanism, the dose, or the

Table 2   Drug Properties Adversely Influencing a Sustained-Release Dosage Form

Property		Explanation
Physical-chemical properties	Dose size	If an oral product has a dose size greater than 0.5 gm, it is a poor candidate for a sustained-release system, since addition of the sustaining dose and possibly the sustaining mechanism will, in most cases, generate a substantial volume product that will be unacceptably large.
	Aqueous solubility	Extremes in aqueous solubility are undesirable in the preparation of a sustained-release product. For drugs with low water solubility, they will be difficult to incorporate into a sustained-release mechanism. The lower limit on solubility for such product has been reported [30] to me 0.1 mg/ml. Drugs with great water solubility are equally difficult to incorporate into a sustained-release system [31]. pH-Dependent solubility, particularly in the physiological pH range, would be another problem because of the variation in pH throughout the GI tract and hence variation in dissolution rate [31].
	Partition coefficient	Drugs that are very lipid soluble or very water soluble, i.e., extremes in partition coefficient, will demonstrate either low flux into the tissues or rapid flux followed by accumulation in the tissues. Both cases are undesirable for a sustained-release system [32,33].
	Drug stability	Since most oral sustained-release systems, by necessity, are designed to release their contents over much of the length of the GI tract, drugs which are unstable in the environment of

		the intestine might be difficult to formulate into prolonged release systems [34]. Interestingly, placement of a labile drug in a sustained-release dosage form often improves the bioavailability picture [31].
Biological properties	Absorption	Drugs that are slowly absorbed or absorbed with a variable absorption rate are poor candidates for a sustained-release system. For oral dosage forms, the lower limit on the absorption rate constant is in the range of 0.25 h^{-1} [31] (assuming a GI transit time of 10–12 h)
	Distribution	Drugs with high apparent volumes of distribution, which in turn influences the rate of elimination for the drug, are poor candidates [31].
	Metabolism	Sustained-release systems for drugs which are extensively metabolized is possible as long as the rate of metabolism is not too great nor the metabolism variable with GI transit or other routes.
	Duration of action	The biological half-life and hence the duration of action of a drug obviously plays a major role in considering a drug for sustained-release systems. Drugs with short half-lives and high doses impose a constraint because of the dose size needed and those with long half-lives are inherently sustained [16,35].
	Therapeutic	Drugs with a narrow therapeutic range require precise control over the blood levels of drug, placing a constraint on sustained-release dosage forms.

route of administration, it might be possible to generate a sustained-release system. Frequently, a seeminly undesirable property of a drug or
dosage form can be overcome or minimized by placement of the drug in a
sustained-release system. For example, low drug bioavailability due to instability may sometimes be overcome by placement in a sustained-release
system [31].

III. FABRICATION OF SUSTAINED-RELEASE PRODUCTS

Having established the desirable concentration versus time profile as depicted in Figure 1, we can now ask two related questions: What approaches can be taken to achieve this type of profile, and how should the sustained-release product be constructed? Our concern, therefore, is to
examine the potential mechanisms available and to describe the general
nature of the dosage form construction.

A. Repeat-Action Release and Continuous Release

To maintain the drug level at a constant desired value, we can employ
frequent dosings of drug to generate a series of peaks and valleys in the
blood level profile, whose mean value lies on the plateau of the ideal case.
This approach is shown in Figure 2. The success of this approach depends on the frequency of the multidoses because, obviously, the more
frequent the dose the smaller the peaks and valleys and the closer the
extreme drug level will adhere to the plateau value. This is the approach
taken with the Spansules, where four dosage units were employed in each
Spansule. One dose unit provided drug in a nonsustained form to establish the initial blood level of drug and the other three doses were intended to release drug at 2-, 4-, and 6-h intervals. Depending on the
drug properties, other intervals can be used, as can a greater number of
repetitive doses, although more than four becomes impractical from a manufacturing standpoint.
    An alternate approach is to employ a continuous release of drug. With
this method, a nonsustained portion of the dosage form is needed to rapidly establish the therapeutic level of drug in the blood, and then by
some suitable mechanism, drug is continuously provided in a zero- or
first-order fashion. In this regard it is appropriate to comment on the
drug concentration versus time profile for a system releasing drug via
first-order kinetics. Contrary to the case where drug is released via
zero-order kinetics, as depicted in Figure 1, first-order release produces
a more or less bell-shaped profile. Whether the bell shape is symmetrical
or skewed and whether it is narrow or wide depends on the drug and
the sustained-release system employed; that is, the kinetics of release.
Examples of this type of profile will be discussed and demonstrated later
in the chapter.

B. Mechanisms of Sustained Release

A zero-order release of drug is needed for the dosage form, which means
that the rate of drug release is independent of drug concentration

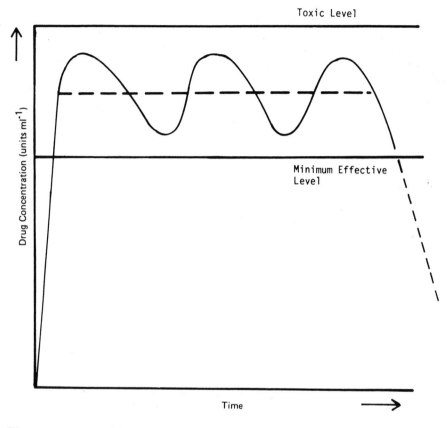

Figure 2 Repetitive release approach to sustained-release. The dotted line represents the ideal sustained-release profile.

$$\frac{dC}{dt} = k_r^0 \qquad (5)$$

or expressed in amounts

$$\frac{dM}{dt} = k_r^0 \qquad (6)$$

At times it is not possible to generate a constant-release product and a slow first-order release of drug is employed. A slow first-order release will approximate a zero-order release as long as only a fraction of drug release is followed [29]; that is, less than one half-life is followed.

To attain a zero-order release rate, we have several mechanisms and dosage form modifications that we can employ. We will restrict our coverage of potential mechanisms to those that can be employed in the coating approach to sustained release.

Diffusion

A number of sustained-release products are based on diffusion of drug.
The following discussion, although somewhat naive, will bring into perspective those properties that should be considered in the diffusion
approach.

Fick's first law of diffusion states that drug diffuses in the direction
of decreasing concentration across a membrane where J is the flux of the
drug in amount/area-time.

$$J = -D \frac{dC}{dx} \tag{7}$$

where D is the diffusion coefficient in area/time, C is the concentration,
and x is the distance. Assuming steady state, equation 7 can be integrated to give

$$J = -D \frac{\Delta C}{\ell} \tag{8}$$

or expressed in more common form when a water-insoluble membrane is
employed

$$\frac{dM}{dt} = \frac{ADK \, \Delta C}{\ell} \tag{9}$$

where A is area, D is diffusion coefficient, K is the partition coefficient of
drug into the membrane, ℓ is the diffusional pathlength (thickness of coat
in the ideal case), and ΔC is the concentration gradient across the
membrane.

In order to have a constant rate of release, the right-hand portions
of equations 8 and 9 must be maintained constant. In other words, the
area of diffusion, diffusional path length, concentration increment, partition coefficient, and diffusion coefficient must be invariant. Usually, one
or more of the above parameters will change in oral sustained-release
dosage forms giving rise to non-zero-order release.

The more common diffusional approaches for sustained drug release
are shown in Schemes 3 and 4. In most cases, the drug must partition
into a polymeric membrane of some sort and then diffuse through the membrane to reach the biological milieu. When the tablet or microcapsule contains excess drug or suspension, a constant activity of drug will be maintained until the excess has been removed, giving rise to constant drug
release. In Scheme 3 the polymer is water insoluble, and the important
parameter is solubility of drug in the membrane, since this gives rise to
the driving force for diffusion. In Scheme 4 either the polymer is partially soluble in water or a mixture of water-soluble and water-insoluble
polymers is used. The water-soluble polymer then dissolves out of the
film, giving rise to small channels through which the drug can diffuse.
The small channels would presumably give a constant diffusional path
length, and hence maintain constant conditions as described earlier. Although diffusion through the channels should be much more rapid than
diffusion through the membrane noted in Scheme 3, it is possible to have
a situation whereby membrane diffusion, being quite rapid in this case,

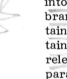

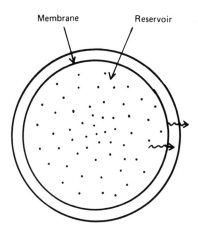

Scheme 3   Diffusion control of drug release by a water-insoluble polymer.

is within an order of magnitude of pore diffusion. In this event, both types of diffusion, membrane and pore, will provide contributions to the overall diffusion rate and the equations would have to be modified to account for these combined effects.

Dissolution

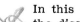

In this case, the drug is embedded (coated) in a polymeric material and the dissolution rate of the polymer dictates the release rate of drug. The

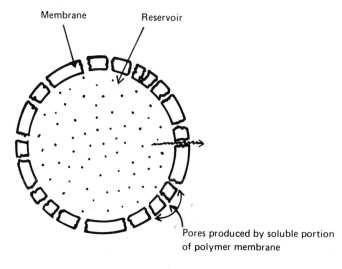

Pores produced by soluble portion of polymer membrane

Scheme 4   Diffusion control of drug release by a partially water-soluble polymer.

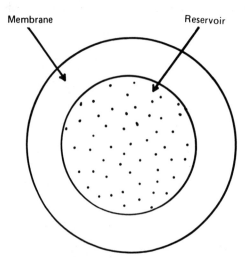

Scheme 5   Dissolution control of drug release via thickness and dissolution rate of the membrane barrier coat.

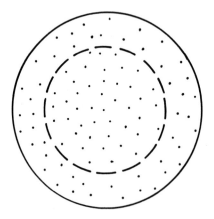

Scheme 6   Dissolution control of drug release via polymer core erosion or polymer-coating erosion. (Note: Although equations are based on spherical tablets, erosion of conventional flattened tablets is similar but there is a combination of various R terms where R depends on the axis being measured. See Ref. 38. It is assumed that diffusion of water, metabolites, or biologically active components is not rate limiting.

drug release rate, if governed by erosion or dissolution, can be expressed as

$$\frac{dM}{dt} = A \frac{dx}{dt} \ f(C) \tag{10}$$

where $(dx)/(dt)$ is the erosion rate, $f(C)$ is the concentration profile in the matrix, and A is area. A constant erosion rate can produce zero-order release kinetics, provided the drug is dispersed uniformly in the matrix and area is maintained constant [36,37]. Oftentimes, swelling of the system or a significant change in area produces non-zero-order release.

The common forms of dissolution control are shown in Schemes 5 and 6. In Scheme 5 we have a barrier coat across a microcapsule or nonpareil seed containing drug, and the release of drug is dictated by the dissolution rate and thickness of the barrier coat. Varying the coating thickness, or layering concentric spheres of coating material and drug reservoir material, gives rise to different release times, producing the repeat action dosage form. Once the polymer has dissolved, all of the drug contained in the capsule or seed is available for dissolution and absorption. In Scheme 6 the drug is either embedded in a polymer or coated with a water-soluble polmyer, which in turn is compressed into a slowly dissolving tablet. The release rate is controlled by the dissolution rate of the polymer or tablet.

Osmosis

Placement of a semipermeable membrane around a tablet, particle, or drug solution, which allows creation of an osmotic pressure difference between the inside and outside of the tablet and hence "pumps" drug solution out of the tablet through a small orifice in the coat, can be used as a sustained-release mechanism. The key component of the system is the ability of a drug solution to attract water through a semipermeable membrane by osmosis. Since the drug solution is contained within a fairly rigid system, drug solution can be pumped out of the tablet or particle at a controlled constant rate if a small hole is created in the coating surface and a constant activity of drug, that is, excess drug, is maintained. Controlling the rate of water imbibition thus controls the rate of drug delivery. This can be seen in the following expression [12]

$$\frac{dV}{dt} = k \frac{A}{\ell} \ (\Delta \pi - \Delta P) \tag{11}$$

where dV/dt is the flow rate of water, k, A, and ℓ are the membrane permeability, area, and thickness, $\Delta \pi$ is the osmotic pressure difference, and ΔP is the hydrostatic pressure difference. Keeping the hydrostatic pressure small relative to the osmotic pressure, equation 11 reduces to

$$\frac{dV}{dt} = k \frac{A}{\ell} \ (\Delta \pi) \tag{12}$$

By maintaining the right-hand side of equation 12 constant, a zero-order release system will result.

COATING METHODS. Coating is a versatile process which imparts
various useful properties to the product. Modifications of drug-release
patterns such as enteric release, repeat-action release, and sustained
release are the most important pharmaceutical applications of coating. Although many coating techniques, for various purposes, have been detailed
in previous chapters, we have elected to discuss the coating methods for
the purpose of modified release.

Pharmaceutical coatings have been classified into four basic categories:
sugar coating, microencapsulation, film coating, and compression coating.
Sugar coating of compressed tablets and granules is regarded as the oldest
process, involving the multistage build up of sugar layers through deposition from an aqueous-coating solution and coating powder. Sugar coating
falls outside the scope of this chapter owing to the inability to control
drug release through a highly water-soluble sugar barrier.

A. Microencapsulation

Microencapsulation is a process in which tiny particles or droplets are surrounded by a uniform coating (so-called microcapsule) or held in a matrix
of polymer (so-called microsphere). A number of microencapsulation techniques, including aqueous phase separation, three-phase dispersion, organic phase separation, and interfacial polymerization, have been used to
encapsulate pharmaceuticals and to retard the liberation of drug from
microcapsules.

Aqueous phase separation methods to prepare microcapsules include the
simple coacervation of hydrophilic colloids with ethanol or sodium sulfate as
dehydrating agents. In addition, one can employ a complex coacervation
of two dispersed hydrophilic colloids of opposite electric charges with subsequent pH change. Aqueous phase separation was patented as an encapsulation process by Green in 1955 [39], and has been used commercially
since that time for numerous applications.

The three-phase dispersion method involves dispersion of the materials
to be coated in a nonsolvent liquid phase containing colloidal or film-
forming materials such as gelatin. This two-phase system is then dispersed in a third phase by emulsification, through spraying or other
means, and the coating material is gelled, usually by cooling. The resulting gelled droplets are then either separated and dried or partially de-
hydrated with an aliphatic alcohol and then separated and dried. Variations on this process have been used commercially to encapsulate oil-
soluble vitamins such as vitamin A. One of the earliest applications of
this method was reported in a British patent in 1938 [40].

Generally, aqueous phase separation and three-phase dispersion methods are used to encapsulate water-insoluble or poorly water-soluble materials which are usually poor drug candidates to incorporate into a sustained-release system. Gelatin is the most commonly used microencapsu-
lating agent for the two processes described above. Even for poorly
water-soluble drugs, gelatin is usually not able to achieve the desired
dissolution profile owing to the hydrophilic properties of gelatin. The use
of formalin in treatment to cross-link the gelatin and/or dual coating of
gelatin microcapsules may be necessary to improve the dissolution profile.
In addition, these encapsulation processes would be precluded for heat-
sensitive materials and substances with a stability and/or solubility problem
at the pH of coacervation.

Nonaqueous phase separation involves dispersion of core material in an organic continuous phase in which the wall-forming polymer has been dissolved. Phase separation is induced by the addition of a nonsolvent, incompatible polymer, inorganic salt, or by altering temperature of the system. The organic phase separation method can be employed in the manufacture of microcapsules using various water-insoluble polymers as coating materials to enclose water-soluble drugs and to slow the drug-release rate.

Encapsulation via interfacial polymerization was pioneered by Chang [41,42] in work designed to produce artificial cells. This method involves the reaction of various monomers, such as hexamethylene diamine and sebacoyl chloride, at an interface between two immiscible liquid phases to form a film of polymer that encapsulates the dispersed phase. Capsules formed by interfacial polymerization usually have relatively thin semipermeable membranes highly suited for artificial cell studies or applications requiring permeable walls. This method may give rise to questions about toxicity of the unreacted monomer, the polymer fragments, and other constituents in the process, instability of the drug in the reaction medium during the polymerization period, fragility of the microcapsules, and high permeability of the coating to low molecular weight species [43]. Various other polymerization procedures, including bulk, suspension, emulsion, and micellar polymerization, have received considerable academic interest to entrap active materials in polymer matrices. However, inherent problems of polymerization procedures such as impurities in the system, limited drug solubility in the monomer, excessive drug degradation caused by reaction with the monomer or initiator, and possible entrapment of drug in polymers may prevent the pharmaceutical industry from actively engaging in this approach to control drug release.

In general, microencapsulation techniques using liquid as a process medium are rather complicated and difficult to control. Several process difficulties such as hardening of the capsule shell, isolating the microcapsules from the manufacturing vehicle, and drying the microcapsules to form free-flowing powder should be solved in order to ascertain batch to batch uniformity. Equipment required for microencapsulation by these methods is relatively simple: It consists mainly of jacketed tanks with variable speed agitation. The process can be carried out on a production scale with good reliability, reproducibility, and control. However, process control, product quality control, and scale-up problems appear to be the limiting factors influencing general acceptance by the pharmaceutical industry.

The most common mechanical microencapsulation process is the spray-drying technique, which consists of rapid evaporation of the solvent from the droplets. Spray-drying techniques may produce monodispersed free-flowing particles which can be directly compressed into tablets, filled into capsules, and suspended in water. However, the microcapsules obtained by spray drying tend to be very porous because of rapid volatilization of the solvent. Spray-congealing techniques accomplish coating solidification by thermal congealing of the molten coating materials such as hydrogenated castor oil, cetyl alcohol, monoglyceride and diglyceride, etc. Spray-congealed coatings are less porous but require coating materials that melt at moderate temperature.

Successful attempts using spray-drying and congealing techniques to control the release of sulfa drugs have been reported [44—47].

B. Film Coating

Film coating involves the deposition of a uniform film onto the surface of
the substrate, such as compressed tablets, granules, nonpareil pellets,
and capsules. Intermittent manual application or continuous spraying of
coating solution onto a mechanically tumbled or fluidized bed of substrates
allow the coating to be built up to the desired thickness. Because of the
capability of depositing a variety of coating materials onto solid cores,
this process has been widely used to make modified-release beads and
tablets in the pharmaceutical industry.

Properly designed film coating can be applied to pharmaceutical products to achieve performance requirements such as rapidly dissolving coatings, sustained- or controlled-release coatings, and enteric coatings. The
polymer(s) used in coating formulations is the predominant factor for the
properties of the film coat. Water-soluble film formers such as methyl cellulose, hydroxypropyl methylcellulose, hydroxypropylcellulose, polyethylene
glycol, polyvinyl pyrrolidone, etc., form a rapidly dissolving barrier.
Enteric materials such as cellulose acetate phthlate, polyvinyl acetate
phthalate, methacrylic acid ester copolymers, etc., form acid-resistant
films. The hydrophobic water-insoluble polymers such as ethyl cellulose,
cellulose acetate, cellulose triacetate, cellulose acetate butyrate, and methacrylic acid ester copolymers are used to extend the release of drug over a
long period of time. Depending upon the physicochemical properties of the
drug and the substrate formulation, several coating approaches have been
employed to regulate drug release.

Partitioning Membrane

Partitioning membranes, continuous hydrophobic polymeric films which remain intact throughout the gastrointestinal tract, can be applied onto the
coating substrate by using a single polymer or a combination of water-
insoluble polymers. Since drug molecules cross the membrane by both a
partition and a diffusion process, solubility of the drug in the polymeric
material is a prerequisite to permeation. The polymeric material should be
carefully selected to have the desired permeability to the drug and water
in order to achieve the desired release profile. In addition to thickness
of membranes, the permeability of the film can also be adjusted by mixing
two water-insoluble polymers in any desired proportion.

Dialysis Membrane

Frequently, the partitioning membrane is too effective to regulate drug release. In other words, the drug within the coating would be released
very slowly or be released not at all for a long period of time. The inclusion of hydrophilic additives within the coating along with hydrophobic
polymer(s) creates pores when the additives are dissolved by water, which
guarantees the penetration of water and elimination of drug entrapment.
When the drug molecule leaves the membrane by diffusing through pores
filled with dissolution media (dialysis mechanism) the size of the drug molecules and solubility of the drug in a dissolution medium are important
factors in transport. Some water-soluble additives such as sodium chloride, lactose and sucrose have poor solubility in organic solvents and may
be micronized and suspended in a solvent-based coating system. Water-
soluble polymers such as methyl cellulose, polyvinyl pyrrolidone, and

polyethylene glycol are commonly mixed with hydrophobic polymers to regulate drug release owing to their excellent film-forming properties and
solubility in organic solvents. In addition to film thickness, the ratio of
soluble components to insoluble polymer in the coating influences the release rate. Porous membranes may also be prepared by incomplete coating
of hydrophobic polymers. However, strict process control is necessary to
ascertain the reproducibility owing to sensitivity to the coating weight.

Fat Wax Barrier

Mixtures of waxes (bees wax, carnauba wax, etc.) with glycerol mono-
palmitate, cetyl alcohol, and myristyl alcohol can be applied onto the substrate to form a barrier by hot-melt coating. Hot-melt coating is the most
economical process owing to elimination of solvent cost and the inexpensive-
ness of the coating materials. However, a higher level of coating, compared to polymeric film coating, is normally required to retard the liberation of the drug.

*Incorporation of Enteric Materials into
the Formulation*

In general, pH-independent dissolution is the ideal attribute of a controlled-
release dosage form. However, most drugs are either weak acids or weak
bases; their release from delivery systems is pH dependent. If the drug
has a higher solubility in acidic than in basic media, enteric material may
be incorporated into the rate-controlling barrier or core matrix to minimize
the effect of pH-dependent solubility. In another approach, physiological
acceptable buffering agents can be added to the core formulation to maintain the fluid inside the rate-controlling membrane to a suitable constant
pH, thereby rendering a pH-independent drug release [48]. Enteric material also can be incorporated into rate-controlling membranes or core
matrices to create pH-dependent release of the drug. The dosage form
with pH-dependent dissolution characteristics may be beneficial in some
cases to improve the extent of absorption by dumping the dose in time
and preventing the unabsorbed dose being entrapped in the stool. Sustained-release preparations overcoated with enteric material can be utilized
as an intestinal delivery system with sustained-release properties. Enteric-
coated dosage forms can be overcoated with a drug layer to form a repeat-
action preparation.

CORE PREPARATION. Very few drug particles possess adequate
physicochemical properties for the usual coating process. These properties
include (1) suitable tensile, compaction, shear, impaction, and attrition
strengths to avoid destruction during the coating process; (2) approximately spherical shape to obtain good flow and rolling properties in the
coating equipment; (3) suitable size and size distribution; and (4) suitable
density to avoid escape of the drug particles during the coating process.
Certainly, different types of coating equipment have their own capabilities
to handle the cores, leading to different requirements of the cores for
various equipment. For the pan coating process, a relatively large particle size (larger than 500 μm) and a spherical shape are generally considered necessary to provide excellent rolling in the coating pan and to avoid
the agglomeration and/or aggregation owing to inefficiency of drying and
long contact time among the cores. Although fluidized-bed coating

systems expanded coating capabilities dramatically, suitable strengths and weight of the cores are needed to avoid excessive attrition of drug particles and suction of drug particles into the filter during the coating process. The major advantages of using pure drug particles as coating substrates are elimination of the core-making process and a less bulky final product. Potassium chloride and acetyl salicylic acid crystals are typical examples which have been satisfactorily coated in a coating pan or a fluidized-bed coating system.

1.   *Compaction process*.   Apparently, tablets are the most common and easiest dosage form to coat. Tablets with excellent friability, hardness, and edge thickness are preferred for coating. However, sustained-release film-coated tablets may prematurely dose dump due to accidental rupture of the coating film. The use of a multiple-unit instead of a single-unit dosage form is a pharmaceutical trend because of the presumed reduction of the inherently large inter- and intrasubject variation linked to gastrointestinal transit time. Tablets of small dimensions have been successfully prepared from polyvinyl alcohol and subsequently cross-linked at the surface to form a quasimembrane-controlled system for a multiple-unit dosage form [49]. In order to achieve high output in large-scale manufacturing, this approach to the preparation of cores may face formulation difficulties and tablet tooling problems; i.e., multitipped punches. The limited size flexibility of the tableting method to manufacture cores for a multiple-unit device is another disadvantage.

Other methods with production capacity, such as slugging, chilsonator, and Hutt Compactor, can be used to produce granules in the compaction mode. However, irregular-shaped granules are commonly observed and extensive sieving is necessary to remove the fines and oversized granules.

2.   *Surface-layering process*.   Another common approach to core production involves the use of substrates and enlargement of the substrates by a surface-layering technique. Thus, nonpareil seeds of various sizes or sugar crystals are used as the substrate. Application of an active substance onto an inert substrate can be carried out by uniform coating in a rotating coating pan in the presence of a suitable adhesive. In detail, the substrate is uniformly wetted by manual spreading of a binding solution, followed by attachment of the active substance to the surface of the substrate. Commonly used adhesives include solutions of polyvinyl pyrrolidone polyethylene glycols, cellulose ethers, natural gums, shellac, zein, gelatin, and sugar syrup. Suitable binder(s) and solvent systems for the binder(s) must be found in order to have smooth production of cores without excessive agglomeration of the cores or separation of the drug particles. Enteric binders, such as cellulose acetate phthalate and shellac, may impart pH-dependent dissolution properties to the final product. Separating agents, such as talcum and magnesium stearate, may be used to eliminate or reduce tackiness of the adhesives. Trituration technique, to blend the potent drug with the auxiliary agents, is usually required to obtain a uniform distribution of the drug onto the substrate surface.

The powder layering process requires a great deal of repetition, and is thus time consuming. Moreover, undesired agglomeration or aggregation and adhesion to the wall of coating equipment can occur. To avoid the labor-intensive powder layering process in a coating pan, a centrifugal-type fluidized bed with a powder feed device (CF-Granulator) has been used to produce high-quality pellets. The stirring chamber of the CF-Granulator consists of a fixed specially curved wall stator and a di- rected rotating plate rotor. Fluidization air, through a gap slit between the stator and rotor, prevents the substrates from falling. The sub- strates are whirled up along the wall of the stator owing to centrifugal force of the rotor and to the upper part of the wall due to the fluidization air. Subsequently, they drop due to gravitational force. During the spiral stirring operation, layering powder is metered to the fluidized bed from a powder feed unit. A binder solution is sprayed from a spraying gun to cause binding of the powder to the substrate surface.

It is also possible to dissolve or to suspend the drug in the binder solution and to apply this liquid uniformly to the surface of the substrate using a coating pan or fluidized-bed system. However, there are several difficulties with this approach, including the tendency to clog the nozzle with the slurry. A large quantity of solvent may be needed to dissolve or suspend the active substance. In addition, drug loss to the air stream and possible adverse aggregation of the cores can occur. Another in- herent disadvantage of the layering process is the possible formation of unduly large pellets owing to the use of nonpareil seeds as a substrate. Small-sized substrates, such as sugar crystals, can be used to eliminate bulkiness of the pellets. The finer the substrate, the finer the drug par- ticle should be and the more difficult the process.

3. *Agglomeration process.* Alternatively, the drug particles in the powder bed can grow by wet agglomeration. The extent of granule growth depends on the amount of granulating solution, the type of binder, the force of agitation, and heat applied. The conventional wet granulation method to prepare the substrate for coating can give rise to problems such as irregular-shaped particles with a coarse and porous surface, soft and pliable particles, and a broad granular size distribution. Application of relatively large amounts of coating material may be required owing to capillary suction of the coating fluid to pores. The porous structure and irregular shape of the granules may lead to an unpredictable sustained- release coating. Additional powder layering to round off the granules into a sphere or to smooth surfaces or perhaps to increase the strength of the pellets may be important. However, Kohnle et al. [50] have suc- cessfully produced microspherules which are suitable for enteric- and sustained-release coating through agglomeration of fine drug particles by using a Twin Shell Blender with an intensifier bar assembly.

The inclined dish granulator or disc pelletizer is well known and high- ly utilized in the fertilizer, iron ore, and detergent industries. It also has been adopted throughout the pharmaceutical, chemical, food, and allied industries. The equipment, known as the nodulizer and pelletizer, are available for continuous production of spherical pellets. The unit normally consists of a shallow cylindrical dish, motor drive, adjustable scrapers, spraying system, and powder feed device. As the pan rotates about an inclined axis, the raw material bed is rolled by centrifugal force and maintained as a uniform deposit of material onto the base of the pan by a plow. Scrapers also prevent buildup of materials on the dish sur- face. Powdered ingredients must be milled, premixed, and deaerated in order to have a uniform chute fed to the unit. Powder materials are continuously metered to the pan at a specific location, normally at a point three-fourths of a radius unit from the top of the dish. The spray angle depends to a large extent on positioning of the sprays and their distance

from the bed powders; commonly, a 60 spray angle is used. The spray
droplet size should be adjusted according to feed size and desired granule
size. In other words, if small granules are desired, a fine droplet spray
should be used and vice versa. Also, the finer the feed material, the
finer the spray droplet.

There are several theoretical equations that can be used to calculate
the rotational speed of the pan. However, appreciable discrepancy exists
in theory and practice. Usually 20–30 rpm seems a reasonable rotation
speed. Following agglomeration, the finished granules are raked over by
the dish rim, and the rim height can be adjusted to control granule size.
Pronounced size segregation is the principal feature of dish granulation.
This ensures almost perfectly spherical pellets with a narrow particle size
distribution. Important parameters in the dish pelletizer include powder
feet rate, position of powder feed chute, spraying rate, position of the
spraying gun, spray nozzle size, angle of inclination, rotational speed, rim
height, powder bed depth, and pan size. These variables interact to
some extent to produce the final granules.

However, the noncontinuous granulation process in which spraying and
drying stages are alternately repeated has been employed to maintain constant moisture levels and to produce high-density granules. A high level
of perfection in shape and size of the granules cannot be obtained by
agglomeration mechanism using a conventional fluidized-bed granulator.
Recently, modified fluidized-bed units, such as the Roto-Processor, the
Spir-A-Flow, and the Glatt Rotor Granulator/Coater, all utilize a rotating
disc at the bottom of a fluidized-bed, replacing the air-distribution plate.
This modification supposedly combines the advantages of the dish granulator and the fluidized-bed granulator. It has been demonstrated that the
rotary fluidizer-bed granulator can be used to produce spherical granules
with high density by an agglomeration mechanism [51]. In general, the
layering mechanism using nonpareil seeds or sugar crystals as a substrate
to build spherical-shaped pellets is relatively easy compared to the agglomeration mechanism.

4. *Extrusion-spheronization process.* Spherical pellets can also be
produced using an extrusion-spheronization process. The main processing
steps include (1) dry blending, (2) wet granulation, (3) kneading, (4)
extrusion, (5) spheronization, (6) drying, and (7) screening. A thoroughly wet granulation containing the drug, diluent, and binder is forced
through a radial or axial extruder with a suitable die design, such as a
perforated die or multiple-hole die, by means of a screw feeder to produce
roughly cylindrical extrudates. The extrudate size and final pellet size
are determined by the size of the die used on the extruder. The pellet
mill, a radial extruder, was initially developed for the agricultural industry to densify and upgrade the particle size of poultry and animal
feeds. In operation, the preconditioned material is fed continuously in a
controlled fashion to the pelleting chamber. The motor-driven outer perforated die ring causes the roller(s), which is mounted inside the die ring,
to turn. The feed, carried by the rotation of the die ring, is compressed
and forced through the holes in the die ring. As pellets are extruded, a
knife, or knives, mounted at the exterior of the die ring, cuts the pellets
to length. Application of the pellet mill to pharmaceutical products has
been extremely limited. However, it deserves special mention owing to its
ability to produce pellets with high density and low friability at a high
output.

The extruded granules can be converted into consistently sized spheres by use of a Japanese device called a marumerizer or an English version of the device called a spheronizer. This device consists of a stationary cylinder with a smooth wall and a grooved rotating disc. The centrifugal and frictional forces, generated by the rough rotating baseplate, spheronize and densify the extruded granule. A typical time for the spheronization process would be approximately 5 min per batch, depending upon the nature of the material. Recently, a unique device called the Roto-Coil has been designed as a continuous spheronizer with no moving parts. This device consists of a spiral-shaped pipe. The extrudate is spheronized by passing through the pipe in a rotation movement with the aid of negative pressure generated by a fluidized-bed system. The advantages of the extrusion-spheronization process include: (1) production of the spherical pellets without using seeds, leading to reduction of the bulk of final product; (2) the ability to regulate size of the pellets within a narrow particle size distribution; (3) the ability to produce high-density, low-friability, spherical pellets; and (4) the ability to achieve excellent surface characteristics for subsequent coating, leading to an homogeneous distribution of coating material(s) onto the spherical pellets.

It is also possible to agglomerate the finely divided solids into spherical matrices from a liquid suspension [52]. In the spherical agglomeration process, fine powders are dispersed in the liquid. With controlled agitation, a small amount of a second liquid, which is immiscible with the first liquid and preferentially wets the solids, is added to induce formation of dense, highly spherical agglomerates. Another approach to prepare spherical matrices in the liquid state is the instantaneous cross-linking of drug-containing droplets of aqueous solution of sodium alginate in a suitable hardening bath, such as calcium chloride solution. This entrapment technique in recent years has become the most widely used method for immobilizing living cells and enzymes. It enjoys several advantages, such as a simple production process, a wide size range of beads, and a narrow size distribution [53]. The spray-drying process has been used to produce a spherical matrix. However, the spray-dried cores may be porous and fluffy because of rapid volatilization of the solvent. The spray-congealing process, also called the prilling process, is well known in the fertilizer industry for production of urea pellets and ammonium nitrate pellets. This process can be defined as the process by which a product is formed into particles, usually of spherical shape, by spraying a melt of the product into a chamber of suitable configuration through which cooling air is passed. The process is fairly restricted to matrix materials having suitable properties; namely, a high melting point and low heats of crystallization [54]. These several techniques may have potential applicability to produce spherical cores containing drug for subsequent sustained-release coating, and thus deserve further investigation. The physical properties of the product, such as pellet size and size distribution, pellet density, strengths, globocity, pore and pore distribution, etc., are different for various methods and may be important for subsequent coating as well as in product performance. Table 3 summarizes the various possible methods to core production and some selected pharmaceutical examples.

LATEX/PSEUDOLATEX COATING. The strict air-quality controls instituted by different federal agencies, spiraling solvent costs, the high price of solvent recovery system, and potential toxicity as well as to some

Table 3 Possible Methods for Core Manufacture and Some Selected Pharmaceutical Examples

Method and example	Equipment	Drug	Carrier binder	Comments and variable studied
Crystallization	Oslo crystallizer	Potassium chloride acetyl salicylic acid, etc.	N/A	Very few drug crystals possess adequate properties for coating.
Compressed tablet	Tablet press	Various	Various	Single-unit device. The accidental rupture of the film barrier may cause premature dumping of drug.
Min-Tablet [49]	Tablet press	Diprophylline	Polyvinyl alcohol	Relatively large matrices for multiunit device.
Granular	Chilsonator, Hutt Compactor	Various	Various	Irregular shaped granules. Extensive screening and recycling of undesired granules.
Layering [55]	CF-Granulator	Theophylline, pseudoephedrine hydrochloride, diphenhydramine hydrochloride	Gelatin, sodium carboxymethylcellulose, Kaolin/ Eudragit E-30D, Povidone	Evaluation of CF-Granulator for pelletization.
Layering [56]	Fluidized-bed coater	Dexamphetamine sulfate	Gelatin	As cores for hot-melt and cellulose acetate phthalate coating to obtain sustained reslease and enteric properties.

Method	Equipment	Drug	Excipient	Remarks
Layering [57]	Coating pan	Sodium salicylate	Ethyl cellulose	As cores for fluidized-bed coating to obtain a product with enteric and sustained-release properties.
Agglomeration [58]	Planetary mixer, high shear mixer	Hydrochlorothiazide	Microcrystalline cellulose	
Agglomeration [50]	P.K. Blender with intensifier bar	Aspirin, caffeine, phenylephedrine hydrochloride, chlorpheniramine maleate	Povidone	Extensive screening and recycling of undesired granules.
Agglomeration [59]	Dish granulator	N/A	Maize starch	Evaluation and studies of operating conditions for the formation of pellets.
Agglomeration [51]	Rotary fluidized bed	Butalbital	Lactose, corn starch, and povidone	Comparison of rotary fluidized-bed granulator with conventional fluidized-bed granulator.
Agglomeration [58]	Rotary fluidized bed	Hydrochlorothiazide	Microcrystalline cellulose	
Extrusion-spheronization [60]	Extruder and marumerizer or spheronizer	N/A	N/A	General description and discussion of extrusion spheronization technology.
Extrusion-spheronization [61]	Extruder and marumerizer or spheronizer	Dibasic calcium phosphate, magnesium hydroxide, sulfadiazine, acetoaminophen	Microcrystalline cellulose	Comparison of extrusion-spheronization process with conventional wet granulation.

Table 3 (Continued)

Method and example	Equipment	Drug	Carrier binder	Comments and variable studied
Extrusion-spheronization [62]	Extruder and marumerizer or spheronizer	N/A	Microcrystalline cellulose, sucrose, lactose	Effect of the spheronization processing variables, dwell time and speed, on the final granule properties.
Extrusion-spheronization [63]	Extruder and marumerizer or spheronizer	Acetoaminophen	Microcrystalline cellulose	Effects of spheronization processing variables including water content, extrusion speed, screen size, spheronizer speed and spheronizer time on tablet hardness and dissolution rate.
Extrusion-spheronization [64]	Extruder and marumerizer or spheronizer	Theophylline, quinidine bisulfate, chlorophenira-mine maleate, hydrochlor-thiazide	Microcrystalline cellulose, sodium carboxymethyl-cellulose	Effect of different diluents and drug-diluent ratio on the final granule properties.
Extrusion-spheronization [65]	Extruder and marumerizer or spheronizer	Acetoaminophen	Microcrystalline cellulose, carboxy-methylcellulose	Use of factorial design to evaluate granulations prepared by extrusion-spheronization.
Extrusion-spheronization [66]	Extruder and marumerizer or spheronizer	N/A	Lactose, dicalcium phoshydrate povidone and microcrystalline cellulose	Elucidation of the factors that influence migration of solvent-soluble materials to the surface of beads made by extrusion-spheronization.

Method	Equipment	Drug/material	Carrier	Comments
Extrusion-spheronization [58]	Extruder and marumerizer or spheronizer	Theophylline, quinidine sulfate, chlorpheniramine maleate, hydrochlorothiazide	Microcrystalline cellulose	Microcrystalline cellulose has excellent binding properties for granulation to be spheronized.
Spherical-agglomeration [52]	Liquid agitator	Sulfamethoxazole, sulfanilamide	White beeswax, ethylcellulose	Parameters affecting the size and release behavior of resultant matrix.
Gellation [53]	Dripping device and calcium chloride solution as a hardening agent	Enzymes and living cells	Calcium alginate	Widely used method for immobilizing living cells and enzymes. Possible pharmaceutical application for pellet making.
Gellation	Dripping device and coolant liquid	Diphenhydramine chloride	Gelation, glycerin	
Spray congealing [67, 54]	Spray congealer	N/A	Materials with high melting point and low heats of crystallization	Variables affecting the spray congealing process, and possible pharmaceutical application for pellet making.

extent explosiveness and danger of these solvents have given pharmaceutical and food supplement processors considerable incentive to remove
organic solvents from the coating process. The most commonly used methods to eliminate organic solvents are presented in Table 4. At present
and in the foreseeable future, latex or pseudolatex coatings appear to be
the best choice to eliminate solvent-based coatings for controlled drug release. Several techniques, including emulsion polymerization, emulsion-
solvent evaporation, phase inversion, and solvent change, can be employed
to prepare suitable latex/pseudolatex dispersion systems. Each method
has advantages and disadvantages based upon ease of preparation, latex
stability, convenience of use, film properties, and economics.

METHODS TO PREPARE LATEX DISPERSIONS

1. *Emulsion polymerization.* Polymerization in an emulsion state can
be applied to a wide variety of vinyl, acrylic, and diene monomers with
water solubility in the proper range, usually 0.001–1.000% [89–91]. The
basic formula used in emulsion polymerization consists of water, monomer,
surfactant, and initiator. The system contains three phases: Water containing small amounts of dissolved surfactant and monomer, monomer droplets stabilized by surfactant, and much smaller surfactant micelles saturated with monomer. The initiator decomposes into free radicals which
react with monomer units at three possible sites for polymerization. The
radicals can react with dissolved monomer in the aqueous phase, or can
diffuse into the monomer droplets or the micelles. Obviously, there is
very little initiation in the aqueous phase owing to low monomer concentration in the water phase. The diffusion rate of the radicals, which is
directly proportional to surface area, is far greater into the micelles, and
thus there is virtually no initiation in the monomer droplets. Free radicals,
from initiator decomposition, begin polymerization in the monomer solubilized
in the micelles. The micelles transform into growing particles. As these
monomer-polymer particles grow, they are stabilized by more surfactant at
the expense of uninitiated micelles, which eventually disappear. The
growing latex particles are continually supplied with monomer by diffusion
through the aqueous phase from monomer droplets. The latter gradually
decreases in quantity as polymerization proceeds, until at a conversion of
about 60%, they disappear completely. All free monomer has then dif-
fused into the latex particles. The polymerization rate decreases as the
monomer in the particles is depleted by further polymerization. The schematic process for emulsion polymerization is shown in Scheme 7.

2. *Emulsion–solvent evaporation technique.* The emulsion–solvent
evaporation technique [92–97] also called emulsion hardening, has been
widely used to prepare microspheres for controlled drug release [98–100].
The technique involves dispersion of drug in an organic polymer solution,
followed by emulsification of the polymer solution in water. After continuous stirring, the solvent evaporates and drug-containing rigid polymer
microspheres are formed. The procedure for preparing pseudolatex is
essentially the same as that described above (Scheme 8). The polymer
emulsion, with droplets so small they are below the resolution limit of the
optical microscope, can be accomplished by subjecting the crude emulsion
to a source of energy such as ultrasonic irradiation or by passing the
crude emulsion through a homogenizer or submicron dispenser. The
polymer solvent is normally stripped from the emulsion at elevated temperatures and pressures to leave a stable pseudolatex. If foaming is not a
problem, the solvent may be removed under reduced pressure.

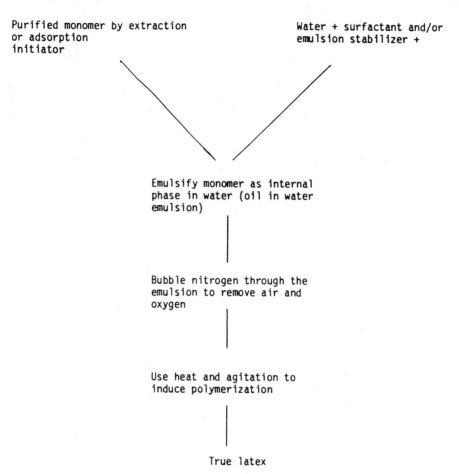

Purified monomer by extraction
or adsorption
initiator

Water + surfactant and/or
emulsion stabilizer +

Emulsify monomer as internal
phase in water (oil in water
emulsion)

Bubble nitrogen through the
emulsion to remove air and
oxygen

Use heat and agitation to
induce polymerization

True latex

Scheme 8

3. *Phase inversion technique.* The phase inversion technique [101–104] involves a hot-melt or solvent gelation of the polymer, which is then compounded with a long-chain fatty acid such as oleic acid, lauric acid, or linoleic acid using conventional rubber-mixing equipment such as an extruder. When the mixture is homogeneous a dilute solution of an alkali is slowly added to the mixture to form a dispersion of water in polymer. Upon further addition of aqueous alkali under vigorous agitation, a phase inversion occurs and a polymer in water dispersion is produced (Scheme 9).

4. *Solvent change and self-dispersible technique.* An ionic water insoluble polymer, which may be generated by acid-base treatment or chemical introduction of functional groups, such as ammonium groups, phosphonium, or tertiary sulfonium groups, may be self-dispersible in water without any need for additional emulsifier [105,106]. Generally, the polymer is first dissolved in a water-miscible organic solvent or in a mixed water-miscible organic solvent system. The pseudolatex can then be obtained by dispersing the polymer solution in deionized water into

Table 4 Common Methods to Eliminate Organic Solvents in the Coating Process

Method	Function	Examples of coating materials	Comments
Compression coating	Compressible materials	Sugars, hydroxypropylmethyl-cellulose, polyvinyl alcohol	Totally eliminates organic solvents. It is not well accepted by pharmaceutical industry owing to complicated mechanical operation and formulation problems.
Aqueous solution	Water-soluble film formers	Methylcellulose, hydroxypropyl cellulose, hydroxypropylmethyl-cellulose	Film formers giving solutions of low viscosity are the most suitable for use. Totally eliminates organic solvents, but unsuitable for controlled drug release.
Mixed organic aqueous system [68]	Enteric materials	Polyvinyl acetate phthalate, carboxylmethylethylcellulose, hydroxypropylmethylcellulose acetate phthalate.	Partially eliminates organic solvents. May be suitable for enteric coating, but not practical for controlled drug release.
Alkali salts [69,70]	Enteric materials	Shellac, hydroxypropylmethyl-cellulose phthalate, cellulose acetate phthalate, cellulose acetate trimellitate.	To form gastric fluid resistant coatings, a volatile neutralizing agent, ammonium hydroxide or morpholine, is preferable to neutralize the enteric materials. Totally eliminates organic solvents.

Hot melts	Materials with low melting point	Organic solvents can be eliminated completely. However, organic solvents may be needed to thin the hot melts, in some cases. Heating devices such as steam jackets or heating tape is needed for the spraying system to avoid solidification of the coating material. Ladle process may be more practical, less troublesome.
	Hydrogenated oil, wax, solid polyethylene glycol	
Aqueous dispersions of waxes and lipids [71]	Waxes and lipids	Totally eliminates organic solvents. Aqueous dispersions of waxes and lipids may not be superior to hot melt coating.
	Castor wax, carnauba wax, Cutina HR, Hoechst Wax E, Durkee 07	
Coating emulsions	Almost all water-insoluble polymers	Partially eliminates organic solvents. Still in their infancy as pharmaceutical coatings.
	Cellulose acetate phthalate, hydroxypropylmethylcellulose	
Latex dispersions [73–80]	Almost all water-insoluble polymers	Totally eliminates organic solvents. Latex dispersions usually have low viscosity and a high solids content. Latex systems have some applications in ophthalmic delivery systems [81], injectable colloidal delivery system [82], and molecular entrapment techniques for sustained-release dosage forms [83–88].
	Ethylcellulose pseudolatex, Eudragit RL/RS pseudolatex, Eudragit E-30D latex	

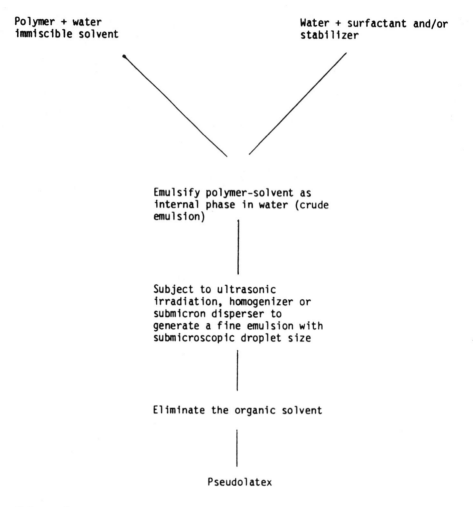

Polymer + water
immiscible solvent

Water + surfactant and/or
stabilizer

Emulsify polymer-solvent as
internal phase in water (crude
emulsion)

Subject to ultrasonic
irradiation, homogenizer or
submicron disperser to
generate a fine emulsion with
submicroscopic droplet size

Eliminate the organic solvent

Pseudolatex

Scheme 8

the polymer solution under mild agitation. The organic solvent(s) is subsequently eliminated from the aquous-organic solution to leave a stable latex (Scheme 10). The absence of emulsifiers has several interesting consequences, such as stability to heat and mechanical shear, and dilutability with organic solvents. Table 5 lists the general features of four commercially available latex-coating systems for controlled drug release. Recently, latex/pseudolatex coating has been further expanded to use cellulose acetate pseudolatex for elementary osmotic pumps [107] and water-based silicone elastomer dispersion for controlled-release tablet coating [108,109].

The aforementioned techniques also can be used to prepare latex or pseudolatex of enteric polymers. Because it is costly to ship aqueous dispersions and some enteric materials are susceptible to hydrolysis, spray- or freeze-drying techniques may be used to dry aqueous polymeric

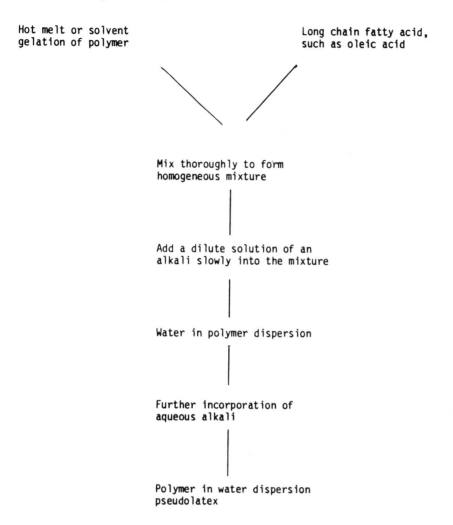

Hot melt or solvent
gelation of polymer

Long chain fatty acid,
such as oleic acid

Mix thoroughly to form
homogeneous mixture

Add a dilute solution of an
alkali slowly into the mixture

Water in polymer dispersion

Further incorporation of
aqueous alkali

Polymer in water dispersion
pseudolatex

Scheme 9

dispersion and form a redispersible aqueous enteric coating system. Table 6 lists the general features of three dispersible aqueous enteric-coating systems.

Basic Considerations in Coating and Accessory Coating Equipment

COATING EQUIPMENT. A perforated pan as well as a conventional coating pan equipped with hot air supply, spray system, pan baffles, and variable coating pan speed can be used for latex coating. However, the relative inefficiency of drying and longer contact time in the coating pan may cause penetration of water into the core and thus discontinuity or irregularity of the film [110]. In the past 10 years, there has been a significant increase in the use of fluid-bed technology to granulate materials for improved compression and to coat cores for desired properties such as controlled drug release, enteric release, appearance, or taste masking. Fluid-bed coating using

Polymer with ionic character,
Polymer undergoes acid-base
treatment to generate ionic
character or polymer undergoes
chemical modification to yield
ionic character + water-
miscible organic solvents   Water

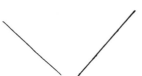

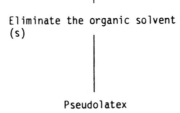

Mix under agitation to form
latex dispersion in aqueous
organic solvent system

Eliminate the organic solvent
(s)

Pseudolatex

Scheme 10

centrifugal-type or Wurster column-type equipment provides ideal conditions, such as rapid surface evaporation, controllable inlet air temperature, and short contact time, for latex coating.

ACCESSORY EQUIPMENT

1. *Nozzle systems.* Characteristics of three different types of nozzle are listed in Table 7 [111]. The ultrasonic nozzle is a relatively new and entirely different type of atomizing nozzle that offers several advantages over conventional nozzles. However, application of ultrasonic nozzles is still in its infancy. Thorough investigations are necessary to dedermine the feasibility of their pharmaceutical applications. Hydraulic guns are sometimes used in place of air-atomizing nozzles for large film-coating processes. The nozzles tend to clog with latex coating because the airless system generates a shear which may coagulate the formulated latex. Pneumatic nozzles have been adapted for fluid-bed systems, and have been shown to be an acceptable nozzle system for latex coating. The atomizing air is exposed to the product and, therefore, must be free of oil and other contaminants.

Table 5 General Features of Four Latex Coating Systems for Controlled Drug Release

Latex system	Method	General features
Eudragit E-30D (Rohm Pharma)	Emulsion polymerization	Poly (ethylacrylate, methylmethacrylate) latex, 30% w/w solid content. No plasticizer is required. May contain residual monomer, initiator, surfactants, and other chemicals used in the polymerization process.
Aqua-Coat (F.M.C. Corp.)	Emulsion-solvent evaporation	Unplasticized ethyl cellulose dispersion. Contains sodium lauryl sulfate and cetyl alcohol as stabilizers. 30% w/w solid content.
Surelease (Colorcon, Inc.)	Phase inversion	Fully plasticized ethyl cellulose dispersion. Contains oleic acid, dibutyl sebacate, fumed silica, and ammonia water, 25% w/w solid content.
Eudragit RS30D and RL30D (Rohm Pharma)	Self-dispersible	Unplasticized poly (ethylacrylate, methylmethacrylate, trimethyl-ammonioethylmethacrylate-chloride) dispersions. Contains no emulsifiers. 30% w/w solid content.

Table 6 General Features of Three Dispersible Aqueous Enteric Coating Systems

Coating system	Method	General features
Aquateric (F.M.C. Corp.)	Emulsion-solvent evaporation followed by spray dry technique	Redispersible cellulose acetate phthalate coating system. Contains polyoxypropylene block copolymer and acetylated monoglycerides. Plasticizer is required.
Coateric (Colorcon, Inc.)	Mechanical means to reduce particle size of the polymer	Completely formulated dispersible polyvinyl acetate phthalate coating system.
Eudragit L-100-55 (Rohm Pharma)	Emulsion-polymerization followed by spray dry technique	Redispersible poly (ethyl acrylate − methacrylate acid) coating system. Contains polyvinylpyrrolidone, polyoxyethylene sorbitan fatty acid ester, and polyethylene glycol. Plasticizer is required.

Table 7　Nozzle Characteristics by Type

	Ultrasonic nozzles	Hydraulic (pressure)	Air atomizing (two fluids)
Principal of operation	Ultrasonic energy concentrated on atomizing surface, causes impinging liquid to disintegrate into a fog of microdrops	Pressurized liquid is forced through orifice. Liquid is sheared into droplets.	High-pressure air or gas mixes with liquid in the nozzle: Air imparts velocity to liquid which is then ejected through an orifice
Average microdrop size	20–50 μ (depending on frequency)	100–200 μ at 100 psi (higher pressure reduces size)	20–100 μ (air pressure from 10–100 psi)
Spray velocity variability flow rate	Low: 0.2–0.4 ms. Infinity variable from zero flow to rated capacity	High: 10–20 m/s ± 10% of specified rating	High: 50–20 m/s. Infinitely variable from 20% of maximum capacity to maximum
Minimum achievable flow rate	0 gph	0.5 gph	0.3 gph
Maximum achievable flow rate	30–40 gph	No limit	No limit
Orifice size/cloggability	Large: up to 3/8"—uncloggable	Very small, usually subject to clogging	Very small, usually subject to clogging

2. *Pumping systems.* Peristaltic or gear pumps are used in combination with nozzles to form a spray system. The ability of a pumping system to deliver the coating liquid at the required rate for the duration of the coating cycle is critical for a uniform coating. A flow integrator can be used to eliminate pulsation of output flow which may cause uncontrolled wetting disruption of the spraying process.

3. *Humidity control.* In order to maximize the drying efficiency of the fluid-bed machine, it may be necessary to dehumidify the inlet air. Furthermore, the amount of moisture in the inlet air can significantly influence batch-to-batch variability of the coating process. Therefore, it is important to control ambient air humidity in the coating operation.

PROCESS VARIABLES

1. *Fluidization air temperature.* Film formation from a solvent-based system is dependent upon the entangling and packing of polymer molecules as the solvent evaporates. Relatively low fluidization air temperatures should be used to prevent spray drying of coating materials because of low heats of vaporization for commonly used solvents. The mechanisms of film formation from a latex system involves the softening of latex spheres caused by plasticization and/or temperature, the contact of latex spheres resulting from loss of water, followed by deformation and coalescence of the latex spheres owing to capillary force and surface tension of the polymer to form a continuous film [112]. The temperature of the inlet air has a dual function; to evaporate water and to soften and coalesce the latex spheres. Latices, as contrasted to aqueous solutions, have a very low affinity for water, and therefore relatively low temperatures can be used to efficiently evaporate water. However, column temperature is critical for latex softening and coalescence. In order to generate a continuous film, the column temperature must be higher than the minimum film-formation temperature. If the temperature is too high, it may cause excessive drying and softening of the latex film, and hence result in electrostatic interaction and agglomeration problems. Minimum film-formation temperature [113] should be used as a guideline to select the temperature of the inlet air. The glass-transition temperature [114] and film-softening temperature [76] can also provide useful information for choosing the column temperature.

2. *Spray rate.* The liquid spray rate affects the degree of wetting and droplet size. At a given atomization air pressure, increasing the liquid spray rate will result in larger droplets and a higher possibility to overwet the coating substrates. Slowing the spray rate may cause electrostatic problems owing to low bed humidity, especially at high temperature settings.

3. *Volume of the fluidized air.* Since a sluggish or vigorous fluidization can have detrimental effects on the coating process, such as side-wall bonding and attrition of core substrates, proper fluidization should be maintained throughout the coating process.

4. *Atomization pressure.* Atomization pressure affects the spraying pattern and droplet size. Excessive high atomization pressure may result in the loss of coating materials and breakage or attrition of the substrates. Excessive low atomization pressure may overwet the core and cause side-wall bonding.

FORMULATION VARIABLES

1. *The nature of the plasticizer.* There are many plasticizers that are compatible with ethyl cellulose and polymethyl methacrylate and can be used for plasticization [115]. For the polymer with a relatively high glass-transition temperature, a plasticizer with a strong affinity to the polymer must be found in order to form a resistant film. Plasticizers with low water solubility are generally recommended for controlled drug release. Dibutyl sebacate, diethyl phthalate, triacetin, triethyl citrate, and acetylated monoglyceride often give satisfactory results.

2. *The amount of the plasticizer.* Experiments should be performed to determine the most favorable proportion of plasticizer. Low levels of plasticizer may not overcome the latex sphere's resistance to deformation and result in incomplete or a discontinuous film. On the other hand, a high proportion of plasticizer may result in seed agglomeration, sticking, and poor fluidization problems caused by excessive softening of the polymer film. The best result generally is obtained with plasticizer concentration in the range of 15–30% based upon the polymer.

3. *Incorporation of plasticizer.* Plasticizer can be incorporated into the latex system during the preparation process which provides more consistent plasticization, more effective use of plasticizer, and a relatively nonseparable plasticized latex system. Plasticizer also can be added to the latex system under mild agitation. Agitation speed, mixing time, and separation of plasticizer during the coating process should be considered in the preparation of the plasticized latex system.

4. *The solids content of the latex system.* Generally, 8–20% solids content give the best results [112]. However, higher or lower solids content can be used to achieve a rapid buildup of film thickness or coating uniformity, respectively.

5. *Additive.* Water-soluble chemicals can be incorporated into the latex film to enhance its dissolution rate. On the other hand, the addition of hydrophobic powder such as talc, magnesium, stearate, or silica in a latex-coating system not only alters drug release, but also facilitates processing by reducing tackiness of the polymer film.

6. *Dual Latex/pseudolatex coating.* Most latice or pseudolatices are stabilized by high surface potential of deflocculated particles arising from ionic functional groups on the polymer or ionic surfactant or stabilizer. For example, the positive charge on Eudragit RS30D and RL30D pseudolatex particles arising from quaternary groups on the polymers and the negative charge on Aquacoat and Surelease pseudolatex particles originated from the anionic surfactants such as sodium lauryl sulfate and oleic acid are the major stabilizing factor. Also, the size of the latex sphere and size distribution are important factors which affect stability, rheological properties, and film properties. Small, monodispersed latex particles are required to have complete coalescence of the latex sphere. Generally, it is not recommended to use dual latex/pseudolatex coating systems because of the possible incompatibility of two latex/pseudolates systems, the different glass-transition temperatures of the polymers, and the different sizes of latex spheres. However, in a British patent, Eudragit E-30D was mixed with Aquacoat to prevent the coated granules sticking together and to

improve the dissolution-retarding effect [116]. It has been demonstrated
that Eudragit RS pseudolatex can be mixed in any proportion with Eudragit
RL pseudolatex. A wide range of release rates for theophylline could be
obtained by changing the ratios of Eudragit RS pseudolatex and Eudragit
RL pseudolatex. The enhancement of theophylline release caused by increasing the amount of Eudragit RL pseudolatex is due to its high permeability to water and theophylline [80].

   7. *Overcoating*. During the curing or storage stage, the pellets
coated with latex or pseudolatex may adhere to one another because of the
softening and tackiness of the film. This could have a detrimental effect
on the dissolution properties of film-coated products. Nevertheless, an
overcoat that is water soluble can solve the problem of tackiness of latex
film without changing the dissolution profile. Immediate mixing of latex-
coated pellets with some separating agents such as talcum, magnesium
stearate, and other diluents also can prevent the formation of clumps of
pellets during storage.

C. Compression Coating and Embedment

Specially constructed tablet presses such as Drycota and Prescota are
available for compressing a polymeric or sugar composition onto a drug-
containing core. This technique has been utilized to create a polyvinyl
alcohol diffusion barrier surrounding a core tablet containing various active
ingredients as described by Conte et al. [117]. In vitro dissolution tests
show that zero-order release kinetics of drug from compression-coated tablets can be achieved as long as the thermodynamic activity of the drug
within the closure and the barrier characteristics are maintained constant.
Salomon et al. [118] coated potassium chloride tablets with a thin layer of
hydroxypropyl methylcellulose by a compression technique for delayed-
release purposes. Such compression-coated tablets release potassium chloride at a constant rate. Enteric coating by a double-compression technique
has been reported [119] using a mixture of triethanolamine cellulose acetate
and lactose as coating materials.

   Other variations of compression coatings such as inlaid tablets and
layer tablets may have application in preparing a sustained-release tablet
with an immediate-release and a separate slow-release portion. In general,
the release rate from compression-coated tablets may be modified by core
composition and characteristics, thickness of membrane layer, composition
of membrane layer, and geometry of core tablet and final tablet. However,
the expense of compression coating and layer tablet production, complicated
mechanical operation, production problems such as multiple granulations,
improper centration, capping, and limited compressible and permeable barrier materials limits its adoption as a popular technique to control drug
release. The compression-embedding technique has received increasing
attention to prepare controlled-release matrix tablets, and intensive research in this area is being conducted by pharmaceutical scientists. There
are three different types of matrix tablets; i.e., hydrophilic matrices,
plastic matrices, and fat-wax matrices, which can be differentiated by the
matrix-building materials.

Hydrophilic Matrix Tablet

Utilization of a hydrophilic matrix as a means to control drug release was disclosed in U.S. Patent 3,065,143. Sodium carboxymethyl cellulose, methyl cellulose, hydroxypropyl cellulose, hydroxyethyl cellulose, polyethylene oxide, polyvinyl pyrrolidone, polyvinyl acetate, carboxy polymethylene, alginic acid, gelatin, and natural gums can be used as matrix materials. The matrix may be tableted by direct compression of the blend of active ingredient(s) and certain hydrophilic carriers, or from a wet granulation containing the drug and hydrophilic matrix material(s). Several commercial patented hydrophilic matrix systems are currently in use, such as the Synchron Technology [120] and hydrodynamically balanced system [121]. The hydrophilic matrix requires water to activate the release mechanism and enjoys several advantages, including ease of manufacture and excellent uniformity of matrix tablets. Upon immersion in water, the hydrophilic matrix quickly forms a gel layer around the tablet. Drug release is controlled by a gel diffusional barrier that is formed and/or tablet erosion. The effect of formulation and processing variables on drug-release behavior from compressed hydrophilic matrices has been studied by a number of investigators [122–134] and can be summarized as follows:

1. The matrix building material with fast polymer hydration capability is the best choice to use in a hydrophilic matrix tablet formulation. An inadequate polymer hydration rate may cause premature diffusion of the drug and disintegration of the tablet owing to fast penetration of water. It is particularly true for formulation of water-soluble drugs and excipients.

2. The amount of hydrophilic polymer in tablet formulations was reported to have a marked influence on the disintegration time and dissolution of the tablet. The disintegration time was extended as polymer content increased. The release rate of drug was decreased when the proportion of polymer was increased but differed quantitatively with different drugs and different matrix-building materials. Slower hydration polymers can be used at higher concentration level to accelerate gel formation or reserved for water-insoluble drug(s).

3. Generally, reduced particle size of the hydrophilic polymer ensures rapid hydration and gel formation, leading to a good controlled release. The impact of polymer particle size on the release rate is formulation dependent, but may be obscured in some cases. The particle size of a drug, within a normal size range, may not significantly influence the drug release from the matrix tablet. Extremes of drug particle size may affect release rate of the drug.

4. Viscosity characteristics of the polymers are of great importance in determining the final release properties of the matrix tablet. Generally, the drug-release rate is slower for a higher viscosity–grade polymer.

5. Commonly, water-soluble excipients in the matrix tablet can increase drug release. However, addition of water-soluble materials may achieve a slower rate by increasing viscosity of the gel through interaction with hydrophilic polymers or by competition with matrix material for water. When water-insoluble nonswellable excipient(s) or drug(s) is used in the matrix system stress cracks can occur upon immersion in water because of the combination of swelling and nonswelling components on the tablet surface.

6. For some hydrophilic matrix building materials, pH may affect the viscosity of the gel which forms on the tablet surface and its subsequent rate of hydration. Under acidic conditions, carboxypolymethylene and sodium carboxymethyl cellulose have little or no retarding effect on the drug-release rate. Gelatin forms gels of higher viscosity in acidic media and is more effective in retarding drug release as compared to a basic media.

7. No conclusions could be drawn as to the effect of compression force on drug-release behavior owing to the different properties of the various hydrophilic matrix materials. However, tablet size and shape can significantly influence drug-release kinetics.

Fat-Wax Matrix Tablet

The drug can be incorporated into fat-wax granulations by spray congealing in air [135 – 138], blend congealing in an aqueous media with or without the aid of surfactants [139 – 142], and spray-drying techniques [44]. In the bulk congealing method, a suspension of drug and melted fat-wax is allowed to solidify and is then comminuted for sustained-release granulations [143]. The mixture of active ingredients, waxy material(s), and filler(s) also can be converted into granules by compacting with a roller compactor, heating in a suitable mixer such as a fluidized-bed and steamjacketed blender, or granulating with a solution of waxy material or other binders. Fat-wax granulations containing drug obtained from all of the above processes may be compressed to form tablet cores or directly compressed into a final tablet form with sustained-release properties.

The drug embedded into a melt of fats and waxes is released by leaching and/or hydrolysis as well as dissolution of fats under the influence of enzymes and pH change in the gastrointestinal tract. Enteric materials such as cellulose acetate phthalate, polyvinyl acetate phthalate, methacrylate copolymer, zein, and shellac may be used to prepare matrix tablets with somewhat a similar drug-release mechanism. In general, the primary constituents of a fat-wax matrix are fatty acids and/or fatty esters. Fatty acids are more soluble in an alkaline rather than an acidic medium. Fatty esters are more suscepitble to alkaline catalyzed hydrolysis than to acid catalyzed hydrolysis. The surface erosion of a fat-wax matrix depends upon the nature and percent of fat-wax and extenders in the matrix [136]. Other factors such as drug particle size and drug concentration affects release of the drug from the matrix system [141]. The addition of surfactants to the formulation can also influence both the drug-release rate and the proportion of total drug that can be incorporated into a matrix [137,142]. Polyethylene, ethylcellulose, and glyceryl esters of hydrogenated resins have been added to modify the drug-release pattern [135].

Plastic Matrix Tablets

Sustained-release tablets based upon an inert compressed plastic matrix were first introduced in 1960 and have been used extensively clinically [144]. Release is usually delayed because the dissolved drug has to diffuse through a capillary network between the compacted polymer particles. Commonly used plastic matrix materials are polyvinyl chloride, polyethylene, vinyl acetate/vinyl chloride copolymer, vinylidene chloride/acrylonitryle copolymer, acrylate/methyl methacrylate copolymer, ethyl cellulose,

cellulose acetate, and polystyrene [145]. Plastic matrix tablets, in which
the active ingredient is embedded in a tablet with coherent and porous
skeletal structure, can be easily prepared by direct compression of drug
with plastic material(s) provided the plastic material can be comminuted or
granulated to desired particle size to facilitate mixing with drug particle.
In order to granulate for compression into tablets the embedding process
may be accomplished by:

1. The solid drug and the plastic powder can be mixed and kneaded
    with a solution of the same plastic material or other binding agents
    in an organic solvent and then granulated.
2. The drug can be dissolved in the plastic by using an organic sol-
    vent and granulated upon evaporation of the solvent.
3. Using latex or pseudolatex as granulating fluid to granulate the
    drug and plastic masses.

Drug release from the inert plastic matrices was affected by varying
formulation factors such as the matrix material, amount of drug incorporated in the matrix, drug solubility in the dissolution media and in the
matrix, matrix additives, and the release media. Since the mechanism of
controlling drug release in the plastic matrix is the pore structure of the
matrix, any formulation factors affecting the release of a drug from the
matrix may be a consequence of their primary effect on apparent porosities
and tortuosities of the matrices. These release factors can be summarized
as follows:

1. The release rate increases as the solubility of the drug increases,
but there seems to be no direct relationship between the two variables.
2. The release rate increases as the drug concentration increases.
An increase in release rate cannot be explained on the basis of increasing
matrix porosity [146]. Rather it has been attributed to changes in matrix
tortuosity with drug concentration [147] and to decreased diffusional resistance by shortening the length of the capillary joining any two drug
particles [148].
3. It is possible to modify the release rate by inclusion of hydrophilic
or hydrophobic additives to the matrix. The release of a sparingly soluble
substance can be increased by the addition of physiologically inert but
readily soluble material such as polyethylene glycol, sugars, electrolytes,
and urea [146,149]. The decrease in the release rate on the addition of
hydrophobic substance may be due to decreased wettability of the matrix
[150].
4. The release rate from plastic matrix tablets could be decreased by
exposure to acetone vapor without changing the release mechanism. The
extent of the reduction was found to be dependent on the amount of
acetone absorbed [147,151]. The tensile strength of the tablets increases
by heating the polymer matrix above the glass-transition temperature.
However, porosity also increases with a marked increase in the release
rate [152,153].
5. The release rate increased as the particle size of the matrix material increased and as the particle size of the drug decreased.
6. Increasing compaction pressure up to the full consolidation point
tends to decrease the pore formed among the polymer particles, resulting
in a slower drug-release rate [154].

Microcapsules, microspheres, or coated pellets also can be compressed into tablets or embedded in a drug-containing matrix. Sustained-release tablets made from individual coated particles may have very different release characteristics than the original coated particles depending upon whether or not the tablets disintegrate to expose the majority of the coated particles to the dissolution environment and whether the coated particles are damaged by the compression process [155]. Generally, nondisintegrating tablets made from ethyl cellulose microcapsules followed matrix-release kinetics are much slower than the uncompressed microcapsules. When compression force was sufficient to prevent breakup of the tablets, greater compression force had little effect on rate of dissolution [156-160]. Apparently, nondisintegrating tablets made from individual coated particles did not provide any advantages over matrix tablets but a more complicated manufacturing process. A dispersible tablet containing individual coated particles distributes the drug-containing coated particles in the gastric content to minimize the high local concentration of drug and to reduce the inter- and intrasubject variation linked to gastrointestinal transit time.

However, the sustained-release properties of the coated particles may be lost due to cracking of the membranes and rupture of the characteristic microcapsule tails. The amount of damage was found to be related to the compressibility and particle size of excipients in the tablet formula as well as to the compression pressure. Large particles led to greater damage as noted by increased dissolution rates of the disintegrating tablets [161]. It also has been found that a combination of microcrystalline cellulose and polyethylene glycol provides maximum protection from the damage of potassium chloride microcapsules by reducing interparticle friction [162]. Matrix particles have the advantage of being very rugged, less subject to dose dumping, and more resistant to compression damage than membrane systems. Little change in the dissolution rate of cellulose acetate butyrate microspheres containing succinyl sulfathiazole has been reported when tableting with microcrystalline cellulose and carboxymethyl starch under compression force between 35 and 350 MPa [163].

IV. SUSTAINED-RELEASE PRODUCTS THROUGH COATING

The preceding discussion has provided the framework for the design of sustained-release products. Application of these principles in the pharmaceutical industry has resulted in varying degrees of success in achieving consistent, nonvarying blood levels of drug from sustained-release dosage forms. It is instructive to examine some of these dosage forms more closely, and to analyze where and why they fail to provide sustained release and whether the failure can be detected in vivo or in vitro. Of course, the reader should keep in mind that these are "failures" only in a relative sense; some forms are very much superior to others, but all do provide some sort of sustained therapy beyond their nonsustained counterparts. Whether this sustained blood or tissue level results in a measurable improvement clinically is often debatable.

It would appear from the earlier sections of this chapter that one can employ the theoretical calculations on release-rate and dosage-form design with great precision to formulate a prolonged-action dosage form. In point of fact, although this has been done in a few studies, the vast

majority of published work has employed these principles and calculations
as a working guideline. The formulator obtains the desired release-rate
constant and size of tablet by suitable calculation and attempts to generate this release pattern by some sustained-release mechanism, such as
coating. If the release rate of drug is dissimilar to the calculated value,
the dosage form is appropriately modified. Since the ideal release pattern,
resulting in a tissue drug concentration–time profile similar to that shown
in Figure 1, is seldom obtained, the formulator will usually be satisfied
with either a bell-shaped profile that has a broad, relatively flat plateau,
or an extension of biological activity. This qualitative approach, which at
times is very empirical, is clearly evident when one reads the literature
dealing with prolonged-action dosage forms. Thus, unless the formulator
has good control over the release mechanism, which is rarely the case, he
or she will be working empirically or semiempirically in preparing the
dosage form. Moreover, because of this lack of control over the release
mechanism, a blood drug profile will usually result that shows simple prolongation rather than the invariant drug level of the sustained type.

In the following discussion, we have arbitrarily classified the approaches used in coating sustained-release products into various subdivisions. A
good argument could be constructed that all of the following subdivisions
are artificial, since all coated sustained-release dosage forms utilize dissolution and diffusion to varying degrees. However, the dosage forms mentioned in each section usually appear to have one major mode of providing
sustained action. These modes can derive from the way the material is
produced, as in the case of microcapsules and bead polymerization, or from
the way the body handles the dosage form, as in the case of soluble coated
granules or impermeable films coated in a tablet. The division has been
created solely for the purpose of organizing the literature in the area and
should not be viewed as being rigid or exclusive.

At the end of some of the subdivisions, the reader will find a section
entitled case study. These sections are intended to provide sufficient experimental detail to allow the novice formulator to initiate preparation of a
prolonged-action dosage form. We will thus examine selected published reports in more detail, providing as much of the experimental methods employed as is practical. In addition, when available, the appropriate equations to describe the release of drug from the dosage form and the type
of in vitro and in vivo profile generated will be noted.

A. Sustained Release Utilizing Dissolution

Dissolution methods in sustained release generally refer to coating the individual particles, or granules, of the drug with varying thicknesses of
coating material so that dissolution of the coat, resulting in release of the
drug contained within, occurs over a long time span owing to the thickness
differences of the coats. These coated particles are then either compressed
directly into tablets (e.g., Spacetabs), or they can be placed in capsules
(e.g., the Spansule or Plateau Cap dosage forms), as shown in Scheme 11.
Alternatively, the dissolution may be that of an exterior tablet coating
where a portion of the drug is placed in the tablet coat and dissolves rapidly to provide enough drug to quickly reach therapeutic levels, whereas
the sustained-release interior of the tablet utilizes some other method, to
be discussed subsequently, to provide controlled, long-term release of

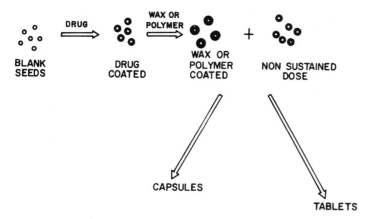

BLANK SEEDS →DRUG→ DRUG COATED →WAX OR POLYMER→ WAX OR POLYMER COATED + NON SUSTAINED DOSE

CAPSULES

TABLETS

Scheme 11

medicament. Exterior tablet coats may also have differentially soluble constituents that dissolve and provide an outer shell to maintain diffusion
path lengths for the drugs contained in the shell. This form of sustained
release is particularly useful for relatively insoluble drugs because it keeps
the dose from disintegrating and being spread out over the gastrointestinal
tract, thus providing some regulation of the dissolution medium and area
for control in maintaining slow release of drug.

Pulsed Dosing

Included in the pulsed dosing category are slowly dissolving coatings such
as the various combinations of carbohydrate sugars and cellulose-based
coatings as well as polyethyleneglycol bases, polymeric bases, and wax-
based coatings. Colbert [164] and Johnson [165] provided a particularly
complete cross section of patents issued since 1960 based on these digestible
bases. These coating materials are used in preparing sustained-release
dosage forms that follow the approach of various thickness coated granules
or seeds combined with uncoated granules which are dispensed in capsule
or compressed tablet form. Examples are the Spansule [166–175] and
Spacetab [176–180] formulations. These coatings vary in thickness and
when they cover a drug granule their digestion by fluids in the gastrointestinal tract results in abrupt release of the medicament at selected
time intervals to provide pulsed dosing for periods up to approximately
12 h.

   With digestible coating materials, the important factors a formulator
must take into account are the dissolution rate of the coating material, the
thickness of the coat, and the changed are for disintegration and dissolution that the increased thickness provides [3–5,10,18,181,182]. As the
drug-coated granules traverse the gastrointestinal tract, the coating is
slowly solubilized by the gastrointestinal fluids. Since the granules have
varying thickness coats, one anticipates a staggered release of drug.
Therefore, by combining a large number of mixes of different thickness
coated granules, a horizontal, or very nearly so, blood drug concentration

versus time curve for extended periods of time should result. In practice, it is often difficult to combine a large number of granules having many different thicknesses of coating, so that the more common approach is to employ one-quarter of the granules in uncoated form, thus providing for immediate release and rapid attainment of therapeutic blood levels of drug, with the remaining three-quarters of the granules being split into three groups of varying coating thicknesses to provide a sustaining effect, through pulsed dosing, over the desired time period. Although the approach of one-quarter uncoated, three-quarters coated is very common, other combinations, such as one-third coated, two-thirds uncoated, have also been employed. The ratio is determined by properties of the coated granules; that is, dissolution rate and derived drug properties such as the elimination rate constant.

CAPSULES. Since the introduction of the Spansule sustained-release dosage form in the early 1950s, there have been numerous studies on the release of active drugs from this type of preparation [172,173,183–198], and also on the clinical effectiveness of these preparations in maintaining therapeutic activity over extended time periods [166–171,174]. Examples of the types of drug formulated as coated granules include antihistamines [166,167], belladonna alkaloids [168,171], phenothiazines [173,174,185,187], combinations of the above [169], antihypertensives [45], cardiac muscle dilators [199–201], anorexigenic agents [175,184,187,192,193], steroid anti-inflammatories [183], and nonsteroidal anti-inflammatories such as aspirin [191].

There are several ways to prepare drug-coated beads or granules. A common procedure is to coat nonpareil seeds with the drug and follow this with either a slowly dissolving wax or polymer coat of varying thickness. Conventional pan-coating or air-suspension coating techniques can be employed for this purpose. Types of coating materials and properties will be discussed later in this chapter. Coatings such as these can also be accomplished through microencapsulation, to be discussed shortly, wherein the drug solution or crystal is encapsulated with a coating substance. The selection of coating material dictates whether pulsed or sustained drug release occurs.

An illustration of this approach is the series of papers by Rosen et al. [189,190] in which they describe the release of ^{14}C-labeled Dextroamphetamine sulfate and ^{14}C-labeled amobarbital from both non-sustained- and sustained-release dosage forms employing wax-coated granules. As can be seen in Figure 3, the amount of drug released in each time period is progressively less as the percentage of wax-fat in the coating increases. This is the expected behavior, and indicates that sustained release can be varied quite readily by changing the makeup of the coating material for the drug granules. Other studies [185,191] along these same lines have indicated that such behavior of coated granules is the general rule. Note in Figure 3 that continuous release of drug occurs. This is because a spectrum of granule size was employed in the study. The dashed line in Figure 3 indicates the release pattern when only a few granule sizes are combined.

The coated granules or seeds can be placed into a capsule for administration to the patient. Actual photographs of the in vivo disintegration and dispersal of coated sustained-release granules in a capsule were provided in a series of papers by Feinblatt et al. [200,201]. Using

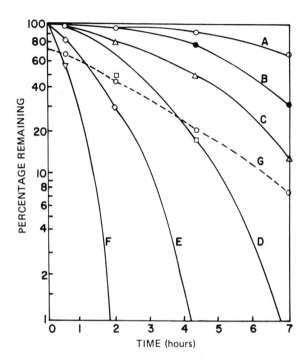

Figure 3   In vitro release pattern of dextroamphetamine sulfate pellets
pan coated with various amounts of wax-fat coating. (A) 17% coating,
(B) 15% coating, (C) 13% coating, (D) 11% coating, (E) 9% coating,
(F) 7% coating, and (G) selected blend of uncoated pellets and coated pellets. (From Ref. 189, used with permission.)

roentgenography, the authors showed that after 10–12 h the coated granules in a sustained-release capsule were well dispersed in the gastrointestinal tract and the active ingredient was completely dissolved.

In a different study concerned with in vitro measurement of drug release from sustained-release coated granules in a capsule, Royal [192] described a modification of the *United States Pharmacopeia* (USP) tablet disintegration apparatus that allowed him to follow the release of drug from
capsule dosage forms. Further modifications [193] allowed him to test different brands of capsules containing a wide range of granule sizes, and
thus be able to compare the brands as to their efficiency in maintaining
continuous release of medicament for extended time periods. Souder and
Ellenbogen [175] described a method for "splitting" (separating) sustained-
release coated granules to ensure an even mix of large and small granules
and to prevent the stratification of such mixes that often occurs when
pooling granules for analysis. They then measured timed release of drug
in a manner differing somewhat from the approach used by Royal. The
results, however, were the same, and indicated that the blending of larger
and smaller coated granules, presumably due to thickness of the sustained-
release coating, was effective in maintaining the characteristics of sustained
drug release. There are several approaches that can be employed for

dissolution testing of coated pellets, and most investigators employ modifications of the rotating vial techniques, such as is described in the *National Formulary* (NF) XIII, or modification of the dissolution test presented in USP XIX.

In clinical evaluations of capsule pulsed dose, prolonged-action dosage form, and sustained-release products, the objectives of the experimental techniques change from that of ensuring that drug release is indeed occurring gradually over a long time to that of (1) showing that the sustained-release dosage form adequately maintains therapeutic blood or tissue levels for extended times [172,173,183,185–188,191], (2) provides relief to the patient over a long period [166–169,171,174], and (3) perhaps reduces the incidence of side effects due to the "peak" effects of non-sustained-release dosing [166,167,169]. Of course, many of the earlier studies were conducted before development of the sophisticated methods now employed in gathering and interpreting blood or tissue drug level data [166,167,169, 171,174], and indeed many such studies were rather qualitative in their assessment of prolonged-action dosage forms. As a result of this lack of sophistication, the focus was either on monitoring some biological response or on urinary receovery of active drug or its metabolites. For example, the reports of Heimlich et al. [172,173] on sustained-release phenylpropanolamine and trimeprazine and of Sugerman and Rosen [188] on sustained-release chlorpromazine present very detailed and thorough urinary analyses of drug content and provide, within the limitations set forth by the authors, a very good analysis of sustained-release characteristics and their worth with respect to administration of these drugs. While results of urinary drug analysis alone can give quantitative information on sustained-release characteristics, it has been pointed out [202] that there are dangers in this approach and comparisons of blood and urine data do not always coincide. When possible, both blood and urine samples should be collected and analyzed.

In the early 1960s, the first really good effort at measuring and analyzing drug levels in the blood began to appear in the literature [183–186]. One of the earliest of these is the study by Wagner et al. [183] on the sustained action of prednisolone in dogs and humans and the comparability of these data to in vitro findings. The work by Rosen and Swintosky [187,189,190] contributed to this field by employing radioactive-labeled drug.

Hollister [186], in a report on sustained-release meprobamate products, presented both urine and blood drug level data and pointed out how they reinforce the interpretation based solely on one or the other.

Of course the nature of the disease state itself can be a major reason for publishing more qualitative results, as was one in some of the earlier work. Those studies measuring relief of symptoms due to sustained-release antihistamines [166,167] have few measurable effects that are easily quantitated, whereas other reports in the area, such as those dealing with ulcer patients and relief of pain, can at least quantitate volume and acidity of gastric acid and digestive juices [168]. The literature is speckled with data that show a sustained effect is operative, but give no indication as to how well it compares to multiple dosing of ordinary tablets.

The question of the bioavailability of sustained-release dosage forms as compared to conventional systems is an important issue. For most drugs placed in a sustained-release system, the bioavailability is less than in conventional dosage forms. There are the occasional drugs that are unstable in gastrointestinal fluid or have absorption problems [31] which become stabilized or show improved absorption when placed in a sustained-release system. A typical example of reduced bioavailability is the study by Henning and Nybert [203] on quinidine, in which the rapidly dissolving tablet was shown to have greater bioavailability than either quinidine Durules or Longacor. Compared to the rapidly dissolving tablet, the Durules had a bioavailability of 76% and the Longacor 54%.

TABLETS. With the tablet dosage form the concern for the thickness and area of granular coating remains, the distinguishing feature of this dosage form being that of tablet disintegration as contrasted to gelatin capsule dissolution. An added problem here may be the influence of excipients used to produce a compressed tablet in the disintegration/dissolution process. Of course, when no fillers or excipients are used, the coated granules alone are compressed and can fuse together, resulting in altered dissolution patterns [18], depending on the properties of the coating material. The role of excipients on the dissolution pattern of compressed coated granules has not been investigated extensively. One would not expect substantial effects on the dissolution process of the individual seeds or granules, but perhaps there would be an influence on fracture or fusing of seeds. Reports using other sustaining mechanisms show, as one would expect, that in compression some of the coated particles are fractured. Green [204], for example, found that in microencapsulated sustained-release aspirin which was subsequently tableted, a small amount of aspirin was immediately released, suggestive of fractured coats. This need not be a problem, since the degree of fracture and immediate release is frequently small and can usually be incorporated into that portion of the dosage form that provides for immediate blood drug levels. Other studies have shown that the dissolution pattern was very much influenced by tablet hardness, so that compression force would be important. These findings were with specific formuations, but they suggest that these variables must be considered.

Because the dissolution patterns of sustained-release coated granules are essentially the same whether the granules are filled into a capsule or compressed with excipients into a tablet, the dissolution studies described earlier are applicable here provided extensive fusing of the granules does not occur in the tableting process.

Here, as in the case of capsules, there has been a wide range of drugs formulated as sustained-release coated granules and compressed into tablets. Antispasmodic-sedative combinations have been investigated [176], as have phenothiazines [172−180], anticholinesterase agents, and aspirin [205,206].

Steigmann and coworkers [176] described the clinical evaluation of Belladenal Spacetabs, a combination of the natural levoratory alkaloids of belladonna and phenobarbital, in patients with peptic ulcer and other gastrointestinal disorders. They measured gastric secretion and bowel motility and found that, for the most part, the results with the Spacetabs formulation were as good or better than those obtained with conventional nonsustained forms, and the convenience to the patient of once or twice a day dosing was recognized.

The treatment of myasthenia gravis with neostigmine bromide formulated as Mestinon Bromide Timespan was examined by Magee and Westerberg

[205]. The need for sustained release is particularly acute here, since with treatment via non-sustained-release dosage forms, the patient generally is very weak upon arising in the morning and remains in this state until the morning tablet dose can be absorbed. A means of maintaining patient strength and comfort throughout the hours of sleep was needed. The results of their study show that the value of this sustained-release dosage form is greatest when taken at bedtime, at times even allowing the patient to arise with sufficient strength to dress before taking morning medication. Results of daytime use were variable, and absorption appeared to be less than optimal in comparison with non-sustained-release tablets.

Probably the largest body of clinical data has been compiled for the phenothiazine tranquilizer thioridazine. Mellinger [177], in an early evaluation of thioridazine formulated as Mellaril Spacetabs, examined serum concentrations following administration of the drug as a liquid concentrate, as tablets crushed in a mortar, as intact tablets, and as the Spacetab sustained-release tablet. He found that the drug persists in the blood for long periods from all the dosage forms studied, and attributed its slow excretion to possible slow metabolism. There were no striking advantages to the sustained-release formulation over that of conventional tablets. This last finding has been reiterated by other workers [178], and as of this time, the Spacetab formulation of thioridazine is not being marketed.

The clinical evaluation and comparison of sustained-release and non-sustained-release aspirin tablets was reported by Cass and Frederik [206, 207]. They measured the duration of analgesic relief obtained via a series of different dosage regimens in patients suffering from a variety of coronic illnesses. In all cases, the sustained release form provided longer and more predictable analgesic relief than any of the other non-sustained-release tablets tested.

Case Study of Slowly Soluble Wax Coating on Nonpareil Seeds [189]. *Prolonged action mechanism.* Pulsed dosing in repeat action fashion. Drug-containing nonpareil seeds were coated with various thicknesses of digestible waxes which were intended to release drug at various times after dosing.

Type and method of coating. A kilogram of medicated non-sustained-release pellets was prepared in a 12-in coating pan. The pellets were composed of 31.2 gm of dextroamphetamine sulfate; 58.8 gm of a 1:1 mixture of starch, USP, and powdered sucrose, USP; and 90 gm of U.S. No. 16 to 20-mesh sugar pellets. The nonpareil seeds were placed in a conventional coating pan and wetted with a water/alcohol/gelatin mixture consisting of gelatin 10% w/v, hydrochloric acid 0.5% v/v, and water 30% v/v, and alcohol 70% v/v (90% ethanol, 10% methanol). When the mixture became tacky the drug diluent was added to the rotating seeds. After a short period of drying, one-fourth of the seeds were removed (these represented the uncoated portion). The remaining seeds were then coated to varying thicknesses with a wax formula consisting of glyceryl monostearate 11% w/w, glyceryl distearate, 16% w/w, white wax 3% w/w, in carbon tetrachloride 70% w/w. Six different groups of pellets with approximately 7, 9, 11, 13, 15, and 17% of wax coating were initially prepared and, through trial and error, a final blend consisting of 25% noncoated pellets, 55% of the 11% wax-coated seeds, and 20% of the 9% wax-coated seeds gave a satisfactory in vitro release pattern. Each group of

Table 8   Blend and Desired in Vitro
Release Patterns, [^{14}C]Dextroamphetamine
Sulfate

	% In vitro release at time interval (h)			
	0.5	2	4.5	7
Blend	34	56	79	92
Desired[a]	39	62	80	90

[a]Average in vitro pattern of 15 commercial
lots of sustained release dextroamphetamine
[190].

pellets was screened through U.S. No. 12 onto U.S. No. 25 standard mesh
sieves to remove lumps and fines.

In vitro test.   In vitro dissolution tests in artificial gastrointestinal
fluids were conducted according to the method of Souder and Ellenbogen
[50].   The dissolution pattern for all six coated seeds is shown in Figure 3, and the results on the blend in Table 8.   A satisfactory prolongation is obtained.

In vivo release.   The in vivo release study was conducted in humans
and employed the following dosage regimens:

1.   15-mg sustained-release dosage form
2.   15-mg nonsustained dosage form
3.   5-mg nonsustained dosage form
4.   5-mg sustained-release dosage form given at intervals of 0, 4, and
     8 h

This particular plan was chosen to determine performance criteria of

1.   Whether the sustained-release formulation provided a prompt initial
     dose
2.   Whether it was similar to 3 times daily drug administration
3.   Whether it was dissimilar to an equivalent nonsustained dose
4.   Whether equal doses in different dosage forms were equally ef-
     fective in making drug available for absorption
5.   Whether there was any significant variability among subjects re-
     ceiving the various regimens

The study was conducted in a crossover sequence, as shown in Table 9.
Blood and urine samples were collected at various times postdosing,
and the results are shown in Figures 4 and 5.   The cumulative urinary
excretion data for human subjects is shown in Table 10.   From the table
the following conclusions were drawn:

1.   In the first 3 h following administration of the drug, the sustained-
     release, 3 times daily regimen, and the 5-mg single dose were

Table 9 Human Study Plan of Various Dosage Regimens

Subject	Initial[a]	1 Week later
1	A	B
2	B	C
3	C	D
4	D	A
5	A	C
6	B	D
7	C	A
8	D	B
9	A	D
10	B	A
11	C	B
12	D	C
13	A	D
14	B	C
15	C	B
16	D	A

[a]A, 15-mg sustained release dosage form given at 0 h; B, 15-mg non-sustained-release dosage form given at 0 h; C, 5-mg non-sustained-release dosage form given at 0 h; D, 5-mg non-sustained-release dosage form given tid, at 0, 4, and 8 h.
Source: From Ref. 189, used with permission.

similar. Thus, the sustained-release formulation did provide a prompt initial dose.

2. The plasma and urine plots for the sustained and 3 times daily regimen were similar, whereas the sustained and 15-mg plain capsule were dissimilar.

3. The sustained-release dosage form made as much drug available as the other two 15-mg regimens.

4. The variation in plasma and urine data is not greater with the sustained-release dosage form than with the 3 times daily regimen.

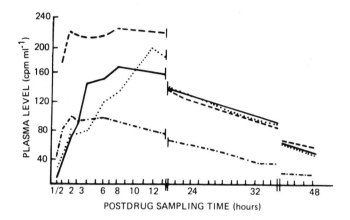

Figure 4 Adjusted average human plasma levels. Each line represents eight subjects per regimen in a balanced incomplete block crossover design. ————, 15-mg dextroamphetamine sulfate sustained-release dosage form; ·······, 5-mg dextroamphetamine sulfate capsule, tid; − − − −, 15-mg dextroamphetamine sulfate capsule; −·−·−, 5-mg dextroamphetamine sulfate capsule. (From Ref. 189, used with permission.)

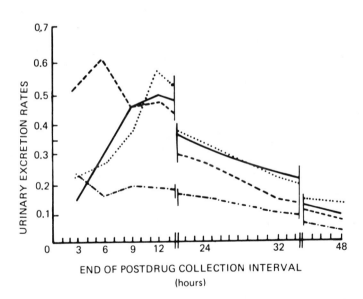

Figure 5 Adjusted average human urinary excretion rates. Radioactive counts are expressed as average milligrams of dextroamphetamine sulfate per collection interval divided by the number of hours in each interval. ————, 15-mg dextroamphetamine sulfate sustained-release dosage form; ·······, 5-mg dextroamphetamine sulfate capsule, tid; − − − −, 15-mg dextroamphetamine sulfate capsule; −·−·−, 5-mg dextroamphetamine sulfate capsule. (From Ref. 189, used with permission.)

Table 10   Adjusted Average[a] Urine Recoveries in Humans, mg of
Dextroamphetamine Sulfate Equivalent

Dosage form	Collection interval (h)		
	0−12	0−24	0−48
5-mg capsule	2.18	3.90	4.89
15-mg sustained-release capsule	4.30[b]	8.24[b]	11.78[b]
5-mg capsule, 3 times each day	4.32	8.48	12.30
15-mg capsule	6.14	9.31	11.86

[a]Each figure is the average for eight humans.

[b]No figure included in a brace is significantly different from any other
figure included in that brace ($p < 0.05$).
Source: From Ref. 189, used with permission.

Sustained Dosing

Although the principal factors controlling drug release are very similar in
this case to those noted in the previous section, they do differ in at least
one important aspect; that is, the drug is made available in a continuous
rather than a pulsed fashion. The continuous release of drug is a result
of the drug being impregnated in a slowly dissolving film; as dissolution
occurs, drug becomes available [10,18,208−210]. This type of coating is
very similar to the embedding of the drug in an insoluble matrix, which
will be described later in this chapter. The difference lies in the fact
that these products are microencapsulations of drug particles or granules,
whereas the matrix tablets are formulated in a different manner.

MICROENCAPSULATION. Tanaka and coworkers [95] investigated the
effects of formalin treatment on the hardness of gelatin microcapsules of
sulfanilamide and riboflavin. As can be seen in Tables 11A and 11B, the
treatment of gelatin micropellets containing sulfanilamide by immersion in
10% formalin/isopropanol for 24 h results in a 10-fold increase in time to
release 100% of the drug. These results were mirrored when sulfanilamide
and riboflavin micropellets were administered to dogs and blood levels of

Table 11A   Dosages and Contents of SA and RF Micropellets[a]

Sample	Dosage and contents
1	Gelatin micropellet containing 33.2% SA
3	Micropellet, treated for 24 h, and containing 10.0% SA

[a]SA and RF refer to sulfanilamide and riboflavin, respectively.
Source: Reproduced with permission of the copyright owner.

Table 11B Percentage of Accumulative SA Recovered in the in Vitro Dissolution Test[a]

Sample 1		Sample 2	
Time	%	Time	%
5 min	32.9	5 min	5.9
10 min	59.5	10 min	9.9
15 min	76.5	20 min	30.7
35 min	80.0	30 min	39.6
1 h	89.6	45 min	53.4
2 h	99.5	1 h	61.5
3 h	99.7	2 h	82.0
		3 h	86.0
		5 h	91.6
		7 h	94.1
		23 h	98.2
		30 h	99.6

[a]SA and RF refer to sulfanilamide and riboflavin, respectively.
Source: Reproduced with permission of the copyright owner.

the drugs versus time were measured. Figures 6 and 7 show that, indeed, sustained blood levels of sulfanilamide and riboflavin were obtained when the micropellets were hardened. Nixon et al. [211,213] studied gelatin coacervate microcapsules of various sulfa drugs and the effect of various coacervating agents on in vitro release of drug. They found that hardened microcapsules gave a more prolonged release of drug in both acid and alkaline pepsin medium. Temperature and pH effects were also investigated, and from the data it was concluded that dissolution was the controlling step rather than diffusion of drug through a microcapsular wall.

The development of the complex form of coacervation as a tool for coating pharmaceuticals was developed by Phares and Sperandio [214]. The technique was further investigated and developed by Luzzi and Gerraughty [217,219] and by Madan et al. [215,216]. They examined the effects of varying starting pH, starting temperature, ratio of solid to encapsulating materials, quantity of denaturant, and final pH. Their results indicate that manipulation of all these variables affects some degree of change in the microcapsules and the resulting drug-release rate. When the drug to be encapsulated by the gelatin/acacia system was a waxy solid, such as stearyl alcohol, the coacervation procedure had to be modified because microscopic examination showed that, in the case of drug particles smaller

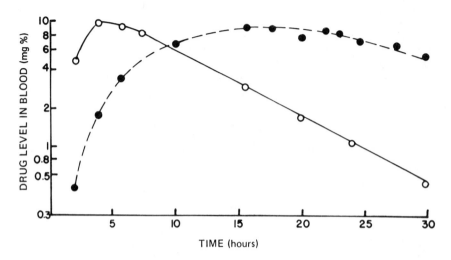

Figure 6 Logarithm of SA levels in blood against time after administration
of SA gelatin micropellets to dogs. ($\circ$) Unitreated micropellets, ($\bullet$) micropellets treated with formalin/isopropanol for 24 h. (From Ref. 213, used
with permission.)

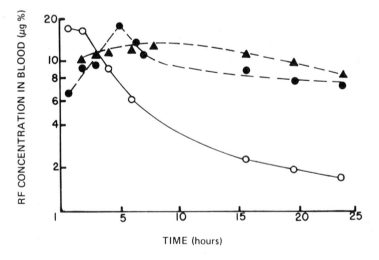

Figure 7 Logarithm of RF concentration in blood after administration of
RF solution and its gelatin micropellets to dogs. ($\circ$) RF solution, ($\bullet$)
untreated micropellets, ($\blacktriangle$) micropellets treated with formalin/isopropanol
for 24 h. (From Ref. 213, used with permission.)

than 250 μm, encapsulation was accomplished by several droplets aggregating and coalescing around the particles rather than by a single droplet as was the usual case. With drug particles larger than 250 μm, they suggested that encapsulation was the result of a direct interaction of gelatin with acacia on the surface of the particles. Scanning electron micrographs lend credence to their suggestion. Merkle and Speiser [218] prepared cellulose acetate phthalate coacervate microcapsules and evaluated them with respect to optimum coacervation and encapsulation conditions. Their findings indicate that while the amount of drug encapsulated had no significant effect on the particle size distribution of the microcapsules, it did influence the release rate. The suggested mechanism for this system is drug diffusion through the shells. When the shells are plasticized in a manner similar to that described earlier, the release rate control is altered from drug diffusion through the shells to dissolution of drug in the microcapsules.

More recently, Birrenbach and Speiser [220] employed polymerized micelles to produce very small particles, termed nanocapsules, to be distinguished from microcapsules. Although this approach is suggested for colloidal solutions to administer antigenic material, it has potential for parenteral drug delivery.

Nylon microcapsules have been examined by McGinity et al. [221], who described an improved method for making them, and by Luzzi et al., who evaluated the prolonged release properties of nylon microcapsules that had been either spray dried or vacuum dried. Both methods of drying produced a large reduction in the dissolution rates of the microcapsules, but since the spray-dried material was free flowing as compared with the vacuum-dried material, the authors felt that spray drying would result in more uniformity and reproducibility of release rates. On the other hand, increased release rates can be obtained by incorporating sucrose into the nylon microcapsules [18]. Interestingly, and perhaps not surprisingly, Luzzi et al. found when compressing these microcapsulated drugs into tablets that the release rate was inversely proportional to the tablet hardness.

Bead polymerization as a technique for preparing sustained-release dosage forms was described by Khanna et al. [222] and further evaluated by Khanna and Speiser [223]. This technique results in drug being embedded in the coating so that its release characteristics are similar to those to be described in the section on the plastic tablet below. By varying the concentration of the α-methacrylic acid content of the polymer solution, the coating can be made to release drug over a wide range of pH values and the release is prolonged for 12–15 h. By combining mixtures of beads with various concentrations of α-methacrylic acid, the correct sustained-release pattern can be made. Seager and Baker [224] described a somewhat different system for making microencapsulated particles in the subsieve size range. These resulted in drug being embedded in an inner core, whereas the outer core was a shellac coating. The release pattern showed good sustained-release properties.

Si-Nang et al. examined the diffusion rate of encapsulated drug as a function of microcapsule size. The influence of the coating on diffusion and the determination of the coating thickness were presented in terms of complex mathematical equations. The equations used were of a general nature and allow a quick estimation of the coating thickness, and thus can be useful in modifying the microencapsulation procedure to attain desired release capabilities.

Crosswell and Becker [225] reported a bead polymerization technique for producing sulfaethylthiadiazole and acetaminophen microencapsulations.

When polystyrene beads were produced in the presence of drug solution, no sustained release was evident; whereas if the beads were produced without drug present and allowed to expand via exposure to n-pentane and subsequent boiling in water, and then the drug solution was allowed to seep into the deep channels produced in the expanded polystyrene beads, the release pattern exhibited good sustaining properties.

The extensive use of polymer-drug interactions to produce sustained-release dosage forms was promoted by Willis and Banker [226]. The drug was made to interact with a cross-linked copolymer such as 1,12-dihydroxy-octadecone hemiester of poly(methylvinylether/maleic anhydride) and the salt that was formed as a result of this exhibited good sustained-release properties upon dialysis testing in artificial gastric and intestinal fluids of tablets and granules fashioned from the polymer-drug salt entities.

Banker and various coworkers [227–231] further studied molecular scale drug entrapment as a means of producing sustained-release dosage forms. Although the technique employed appears to be similar to bead polymerization, it is not clear whether each drug particle was coated (entrapped) within the polymer or whether the drug was actually chemically bonded to the polymer. For purposes of this discussion, the results are similar to those obtained via bead polymerization processes, so they are included here. The authors prepared and tested cationic drugs such as methapyrilene hydrochloride, chlorpromazine hydrochloride, atropine sulfate, etc., for their amenability to the entrapment procedures. The subsequent increases in sustained-release properties were tested and reported.

Further exploration revealed that additives such as organic acids could greatly facilitate drug entrapment by increasing the degree of interaction between the drug and the polymer, and could provide more control over the sustained-release characteristics. Other variables, such as flocculation pH, rate of agitation, use of different polymers, etc., can exert significant effects on sustained-release properties. Some of the important variables and their influences are described in Table 12.

Anionic drugs, such as sodium phenobarbital, sodium salicylate, chloral hydrate, etc., were also entrapped via coagulated (gelled) polymer emulsion systems. These polymer-drug products were tested in a manner similar to that employed for the cationic drugs and the increase in and reproducibility of the sustained-release products was noted. The authors make special mention of the fact that their procedures result in a highly uniform distribution of drug throughout the polymeric system and no drug segregation, with resultant variability in blood levels of drug after dosing, was evident upon scale-up processing and blending for incorporation into sustained-release dosage forms.

All the procedures mentioned thus far in this section are at least loosely related via their production of microencapsulated drug particles that employ slowly soluble films or coatings as the encapsulating material. A good portion of the literature in this area is experimental, usually resulting in statements that reflect how well these methods might be for actually producing commercial sustained-release products. As was mentioned earlier, very few products, aside from aspirin, have been actually formulated from these microencapsulated particles, and thus there is a scarcity of clinical evaluations in the literature. In in vitro evaluation of sustained-release systems, one would like to have linearity in drug release versus time up to 60–70% or more of drug content. However, it is

Table 12 Summary of Effects Produced by Variables on the Molecular Scale Drug Entrapment Method of Banker and Coworkers

Variable studied	Effect on entrapment	Ref.
Methapyrilene base and hydrochloride salt	No appreciable difference in equilibrium dialysis release rates between free base and hydrochloride salt, either as solutions or as solids. Prolongation of release of drug from granular and tableted forms in vitro was shown.	226
Entrapment of cationic drugs by polymeric flocculation	The flocculation of highly concentrated colloidal polymeric dispersions (latices) in the presence of the drug in solution which is to be occluded provides the entrapment mechanism. Significant increases in duration of action and reduction in acute toxicity were demonstrated.	227
Addition of a suitable organic acid to the system described in Ref. 227	Excellent control of sustained-release characteristics. Drug entrapped as the carboxylate salt or in conjunction with the appropriate dicarboxylic acid, while demonstrating substantially complete drug dissolution release in intestinal fluid, could be maintained in the entrapped form in aqueous suspensions during storage periods in excess of 1 month. Greater binding of drug was also shown.	228 229
Flocculation pH and rate of agitation	Effect of an increase in flocculation pH was twofold. It increased both the amount of drug bound and the rate at which drug was released. Increase in the stirring rate during flocculation resulted in an increase in the amount of drug bound to the polymer.	229
Entrapment of anionic drug by polymeric gelation	The phenomenon of gelation of the polymer emulsions by the addition of divalent cation (Mg^{2+}) was utilized for the entrapment of various anionic drug materials. Good control both in vitro and in vivo sustained release characteristics were shown. With increases in drug concentration, release was rapid and a poor release pattern resulted. With diminished drug concentration, too small an amount of drug was released initially to provide therapeutic levels. Smaller size gel particles resulted in more rapid and complete release of	230

Table 12   (Continued)

Variable studied	Effect on entrapment	Ref.
	drug. This suggests mixing gel particle sizes to get a particular release pattern.	
Uniformity of distribution of amine drug in solid dispersions	Excellent reproducibility of drug content throughout the entire entrapment product as demonstrated in both flocculated (high drug levels) and defloccu-lated (low drug levels) systems. Dry blending was inferior to molecular scale drug entrapment in distributing small quantities of drug uniformly.	231

common to see studies showing linearity in the sustained effect for only 30-40% of the system. The study by Nixon and Walker [211] using gelation coacervate showed linearity up to 60% release.

Of the clinical evaluations reported, microencapsulated aspirin has received the lion's share of attention. Bell et al. [232] pointed out the need to monitor blood levels of both acetylsalicylic acid (ASA) and its metabolite, salicylic acid (SA). The need for this is obvious because ASA is reportedly far more potent as an analgesic than SA, so that modification of sustained-release products to provide more ASA and protect it from metabolism to SA become very important. The Bell study compared sustained-release aspirin versus regular aspirin administered as a single dose and in divided doses and analyzed the blood levels of ASA provided by each dosage form or regimen. This resulted in statements to the effect that sustained-release aspirin gave greater analgesic effects than regular aspirin because the ASA blood level remains higher for longer periods of time. When total salicylate blood levels are measured all salicylates presumably producing and contributing to the anti-inflammatory effect of aspirin, the sustained-release product still gave release rates that were too small for sustained-release aspirin. Optimum levels were achieved with about 3% of the drug in the encapsulated material.

Green [80] investigated sustained-release aspirin tablets formulated from microencapsulated particles and found the blood level curves of salicylate to be virtually flat with repeated dosing as opposed to a saw-tooth effect exhibited with repeated dosing of regular aspirin. No conclusion was drawn from this observation, but the influence is that a flat blood level curve represents better control over the therapeutic regimen.

Rotstein et al. [233] examined sustained-release aspirin for use in the management of rheumatoid arthritis and osteoarthritis. In short-term double-blind crossover studies, the doses employed were large enough that the patients received relief from both regular and sustained-release aspirin and observable differences between the two were obscured. However, in long-term usage studies, all the patients who had been on any type of previous salicylate therapy preferred the sustained-release aspirin formulation because it reduced the frequency of dosage and supplied more medication during the night hours, thus relieving the morning aches and pains of arthritis. In both studies the incidence of side effects was significantly lower with sustained-release therapy. These clinical studies have thus established that microencapsulation of aspirin formulated into sustained-release dosage forms is an attractive and effective alternative to nonsustained dosage forms.

IMPREGNATION. There are two general methods of preparing drug-impregnated particles with wax: (1) congealing and, (2) aqueous dispersion. In the congealing method, the drug is admixed with the wax material and either screened or spray congealed. The aqueous dispersion approach is simply spraying or placing the drug-wax mixture in water and collecting the resulting particles.

In a series of papers by Becker and associates [225,234-239], the formulation and release characteristics of wax impregnations of sulfaethyl-thiadiazole were thoroughly investigated. The authors looked at dispersant concentration, effects of surfactant addition, effects of different waxes and modifiers, etc., as to their effect on release rate and proportion of total drug constituting the prolonged-release fraction. As might be expected, the size of the microcapsules produced and the physical properties of the various wax coating materials had profound effects on the release patterns reported. When the spray-congealed formulations of wax and sulfaethyl-thiadiazole were compressed into tablets the release mechanism appeared to be due to erosion, solubilization, and leaching of the drug from the tablet. No one model could describe the release pattern over the 48-h period of the study. It has been reported, in general terms, that the aqueous dispersion method gives higher release rates for all waxes tested, presumably due to increased area and perhaps the physical entrapment of water. Further, with aspirin as the test drug, the dissolution rate increases in the order stearic acid > spermaceti > hydrogenated cottonseed oil.

Case Study of Slowly Soluble Wax Microencapsulation [234]. *Prolonged action mechanism.* Drug is impregnated in a slowly dissolving wax.

Type and method of coating. Bleached beeswax or glycowax S-932 is mixed with drug, in a ratio of 1 part drug to 3 parts wax, and heated on a water bath to 75°C. Typical amounts were 24 gm beeswax and 8 gm sulfaethylthiadiazole (SETD). In a separate container heated to 80°C was 1 ml sorbitan mono-oleate and 1.15 ml polysorbate 80 in 400 ml of distilled water. The aqueous phase was slowly added to the wax mixture with continuous stirring at a predetermined speed until the mixture cooled to approximately 45°C. Stirring at around 300-400 rpm produced particles that were primarily in the size range of 30-100 mesh. The drug-wax particles were separated from the aqueous phase by filtration, washed with distilled water, and dried. Fractionation of the resulting particles into three mesh sizes 16-20, 30-40, and 50-60 was accomplished with USP sieves, and only the 50- to 60-mesh particles were retained for in vitro and in vivo testing.

In vitro test. Dissolution tests were conducted in a modified USP disintegration apparatus, and the results are shown in Figures 8(a) and 8(b). Drug release during the first 15 min was in direct relation to the specific surface, since the particles were assumed to have a uniform distribution of drug on the surface. After the first 15 min period, the rate of drug release varied as a function of mesh size and appeared to follow

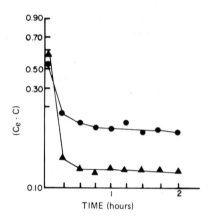

(a)

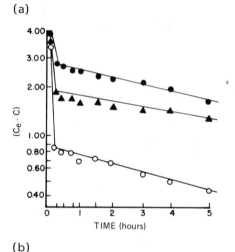

(b)

Figure 8   (a) In vitro dissolution rates of SETD from various mesh sizes of
SETD-glycowax particles in 0.1 N HCl.   (●) 16−20 mesh, (▲) 30−40 mesh,
$C_e - C = 0$.   (b) In vitro dissolution rates of SETD from various mesh sizes
of SETD-glycowax particles in alkaline pancreatin solution.   (●) 16−20
mesh, (▲) 30−40 mesh, (○) 50−60 mesh.   (From Ref. 234, used with
permission.

first-order kinetics.   The first-order dissolution appears to be due to the
changing surface area.
    In vivo release.   Urinary excretion rates of SETD-glycowax, 50−60
mesh size range, were compared to rates for plain SETD in four humans.
The 50−60 mesh size was selected because the in vitro release data were
most similar to the in vitro release of a similar commercial prolonged-
release SETD product.   Figure 9 shows the comparison of the excretion
rates for the plain SETD and the prolonged release form.   The SETD-
glycowax particles released 50% less drug during the first 3 h, and then
the rates increased so that at the end of 24 h, 71% of the total SETD had
been excreted as compared to 85% for plain SETD.   Over 72 h, the

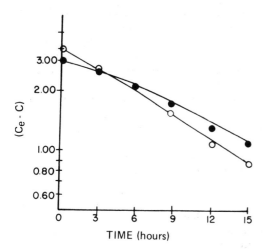

Figure 9 Average urinary excretion rates of free SETD for four humans receiving a 3.9-gm oral dose of SETD in (a) plain form and (b) SETD-glycowax combination. (●) plain SETD, (○), SETD-glycowax combination. (From Ref. 113, used with permission.)

in vivo SETD-glycowax release gave 85% excreted versus 81% in the in vitro experiment.

B. Sustained-Release Utilizing Diffusion

This section describes coated sustained-release systems that are distinguished from those in the previous section primarily by their mechanism of action (i.e., diffusion), as well as by their means of application and by the appearance of the final dosage form. Some of the microencapsulated materials discussed earlier released drug via a diffusion process, but the bulk of the diffusion systems will be discussed here. In the case of slowly soluble films and coatings, the reader will recall that these were generally applied via pan-coating techniques or by some form of polymerization with the end result being coated pellets or granules or microspherules that could then be compressed into tablets or placed in a capsule. The products in this section are, for the most part, press-coated films whereby a core is fed into the die and the coating material is then pressed onto it, resulting in a single-coated tablet, or they are whole tablets or particles that have been coated via air-suspension techniques. As in the previously described cases, the area and the thickness of the coating are important parameters, but they take on added importance here because diffusion of drug, either from the core or from the coating itself, must pass through the barrier represented by the coating or film. Insoluble films will thus present a rigid barrier that will act to keep the diffusion path length of drug from the tablet interior to the absorption site (outside of tablet) relatively constant. Some of the films described below are also slowly soluble, but their maintenance of constant path length is still the most important activity.

As might be expected, a lot of the research in this area has to do with the mechanics of the coating process itself, in addition to the research on developing new coatings and measuring the efficacy of administering drugs in this manner. Of course, the patent literature is filled with polymeric systems that can be used via press-coating or air-suspension techniques [154,165,240,241], and the research literature likewise [242–250]. However, since the press-coating and air-suspension processes are utilized in the pharmaceutical industry, a body of research has been developed to overcome some of the manufacturing difficulties presented by these techniques [251–254].

The original work that developed the air-suspension technique has been reported by Wurster [255,256]. This patented process is now widely used in the industry, since it is a fast, efficient way of making uniform coatings on granules and core tablets. The use of the technique for coating aspirin granules has been described by Coletta and Rubin [257]. Wood and Syarto [258] continued the same line of work involving coating aspirin with various ratios of ethylcellulose to methylcellulose. As the methylcellulose dissolved, whereas the ethylcellulose did not, the shell left behind presumably provided a restraining barrier for keeping the ASA diffusion path length constant. These authors attempted to correlate the in vitro dissolution pattern with that obtained in vivo, as shown in Figure 10. As can be seen from the correlation lines, with high-content ethylcellulose the in vitro/in vivo correlations are good. As the percent of methylcellulose in the coating is increased, the correlation falls off, and this points out the fallacy of using in vitro data alone to predict in vivo performance of these tablet coatings.

Many researchers have, of course, looked at the polymeric materials used in the coating processes with an eye to developing better, more durable, and more easily applied coats. Polyvinylpyrrolidone-acetylated monoglyceride [244], styrenemaleic acid copolymer [245], hydroxypropyl-cellulose-polyvinylacetate [259,260], and many other polymers have been studied for their value as enteric coatings [243,248,250] and for use in developing sustained-release preparations [246–248]. Enteric coating is a subject dealt with elsewhere in this text, but the application of enteric coats can be accomplished via press-coating and air-suspensions techniques just as described here.

Donbrow and Friedman [259] reported the release of caffeine and salicylic acid from cast films of ethylcellulose and the release rates were found to agree with both the classic first-order equation (log drug retained in film versus time) and with the diffusion-controlled release models (drug release linearly related to square root of time) as developed by Higuchi [260]. More stringent mathematical treatment of their data resulted in the diffusion-controlled release model being most appropriate to describe their data. Borodkin and Tucker [261,262] also used cast films of drug in hydroxypropylcellulose, studying the release of salicylic acid, pentobarbital, and methapyrilene. These drugs were released according to the same diffusion-controlled model described above. Further work to modify the system resulted in zero-order drug release obtained by laminating a second film without drug to the releasing side of the film containing drug. Thus, the nondrug layer functions as a rate-controlling membrane, and the drug-containing film serves as a reservoir. In vitro zero-order drug release for the three species mentioned was demonstrated using this technique.

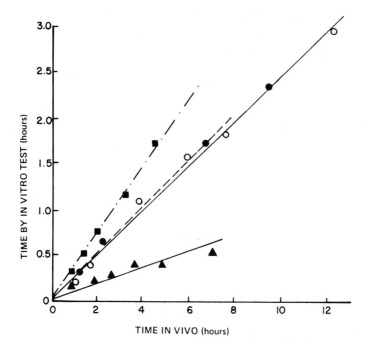

Composition and Characteristics of Test Delayed-Release Aspirin Products
Used in This Study

	Code			
	134B	134C	152	138
Ratio ethyl to methylcellulose	75/25	25/75	82.5/17.5	100/0
Aspirin mesh size	−20	−40	−20+40	−20+40
Amount of coating (wt %)	2.7%	4.8%	6%	6%
Tablet disintegration time (sec)	40−60	25−35	3	3
Aspirin content	5 gr	5 gr	5 gr	5 gr
Cornstarch	0.87 gr	0.90 gr	0.96 gr	0.96 gr
Talc	−	−	0.13 gr	0.13 gr

Figure 10 Correlation between in vivo absorption and in vitro release
rates for corresponding fractions of total salicylate considered. (■) 152,
(●) 138, (▲) 134C, (○) 134B. (From Ref. 258, used with permission.)

Since the technique described in this section can be used to coat core tablets or granules, it is conceivable that many of the clinical studies described earlier could be applicable in this case. However, a very good clinical study of the Sinusule sustained-release dosage form has been described [263]. This product is somewhat different from the others examined thus far in that the film applied to the granules actually functions as a microdialysis membrane. Thus, one need not worry about the acidity of the gut, the digestive process, nor the contents of the gut. The only requirement is that there be fluid in the gut. The fluid, primarily water, passes through the dialysis membrane into the sphere and dissolves the granule of drug. This drug then diffuses through the intact membrane at a rate proportional to the permeability of the membrane, the mobility of the drug molecule, and the concentration of the drug within the hydrated microdialysis cell. When this product was tested in patients having hay fever, upper respiratory infection, and miscellaneous respiratory allergies, good to excellent results with a minimum of side effects were reported for a large majority of the test population. This novel sustained-release dosage form is not marketed anymore.

Case Study of Duffusion-Controlled Coating [261]

PROLONGED ACTION MECHANISM. Drugs are dispersed in a water-soluble polymeric coating which, when subjected to an aqueous environment, allows slow diffusion of drug into the leaching fluid.

TYPE AND METHOD OF FILM FORMATION. Hydroxypropylcellulose, average molecular weight of 100,000, having viscosity 75−150 cps as a 5% water solution, and polyvinylacetate, average molecular weight 500,000, having viscosity 90−110 cps as an 8.6% benzene solution, were used. Drugs were pentobarbital, salicylic acid, and methapyrilene. The films were cast from a solution containing 10% solids (drug plus polymer), using methylene chloride/methanol mixture (9:1) as the solvent. The polymers were added as dry powders, as was salicylic acid, while the pentobarbital and methapyrilene were added from stock methylene chloride solutions. Films were cast from the solutions at various wet thicknesses (0.64−2.54 mm) using a knife on Teflon-coated plate glass. The films were allowed to air dry at least 48 h before evaluation. The percent drug in the dry film was calculated from the ratio of drug and polymer weights used.

MECHANISM OF DRUG RELEASE. Release of drug from a matrix can be either via a first-order process or via a diffusion-controlled process. Which release is operative can be ascertained by appropriate data treatment. First-order release would be a linear plot following the normal first-order equations, whereas a diffusion-controlled process should result in an S-shaped curve following the equation

$$Q = \sqrt{\frac{D\varepsilon}{\tau}(2A - \varepsilon C_s)C_s t} \tag{13}$$

where Q = amount of drug released per unit area of tablet exposed to solvent

D = diffusion coefficient of drug in the permeating fluid

ε = porosity of the matrix

τ = tortuosity of the matrix

A = concentration of solid drug in the matrix

C_s = solubility of drug in the dissolution medium

t = time

The above equation is more commonly expressed as

$$Q = k_H t^{1/2} \qquad (14)$$

where $k_H = \Sigma D[(2A - C_s)C_s]^{1/2}$ for plotting purposes.

IN VITRO TEST. Rectangular films measuring 2.2 × 4.0 cm (8.8 cm^2) were cut using a razor blade with a microscope cover glass as a template. The film was weighed and its thickness was measured at all four corners and the center with a micrometer. A thin coating of high-vacuum silicone lubricant was applied to a 2.54 × 7.62 cm microscope slide and the film was pressed into the slide, making sure that all edges adhered and no lubricant touched the exposed surface. The slide was placed at an angle into a 250-ml beaker in a 37°C-water bath containing 200 ml of pH 7 buffer preheated to 37°C. A nonagitated system was used to eliminate turbulence effect on release rate and to maintain film integrity. Periodic assay samples (~ 10 min^{-1}) were obtained by removing the slide, stirring the solution, and pipetting a 5-ml sample, and then reimmersing the slide with film into the buffer solution. Beakers were covered throughout the length of the runs (7 h at least and 31 h in the extreme for slow-releasing films) to prevent evaporation. The samples were assayed by ultraviolet (UV) spectrophotometry at 240 nm for pentobarbital in 0.1 N NH$_4$OH, at 312 nm for methapyrilene in 0.1 N HCl, and at 297 nm for salicylic acid in 0.1 N NaOH.

Table 13 shows the results of comparing the drug release to first-order and square root of time equations. When these data were evaluated to determine which equation gave best fit, the correlation coefficients for the best statistical lines and the lag times (time intercept extrapolated to Q = 0) were used as the principal criteria. Although the correlation coefficients looked good for either mechanism, when these types of data are plotted out, as is shown in Figure 11, the curvature in the first-order mechanism was evident. This indicated that the Q versus $t^{1/2}$ relation more readily described the mechanism. Correlation coefficients were generally greater than 0.995 for this type of plotting and deviations, when they occurred, were random rather than the result of curvature. Linearity in release held through 75−80% of drug release when a constant concentration gradient was operative.

The effect of film thickness on the rate of drug release for pentobarbital is shown in Table 14. These results indicate that the release rate constant, k_H, is independent of film thickness. However, film thickness will affect the duration of drug release, as is shown in the last column where $t_{1/2}$ represents the time, in minutes, for 50% of the drug in each particular film to be released.

Tables 15−17 show the effects of varying polymer ratio on the release rate, k_H, for the drugs methapyrilene, salicylic acid, and pentobarbital, respectively. In general, an acceleration of release rate can be obtained

Table 13 Comparison between First-Order and Q versus $t^{1/2}$ Treatments of Pentobarbital Release Rate Data

Drug concentration (%)[a]	Hydroxypropylcellulose/ polyvinylacetate ratio	Number of runs	First-order		Q versus $t^{1/2}$	
			t_{lag} (min)[b]	Correlation coefficient	t_{lag} (min)[b]	Correlation coefficient
36.4	10:0	4	−3.2	0.996	3.1	0.997
18.2	10:0	4	−14.0	0.957	2.6	0.993
18.2	9:1	2	−9.8	0.986	2.8	0.996
18.2	8:2	2	−6.5	0.986	2.3	0.993
18.2	6:4	2	−84.0	0.982	1.4	0.996
18.2	4:6	4	−142.0	0.983	0.3	0.998
18.2	2:8	4	−176.0	0.981	0.6	0.998
18.2	1:9	4	−176.0	0.982	0.7	0.998
18.2	0:10	3	−214.0	0.979	1.0	0.997
9.1	0:10	4	−199.0	0.981	1.3	0.990

[a]Weight of drug per weight of dry film.
[b]All t_{lag} and correlation coefficient values expressed are mean values.
Source: From Ref. 259, used with permission.

Table 14 Effect of Film Thickness on Pentobarbital Release Rate Constant and Half-Life

Drug concentration (%)[a]	Hydroxypropylcellulose/ polyvinylacetate ratio	Wet film thickness setting (mm)	Dry film thickness (μm)[b]	k_H (mg cm^{-2} min$^{-1/2}$)	Correlation coefficient	$t_{1/2}$ (min)
36.4	10:0	0.64	44.0 ± 1.1	0.33	0.996	14.8
		1.27	56.2 ± 2.1	0.29	0.996	25.2
		1.91	100.2 ± 4.6	0.33	0.998	49.8
		2.54	109.3 ± 3.3	0.32	0.998	60.2
18.2	4:6	0.64	61.4 ± 4.9	0.032	0.999	360
		1.27	113.2 ± 9.9	0.034	0.999	1,280
		1.91	145.0 ± 8.0	0.034	0.999	2,850
		2.54	204.2 ± 3.1	0.037	0.997	3,850
18.2	1:9	0.64	76.8 ± 1.2	0.0101	0.996	8,520
		1.27	118.4 ± 2.6	0.0102	0.999	19,200
		1.91	202.8 ± 2.2	0.0101	0.998	50,900
		2.54	268.0 ± 2.4	0.0102	0.998	83,600

[a]Weight of drug per weight of dry film.

[b]Thickness = mean ± standard deviation of five measurements.

Source: From Ref. 259, used with permission.

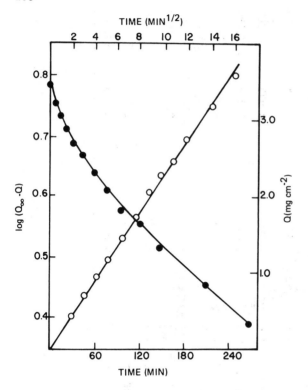

Figure 11 Comparison between first-order release treatment and Q versus $t^{1/2}$ treatment of data from a film containing 26.3% methapyrilene at a 5:5 ratio of hydroxypropylcellulose/polyvinylacetate. (●) log $(Q_\infty - Q)$ versus t, and (○) Q versus $t^{1/2}$. (From Ref. 259, used with permission.)

by increasing the proportion of hydroxypropylcellulose to polyvinylacetate. The large variations in the $t_{1/2}$ values reflect the changes in the polymer ratio and, in addition, the changes in film thickness.

C. Sustained-Release Utilizing a Combination of Dissolution and Diffusion

The products to be discussed in this section are those that provide the sustaining portion of the dose in some sort of relatively insoluble core that has been impregnated with the drug. This core is almost always coated and the coat contains that portion of the dose meant for immediate release upon dissolution of the coat in the stomach. Once this occurs, the gastro-intestinal fluids are free to permeate the core and thus slowly leach out the drug. Of course, the possibility exists that the core material can sometimes be dissolved slowly to provide drug, but this is usually not the the case. The diffusion of drug out of the core is the major mechanism for providing drug in sustained release form. In these preparations the area over which diffusion cocurs remains relatively constant (especially if no core dissolution occurs) and the amount of drug is in excess. The

Table 15 Effect of Hydroxypropylcellulose/Polyvinylacetate Ratio on the Release Rate from Films Containing 26.3% Methapyrilene

Hydroxypropyl- cellulose/ polyvinylacetate ratio	Dry film thickness (μm)[a,b]	k_H (mg cm^{-2} min$^{-1/2}$)	Correlation coefficient	$t_{1/2}$ (min)
10:1	210 ± 7.4	0.549	0.999	33
9:1	210 ± 6.5	0.593	0.997	28
8:2	216 ± 9.1	0.497	1.000	42
7:3	181 ± 7.8	0.272	0.995	99
6:4	218 ± 4.4	0.217	0.998	226
5:5	208 ± 4.6	0.225	0.999	190
4:6	142 ± 4.5	0.191	0.997	124
3:7	157 ± 3.3	0.094	0.998	630
2:8	136 ± 3.3	0.089	0.999	523
1:9	131 ± 6.0	0.075	0.998	681
0:10	185 ± 0.9	0.074	0.996	1404

[a]Thickness = mean ± standard deviation of five measurements.

[b]All films cast using a wet thickness setting of 2.54 mm.
Source: From Ref. 259, used with permission.

factor that changes, in this case, is the path length term in Fick's first law. As more drug diffuses out of the core, the permeating gastrointestinal fluid must travel an increasingly longer and more tortuous path to get to the remaining drug. The dissolved drug, in turn, has to diffuse out via the same altered pathways. Thus, a tortuosity factor must be included in the equation to describe release.

One of the earliest of these core-type products to be described was Duretter, developed by Sjogren and Fryklof [264] in Sweden. It differs from other core-type tablets, such as Ciba's Lontab, in that the core is produced by directly compressing a granulate of the drug and an insoluble plastic material so that a coherent, porous skeleton of the matrix material forms around the drug. In core tablets such as Lontab, on the other hand, the drug is incorporated into the melted matrix material and this is then spread out to dry. After drying it is granulated, and this granulation is then compressed into the core tablet [265]. In the final result the differences in manufacturing are not evident, and the release patterns of drug from these species are similar in many respects.

The release rate and absorption characteristics of various drug incorporated into a plastic matrix type of tablet have been extensively studied. Sjogren and Ostholm [266] studied the release of nitroglycerin, lobeline hydrochloride, [82]Br-labeled ammonium bromide, creatinine, potassium

Table 16   Effect of Hydroxypropylcellulose/Polyvinylacetate Ratio on the
Release Rate from Films Containing 20.0% Salicylic Acid

Hydroxypropyl- cellulose/ polyvinylacetate ratio	Dry film thickness (μm)[a,b]	k_H $(mg\ cm^{-2}\ min^{-1/2})$	Correlation coefficient	$t_{1/2}$ (min)
10:0	189 ± 2.8	0.403	0.997	28
9:1	223 ± 5.6	0.336	0.997	57
8:2	210 ± 0.9	0.328	0.993	53
7:3	229 ± 2.5	0.241	0.998	116
6:4	209 ± 6.6	0.216	0.984	120
5:5	204 ± 7.9	0.175	0.997	175
4:6	145 ± 0.5	0.115	0.997	206
3:7	156 ± 3.4	0.122	0.997	210
2:8	181 ± 7.9	0.112	0.998	338
1:9	222 ± 4.3	0.073	0.998	1190
0:10	172 ± 1.8	0.057	0.996	1040

[a]Thickness = mean ± standard deviation of five measurements.

[b]All films cast using a wet thickness setting of 2.54 mm.
Source: From Ref. 259, used with permission.

penicillin V, and dihydromorphinone hydrochloride both in vitro and in vivo,
in cats and humans. They noted good correlations between in vitro and
in vivo results, both in blood levels of active drug, and also when monitoring a particular pharmacological effect produced by the drug, although of
course in vivo determination of release rate was much more difficult to estimate. In a continuation of this type of study, Sjogren and Ervik [267]
developed an automatic spectrophotometric method for studying continuous
release rates of quinidine bisulfate and ephedrine hydrochloride from
Duretter plastic matrix tablets and obtained highly reproducible results.

The complex interplay between the processes of release and degradations of substances dispersed in polymeric matrixes has been described in
great detail by Collins and Doglia [268]. Although their discussion is of
general nature, the analogy to drugs and pharmaceutical systems is apparent. El-Egakey et al. [269] and Asker et al. [270–272] have delved
into the in vitro release of drugs from polymeric matrixes and granulations.
In the case of water-soluble drugs, merely granulating the drug with the
melted matrix material will provide suitable sustained release of drug,
whereas with more water-insoluble drugs, a coating providing drug for
immediate release and absorption takes on increasing importance as the
degree of water solubility decreases. Obviously, the limiting case here is
a drug with virtually no water solubility. This drug would not need to

Table 17 Effect of Hydroxypropylcellulose/Polyvinylacetate Ratio on the Release Rate from Films Containing 18.2% Pentobarbital

Hydroxypropylcellulose/ polyvinylacetate ratio	Wet thickness setting (mm)	Dry film thickness (μm)[a]	k_H (mg cm^{-2} min$^{-1/2}$)	Correlation coefficient	$t_{1/2}$ (min)
10:1	1.27	98 ± 5.4	0.225	0.995	20
9:1	2.54	163 ± 3.4	0.224	0.995	57
8:2	1.27	87 ± 6.4	0.178	0.987	25
6:4	2.54	236 ± 7.1	0.0767	0.997	1.010
4:6	1.91	145 ± 8.0	0.0342	0.999	2.280
2:8	1.27	94 ± 1.9	0.0161	0.999	3.630
1:9	1.27	118 ± 2.6	0.0102	0.999	19.200
0:10	1.91	210 ± 15.5	0.0260	0.998	6.960

[a]Thickness = mean + standard deviation of five measurements.
Source: From Ref. 259, used with permission.

be placed in a special sustained-release dosage form, since it is inherently long acting by nature of its poor aqueous solubility. Of course, the method of preparation of the granulating materials, the choice of in vitro dissolution media, and the plastic matrix material chosen will all have an influence on release of the drug from the sustained-release dosage form.

Water-soluble drugs dispersed in hydrophilic matrixes were studied by Lapidus and Lordi [273]. Their results indicate that chlorpheniramine maleate dispersed in methylcellulose is release-rate controlled mostly by drug diffusivity rather than by polymer dissolution and water permeability. Thus, even for drugs formulated in a water-soluble matrix, one which would itself be subject to erosion and absorption in the body, the determining factor in providing sustained release is still diffusion of the drug out of the matrix. This important fact was further elaborated on by Huber et al. [274] for hydrophilic gums versus the matrix material. In this case, the mechanism of prolonged release was determined to be drug diffusion from, and eventual attrition of, a gel barrier at the periphery of the tablet core.

A modification of this type of matrix tablet was described by Javaid et al. [275]. They used a lipase-lipid-drug system to provide sustained release whereby the erosion of the matrix due to the hydrolytic action of lipase on the substrate was the desirable first step in obtaining release of the drug for absorption. Accelerators of lipase activity, such as calcium carbonate or glyceryl monostearate, could be used to tailor make a sustained-release tablet to provide a desired release profile. Javaid and Hartman [276] then tested these enzyme-substrate-drug tablets in dogs, and the action of lipase to control drug release was confirmed. Tablets containing lipase consistently gave higher and more uniform blood levels of drug than those without, as is evident in Figure 12. It is apparent that the enzyme-substrate type of matrix tablet has potential for commercial use in providing sustained release.

The type of plastic matrix sustained-release dosage form that has been investigated the most extensively is undoubtedly that of a drug dispersed in an insoluble, inert matrix [3-5,10,15,18,278-285]. The kinetics of release and the methods of treating the matrix tablets have been reported

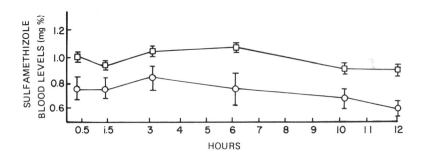

Figure 12   Average sulfamethizole blood levels (mg%) in dogs after receiving tablets containing 100% drug in drug-lipid granules with 5% glyceryl monostearate. (□) tablets with lipase and (○) tablets without lipase. Standard errors are plotted around the averages. (From Ref. 276, used with permission.)

by Farhadieh and coworkers [277,279] for drugs dispersed in a methyl acrylate-methyl methacrylate matrix. As seen in Table 18, treatment of the tablets by exposure to acetone vapor results in a significant decrease in the release rate of drug from the matrix. This, coupled with control of the treatment temperature, allowed production of sustained release tablets with highly reproducible release rates. An investigation of the problems that could result from chewing an insoluble matrix was the subject of a paper by Ritschel [280]. If the drug is incorporated in the pores and channels of a matrix tablet, potential toxicity could occur if the tablet was inadvertently chewed by the patient, since this would result in the release of large quantities of the drug. For drugs with a narrow therapeutic range, such as nitroglycerin, this could be a problem. When the drug was dissolved directly into the plastic matrix material, the problem is alleviated since even with mastication the drug is not free to be absorbed.

Sjuib et al. [281,282] continued the work of Higuchi on the study of drug release from inert matrixes. The original physical model described by Higuchi and coworkers [286−294] was tested for binary mixtures of acidic drugs and also for binary mixtures of amphoteric drugs. Analysis showed that the physical model could describe the experimental data quite well and also pointed out that the precipitation of the drug in the matrix during release into alkaline media, such as might be encountered in the intestinal fluids, has to be considered more important than theories involving supersaturation of the drug in the matrix. The mathematics of both matrix-controlled and partition-controlled drug release mechanisms were elucidated by Chien et al. [285]. They pointed out that the transition that occurs between the two processes is dependent on the magnitude of the solution solubility of the drug and, via a series of equations, indicated that this term dictates the mechanism and rate of drug release from the polymer matrix.

Other research in the area of drug release from insoluble matrix tablets has found that the square root of time relation originally proposed by Higuchi [260] described the advance of the solvent front into the tablet [283]. Compression force was not a major factor and drug release was, of course, proportional to the total surface area.

As can be seen from the above cited work, a tremendous amount of time and effort has been expended to elucidate and quantify the factors that are important in obtaining controlled-release from plastic matrix-type tablets. The perturbations introduced by varying diluents, matrix material, and so on are all important in describing the in vitro release of drug from these tablets, and presumably are equally important in describing the in vivo release rates. However, we would be remiss if the clinical evaluation of these types of dosage forms are not included here, since the literature is full of examples in which systems showing good in vitro possibilities were unsuccessful in an actual clinical trial.

The effects of gastric emptying time and intestinal peristaltic activity on the absorption of aspirin from a sustained-release tablet containing coated particles in a hydrophilic gel type matrix and conventional aspirin tablets were described by Levy and Hollister [295]. The lag times in the absorption profiles reported were undoubtedly due to the time required for transfer of the dosage form from the stomach to the intestine. The authors point out the pitfalls of plotting averaged individual absorption data versus time and how this could lead to erroneous assumptions about whether a dosage form is a good candidate for sustained release or not.

Table 18 Effect of Acetone Vapor Pressure on the Release Rate of Drug from 100-mg Sodium Pentobarbital Tablets at Three Different Temperatures

Temperature	Acetone vapor pressure (mmHg)	Acetone absorbed (mg/tablet)	ε	τ	$k \times 10^1$ (g cm^2 sec$^{-1/2}$)	$t_{1/2}$ (hr)
Untreated tablets		0	0.575	9.24	5.38	3.38
37°	217	16.2	0.567	11.5	4.93	4.03
	244	19.0	0.559	13.3	4.64	4.54
	267	25.3	0.559	19.7	3.87	6.52
	307	30.7	0.535	52.2	2.44	16.4
	347	44.9	0.530	154.9	1.43	47.8
34°	217	18.4	0.560	12.2	4.79	4.26
	244	22.5	0.51	16.6	4.19	5.57
	267	27.9	0.539	43.2	2.67	13.7
	307	39.7	0.534	198.2	1.26	61.5
31°	217	26.1	0.551	18.6	4.01	6.08
	244	29.3	0.540	36.4	2.91	11.5
	267	32.8	0.528	86.2	1.93	26.2

Source: From Ref. 277, used with permission.

Individual absorption data that results in a first-order plot can often appear to be zero-order, indicating good sustained release, when such data are averaged. Thus, it is necessary to look at the data for each individual in the test population when assessing sustained-release characteristics.

Nicholson et al. [296] described the blood and urine levels obtained in humans following ingestion of sustained-release tablets. It was noted that the sustained-release tablets gave less variation between maximum and minimum blood level concentrations and more uniform urinary excretion rates than conventional release tablets. Theophylline aminoisobutanol, administered in a tablet containing a sustained-release core having a matrix of hydrophilic gums, a delayed barrier coat on the core, and an outer coat containing the drug for immediate release was investigated by Kaplan [297]. Both in vitro and in vivo results were obtained and the blood level data correlated well. Although differences were noted in the urinary data, no explanation was tendered other than noting that these differences have been reported previously. The in vivo absorption and excretion of radioactively tagged [10-^{14}C]pentylenetetrazol was studied by Ebert et al. [278]. Human volunteers were given either a single dose of sustained-release insoluble matrix tablets or three divided doses of conventional tablets. It was shown that the sustained-release form gave absorption and excretion patterns similar to those obtained in the divided dose case.

As noted earlier in the section on coated granules, the earliest commercially available sustained-release preparations available for clinical trials seem to be those providing antihistamines [166,167,298,299]. Such research has led to clinical trials of sustained-release triethanolamine trinitrate [300] for use in angina pectoris. The drug was provided in a plastic matrix that leached out drug over a 7- to 8-h span. Patients reported no undesirable side effects and the frequency and severity of attacks were diminished in 80% of those tested.

De Ritter [301] used urinary excretion rates to evaluate nicotinic alcohol tartrate administered to humans via Roche's Roniacol Timespan matrix tablets. This dosage form uses a coating containing drug to provide the immediate release portion of the dose and the sustaining portion is provided by erosion and/or leaching of the insoluble matrix in the gastrointestinal tract. The results indicate good correlation of in vitro and in vivo release rates, and the drug is as completely available in this form as in conventional tablets. In addition, the intense flushing caused by non-sustained-release tablets is absent with the sustained release form.

The tension-relieving and sedative properties of pentobarbital sodium, administered via conventional capsules and Abbott's Gradumet plastic matrix sustained-release form, were clinically evaluated by Cass and Frederik [302]. Although the grading system employed was qualitative in nature, the results indicated that the Gradumet form was useful in providing daytime tranquilization and it was virtually free of untoward side effects.

The Gradumet matrix dosage form has also been evaluated for treatment of iron deficiency anemia via the sustained release of ferrous sulfate [303,304]. In all cases, the hematocrit and hemoglobin responses were virtually identical whether the non-sustained-release form or the matrix tablet was administered. However, the incidence of reported gastrointestinal upset due to ferrous sulfate, an important problem because more iron is absorbed by fasting patients while at the same time causing more gastrointestinal distress, was greatly diminished when the dose was given as a sustained-release tablet. Crosland-Taylor and Keeling [305] formulated their own sustained-release ferrous sulfate tablets in an inert polymer matrix and they added [^{59}Fe]SO$_4$ as a marker to aid in evaluation. They point out that the previously mentioned hematocrit and hemoglobin responses are relatively insensitive means for comparing conventional and sustained-release tablets, and their results indicate variable absorption from sustained-release forms. They found no real advantage, even in the area of management of side effects, to the use of sustained-release forms of ferrous sulfate. It is not clear, then, whether there is any significant advantage to providing oral hematinics in sustained-release form.

Owing to the many unpleasant side effects of oral potassium supplementation, such as extremely salty taste and severe gastrointestinal upset, the past few years have seen a need for a slow-release potassium-providing product. Slow-K, marketed by Ciba, is the best example of this type of product. The sugar-coated wax matrix contains 600 mg of potassium chloride that leaches out gradually over a 4- to 6-h period. Tarpley [306] studied the patient acceptability of this product as well as its ability to maintain normal serum potassium levels in clinical trials comparing it to oral potassium liquid preparations. His findings indicate that both types of products maintain serum K$^+$ levels, but the sustained-release tablet gives much less incidence of nausea, abdominal pain, cramps, diarrhea, etc., and, of course, since it has little or no taste before being swallowed, it was much more palatable and acceptable to all the patients involved.

As was noted earlier, aspirin has been tested for delivery via every new dosage form developed for the past 20–25 years. Here, as in the case of oral antihistaminics, the simple arithmetic of profit and loss statements has compelled pharmaceutical firms to develop sustained-release aspirin preparations [307]. The market is largely due to the vast numbers of arthritics who need a preparation that will provide aspirin throughout the night and eliminate morning stiffness, the most common plight of arthritis sufferers. Many products have been extensively tested in clinical trials as well.

Wiseman and Federici [308] have developed a sustained-release aspirin tablet utilizing the matrix principle. By carefully monitoring both in vitro and in vivo data, the authors were able to fashion a product that gave constant plasma salicylate concentrations on chronic administration. Wiseman [309] then extended the tests to the clinic where highly reproducible, stable plasma salicylate concentrations were attained that overcame the fluctuations due to multiple dosing of conventional tablets. The stable levels do not exhibit the peaks in serum salicylate levels shown by conventional tablets; therefore the incidence of gastrointestinal upset was reduced and the valleys, or low points, were eliminated, thus providing therapeutic levels of salicylate throughout the night. Harris and Regalado [310], however, compared conventional and sustained-release aspirin for their ability to provide relief to patients in order that the latter might perform simple tasks requiring phalangeal dexterity. They reported no difference between the two types of tablets, but a majority of the patients preferred the sustained-release form. The inference here is that the sustained-release product gave relief throughout the night and did not cause the unpleasant gastrointestinal side effects, thus contributing to the patient's preference. Also, the convenience of eliminating frequent daytime doses was significant in the preference for sustained-release aspirin.

These are just a few examples of the benefits obtained from providing aspirin in a sustained-release matrix tablet and of sustained-release dosage forms for administering aspirin, in general. The recent flourish of timed release and double- or triple-strength aspirin tablets to the market attests to the desirability and, consequently, the profitability of long-acting aspirin preparations.

Case Study of Combination Dissolution – Diffusion
Coating [280]

PROLONGED ACTION MECHANISM. Coated or uncoated plastic matrix tablets. Solvent dissolves the coat containing the initial dose and drug is leached out of the plastic core to maintain therapeutic levels. A diagrammatic structure of the tablet is shown in Figure 13 for the drug combination nitroglycerin and proxyphylline.

Complete Depot Dosage Form

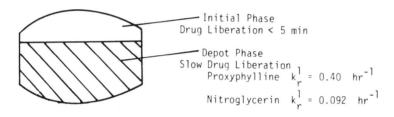

Initial Phase
Drug Liberation < 5 min

Depot Phase
Slow Drug Liberation
Proxyphylline $k_r^1 = 0.40 \; hr^{-1}$

Nitroglycerin $k_r^1 = 0.092 \; hr^{-1}$

Structure of Depot Phase

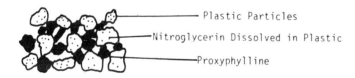

Plastic Particles

Nitroglycerin Dissolved in Plastic

Proxyphylline

Drug Release from Depot Phase

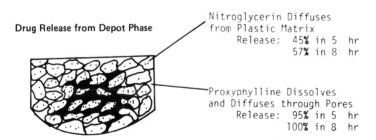

Nitroglycerin Diffuses
from Plastic Matrix
Release: 45% in 5 hr
57% in 8 hr

Proxyphylline Dissolves
and Diffuses through Pores
Release: 95% in 5 hr
100% in 8 hr

Figure 13 Diagrammatic structure of the peroral sandwich tablet with timed release and its release characteristics. (From Ref. 280, used with permission.)

Table 19 Pharmacokinetics of Proxyphylline in a Timed-Release Tablet into Which Nitroglycerin Was to Be Incorporated

Biological half-life	$t_{1/2}$ = 4.3 (h)
Absorption rate constant	K_a = 1.3 (h^{-1})
Elimination rate constant	K_{el} = 0.163 (h^{-1})
Time to reach peak	T_p = 2.5 (h)
Therapeutic concentration to maintain for 12 h	B_D = 0.8 (mg/100 L)
Single dose producing desired blood level	D_B = 0.48 (g)
Liberation constant from depot phase	k_r^1 = 0.4 (h^{-1})
Equation for plasma concentration	$C = 11.5 \cdot e^{-0.153t} - 12.5 \cdot e^{-1.3t}$
Percent absorbed relative to the amount ultimately absorbed	$\dfrac{AT}{A}$, $100 = CT + K_{el}TC_{DT}$

$$
\begin{array}{rrl}
\text{Percent after } 0.25 \text{ h} &=& 35.6 \\
0.5 \text{ h} &=& 45.5 \\
1.0 \text{ h} &=& 74.4 \\
1.5 \text{ h} &=& 100.0
\end{array}
$$

Maintenance dose

$$D_M = \frac{K_{el}B_D}{k_r^1} = 0.312 \text{ (g)}$$

Initial dose

$$D_i = D_B - D_M \cdot (k_r^1 T_p) = 0.177 \text{ (g)}$$

Total dose per tablet

$$W = D_B - D_M \cdot (k_r^1 T_p) + \frac{K_{el}B_D}{k_r^1} = 0.489 \text{ (g)}$$

Source: From Ref. 280, used with permission.

EXPERIMENTAL DESIGN. The pertinent design variables for this dosage form are shown in Table 19. Nitroglycerin was dissolved in 1:1 alcohol/acetone solvent and was then impregnated in plastic granules of either polyvinylchloride, ethylcellulose, polyamide, polyvinylacetate, or polyacrylate. The plastic granules must be partly soluble in the alcohol/acetone solvent. The solvent was evaporated and the plastic mass containing nitroglycerin with screened to particle sizes of 0.5−1.0 mm. These particles were then mixed with proxyphylline and compressed into tablets. The final two-layered tablet contained 0.2 mg nitroglycerin and 180 mg proxyphylline in the immediate-release coat and 5 mg of nitroglycerin, in a solid−solid solution matrix with the plastic material, and 310 mg of proxyphylline in the matrix pores, constituted the sustaining section.

IN VITRO TEST. The results of in vitro testing of the tablet are shown in Figure 14. The solid and open circles indicate that good sustainment is achieved with this tablet and that if accidental mastication occurs, as illustrated by the other lines in the figure, some of the sustaining effect is lost. Proxyphylline was released with an apparent first-order rate of $k_r^1 = 0.40$ h^{-1} and nitroglycerin had $k_r^1 = 0.092$ h^{-1}. The data indicate that the proxyphylline, incorporated into the pores of the matrix, dissolves as soon as the artificial gastrointestinal fluid enters the pores resulting 95% release within 5 h. Nitroglycerin, because it is dissolved into the plastic matrix as a solid−solid solution, must diffuse through the plastic material into the artificial gastrointestinal fluid. Consequently, its release is much slower, resulting in only about 45% being released within 5 h.

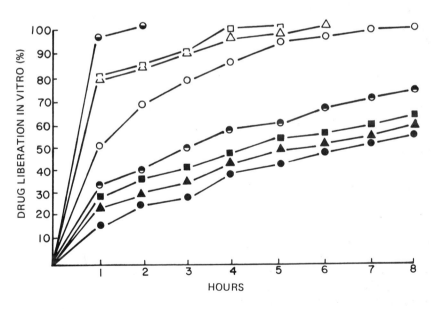

Figure 14 In vitro drug liberation. Proxyphylline: (○) intact tablet, (△) cut into two parts, (□) cut into four parts, (◒) powdered. Nitroglycerin: (●) intact tablets, (▲) cut into two parts, (■) cut into four parts, (◓) powdered. (From Ref. 280, used with permission.)

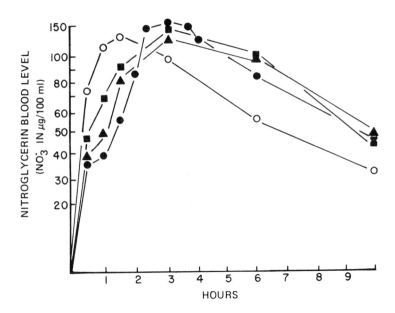

Figure 15 Nitroglycerin blood level after peroral administration. (●) intact tablet, (▲) cut into two parts, (■) cut into four parts, and (○) powdered and masticated. (From Ref. 280, used with permission.)

Although the in vitro release study showed that in divided tablets the prolonged activity was essentially lost for proxyphylline, the nitroglycerin still maintained its sustaining activity.

IN VIVO TEST. Figure 15 shows the results of the in vivo testing for sustained release of nitroglycerin in these products. These are the mean curves from three human subjects. As stated by the author, three subjects is too small a population to generate definitive statistics, so that this study should be repeated with more subjects. The results did indicate good sustained release of nitroglycerin and served as a useful experimental guide.

D. Sustained Release Utilizing Osmosis

An example of sustained release through osmosis is the so-called osmotic tablet [11,12,311]. The coating in this case is just a semipermeable membrane that allows penetration of water, but not drug, to dissolve its contents. The dissolved drug plus diluents establishes an osmotic pressure and forces drug solution to be pumped out of a small hole in the tablet coating. The rate of this drug pumping can be controlled through core composition, coating material, and delivery orifice. A pictorial representation of the osmotic tablet is shown in Figure 16.

The tablet imbibes fluid through its semipermeable membrane at a constant rate determined by membrane permeability and by osmotic pressure of the core formulation. With the system at a constant internal volume, the

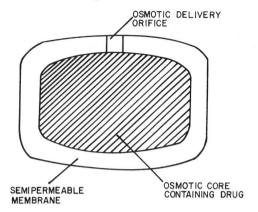

Figure 16   Elementary osmotic pump cross section. (From Ref. 12, used with permission.)

tablet will delivery, in any time interval, a volume of saturated solution equal to the volume of solvent uptake. The delivery rate is constant as long as an excess of solid is present inside the device, declining parabolically toward zero once the concentration falls below saturation, as is shown in Figure 17.

The principles upon which this device is based were presented earlier in this chapter. A key factor in proper drug delivery is the size of the

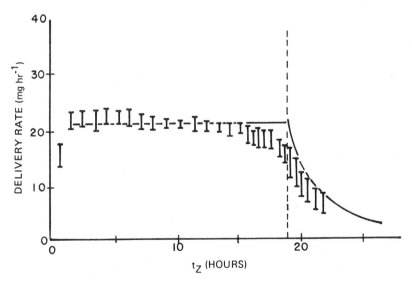

Figure 17   In vitro release rate of potassium chloride from elementary osmotic pump in water at 37°C. (I) range of experimental data obtained from five systems, (———) calculated release rate. (From Ref. 12, used with permission.)

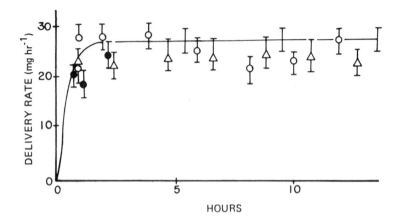

Figure 18   In vitro and in vivo release rate of potassium chloride from elementary osmotic pumps.   (———) average in vitro rate from systems of the same batch; and ($\triangle$), ($\circ$), ($\bullet$) average release rate in one system in the GI tract of dogs 1, 2, and 3, plotted at the total time period each system resided in the dog.   (From Ref. 12, used with permission.)

delivery orifice.   Two conditions must be met, relative to the size of the delivery orifice, in order for it to be successful.

1.   It must be smaller than a maximum size, A_{max}, to minimize the contribution to the delivery rate made by solute diffusion through the orifice.
2.   It must be sufficiently large, above a minimum size, A_{min}, to minimize hydrostatic pressure inside the system that would affect the zero-order release rate.

Too small a hole will depress the delivery rate below that of the desired constant delivery.

In vivo tests in three dogs are shown in Figure 18.   That zero-order release is maintained for long periods is evident.

It should be quite obvious from the mechanistic description of this apparatus that drug delivery would be independent of stirring rate and independent of pH.   These are sizable advantages to a sustained release system and have indeed been shown operable both in vitro and in vivo.

V.   COATING MATERIALS

Other sections of this text have dealt with coating substances insofar as describing their properties, coating technology, quality control, etc. Some of these coating materials, for conventional coating purposes, can be employed to produce sustained-release products depending on the thickness of coat employed as well as addition of fillers to the coating substance.   Table 20 lists some of the more common coating substances and their properties.   This listing is not intended to be comprehensive, but

Table 20 Coating Materials and Their Properties

Type of coating	Most suitable dosage form(s)	Examples	Probable release mechanisms	Properties
Barrier coating (includes microencapsulation)	1. Film-coated tablets	Various shellacs [18]	1. Diffusion and dialysis	1. Slow or incomplete release
	2. Film-coated pellets or granules placed in gelatin capsules	Beeswax [18]	2. Some disintegration possible	2. Coating is subject to fracture during compression
	3. Compressed tablets containing mixtures of barrier-coated particles with filler particles	Glyceryl monostearate [18]	3. Also have had pH-dependent dissolution and some enzymatic breakdown incorporated into some films, but these are, therefore, poor "barriers"	3. Release depends on solubility of the drug and pore structure of the membrane
	4. Compressed tablets containing only barrier-coated particles forming a matrix	Nylon [18]		4. Obtain constant release when water or GI fluids pass through barrier to dissolve drug and form a saturated solution within the tablet
		Acrylic resins [18]		
		Cellulose acetate butyrate [20]		
		dl-Polylactic acid [20]		
		1,6-Hexanediamine [20]		
		Diethylenetriamine [20]		
		Polyvinylchloride [20]		
		Sodium carboxymethylcellulose [243]		
		Various starches [244]		
		Polyvinylpyrrolidone [245]		
		Acetylated monoglycerides [245]		
		Gelatin coacervates [211]		
		Styrene/maleic acid copolymer [245]		

Table 20 (Continued)

Type of coating	Most suitable dosage form(s)	Examples	Probable release mechanisms	Properties
Barrier coating (includes microencapsulation) (cont)		Gelatin coacervates [88] Styrene/maleic acid copolymer [124]		1. Slow or incomplete release 2. Difficult to control release pattern due to variations in pH and enzyme content of the GI tract
Embedment into a fatty coating (similar to embedding in a matrix of fatty materials)	1. Compressed granules into a tablet 2. Compressed granules placed in a gelatin capsule 3. Multilayered tablets 4. Compression-coated tablets	Glycerol palmitostearate [18] Beeswax [18] Glycowax [18] Castor wax [18] Carnauba wax [18] Glyceryl monostearate [18] Stearyl alcohol [18]	1. Gradual erosion of the coat, aided by pH and enzymatic hydrolysis of the fatty acid esters 2. Coating may contain portion of the dose for quick release upon hydrolysis with subsequent slow release from erosion of core	
Repeat action coatings	1. Sugar coating of an enteric-coated core tablet 2. Compression coating of an enteric-coated core tablet	Cellulose acetate phthalate [18] (Many of the examples listed for "Barrier Coating" apply here also)	1. pH-Dependent dissolution and enzymatic breakdown 2. Outer coating releases first dose rapidly in stomach fluids, inner enteric-coated core releases a second dose at	1. Variations due to changing stomach emptying times 2. Not a "true" sustained form as defined in text

	Dosage forms	Polymers	Drug-release process	Characteristics
			some later time in intestinal fluids	
Coated plastic matrix	1. Multilayer tablets 2. Compression-coated tablets	Polyethylene [18] Polyvinylacetate [18] Polymethacrylate [18] Polyvinylchloride [18] Ethylcellulose [18] Silicone devices [20] Methylmethacrylate [20] Ethylacrylate [20] 2-Hydroxyethylmethacrylate [20] 1,3-Butyleneglycoldimethacrylate [20] Ethyleneglycoldimethacrylate [20]	1. Outer coating containing active drug dissolves rapidly to provide drug for immediate absorption 2. Above process is followed by leaching of drug from inert matrix via penetration of GI fluids into pores of the matrix	1. Slow or incomplete release 2. Only water-soluble or fairly water-soluble drugs can be used 3. Plastic matrix skeleton is excreted in its original shape in the feces 4. Drug liberation depends only on solubility in GI fluids, completely independent of pH, enzyme activity, concentration, or GI motility
Coated hydrophilic matrix	1. Multilayer tablets 2. Compression-coated tablets	Carboxymethylcellulose [18] Sodium carboxymethylcellulose [18] Hydroxypropylmethylcellulose [18] Methacrylate hydrogels [19] Polyethyleneglycols [106]	1. Outer coating containing active drug dissolves rapidly along with rapid dissolution from the surface of the matrix to provide drug for immediate absorption	1. Drug liberation rate is dependent on type and amount of gum used 2. High water solubility of the drug is absolutely necessary

Table 20 (Continued)

Type of coating	Most suitable dosage form(s)	Examples	Probable release mechanisms	Properties
Coated hydro-philic matrix (cont)			2. Above process continues until a viscous gelatinous barrier is formed around the matrix surface 3. Once the gelatinous barrier has formed, diffusion and dissolution, via erosion, occur at a slow, controlled rate	3. Release is controlled by drug diffusivity more than by gum dissolution or water penetrability as long as the hydrated gelatinous layer remains intact

rather is a starting point for the formulator interested in preparing a sustained-release product through coating.

VI. SUMMARY

During the past several years we have witnessed an increased number of publications dealing with polymer coatings as a means of sustained drug action. Most of these approaches have been aimed at the parenteral or specialty areas and as yet many have not been brought to the market stage, but their potential utility is apparent. Our ability to manipulate film properties gives us a powerful tool by which to prolong drug delivery and produce variable drug release rates. It seems reasonable to conclude that we are limited in attempting to produce variable release rates from conventional tablets or pellets if we rely strictly on dissolution rates and shape factors, but the addition of polymer coatings with variable properties gives us considerable latitude in producing sustained-release products with varying release rates.

REFERENCES

1. Lipowsky, I., Australian Patent 109,438, Filed November 22, 1938.
2. Williams, A., *Sustained Release Pharmaceuticals*. Noyes Development Corp., Park Ridge, New Jersey, 1969.
3. Eriksen, S., Sustained action dosage forms. In *The Theory and Practice of Industrial Pharmacy*, 1st Ed. (L. Lachman, H. A. Lieberman, and J. L. Kanig, eds.), Lea & Febiger, Philadelphia, 1970.
4. Grief, M. and Eisen, H., Prolonged action oral medication. *Am. Prof. Pharmacist*, *25*:93 (1959).
5. Hanselmann, B. and Voight, R., Wirkungsverlangerung von arzneimitteln unter besonderer berucksichtigung der operoralen depot-arzneiform. *Pharmazie*, *26*:57 (1971).
6. Lazarus, J. and Cooper, J., Absorption, testing, and clinical evaluation of oral prolonged action drugs. *J. Pharm. Sci.* *50*:715 (1961).
7. Lazarus, J. and Cooper, J., Oral prolonged action medicaments: Their pharmaceutical control and therapeutic aspects. *J. Pharmacol.*, *11*:257 (1959).
8. Robinson, M. J., Making sustained-action oral dosage forms. *Drug Cos. Ind.*, *87*:466 (1960).
9. Stempel, E., Patents for prolonged action dosage forms. 1: General products. *Drug Cos. Ind.*, *98*:44 (1966); 2: Tablets. *Drug Cos. Ind.*, *98*:36 (1966).
10. Parrott, E. L., *Pharmaceutical Technology: Fundamental Pharmaceutics*. Burgess, Minneapolis, 1970, pp. 100−103.
11. Theeuwes, F. and Higuchi, T., U.S. Patent 3,845,770 (1974) (assigned to Alza Corp., Palo Alto, California).
12. Theeuwes, F., Elementary osmotic pump. *J. Pharm. Sci.*, *64*:1987 (1975).

13. Theeuwes, F., Ashida, K., and Higuchi, T., Programmed diffusional release rates from encapsulated cosolvent system. *J. Pharm. Sci.*, 65:648 (1976).
14. Cooper, J. and Rees, J. E., Tableting research and technology. *J. Pharm. Sci.*, *61*:1511 (1972).
15. Sjogren, J., Studies on a sustained release principle based on an inert plastic matrix. *Acta Pharm. Suecica*, *8*:153 (1971).
16. Nelson, E., Pharmaceuticals for prolonged action. *Clin. Pharmacol. Ther.*, *4*:283 (1963).
17. Edkins, R. P., The modification of the duration of drug action. *J. Pharm. Pharmacol.*, *11*:54T (1959).
18. Ritschel, W. A., Peroral solid dosage forms with prolonged action. In *Drug Design*, Vol. IV (E. J. Ariens, ed.), Academic Press, New York, 1973, pp. 37–73.
19. Andrade, J. D., *Hydrogels for Medical and Related Applications.* ACS Symposium Series 31, American Chemical Society, Washington, D.C., 1976.
20. Paul, D. R. and Harris, F. W., *Controlled Release Polymeric Formulations.* ACS Symposium Series 33, American Chemical Society, Washington, D.C., 1976.
21. Robinson, J. R., Controlled release pharmaceutical systems. In *Symposium on Economics and Market Opportunities for Controlled Release Products.* 172nd National Meeting of the American Chemical Society, San Francisco, August 29–Sept. 3, 1976, pp. 210–226.
22. Hall, H. S. and Hinkes, T. M., Air suspension encapsulation of moisture-sensitive particles using aqueous systems. In *Microencapsulation: Processes and Applications* (J. E. Vandagaer, ed.), Plenum, New York, 1974.
23. Lehmann, K., Acrylic resin coatings for drugs: Relations between their chemical structure, properties and application possibilities. *Drugs Made in Germany*, *11*(34):145–153 (1968).
24. Lehamnn, K. and Dreher, D., Permeable acrylic resin coatings for the manufacture of depot preparations of drugs. 2: Coatings of granules and pellets and preparation of matrix tablets. *Drugs Made in Germany*, *12*:59 (1969).
25. Hall, H., personal communication.
26. Kwan, K. C., Pharmacokinetic considerations in the design and evaluation of sustained and controlled release drug delivery systems. In *Sustained and Controlled Release Drug Delivery Systems* (J. R. Robinson, ed.), Marcel Dekker, New York, 1978.
27. Levy, G., Pharmacokinetic aspects of controlled drug delivery systems. In *Temporal Aspects of Therapeutics* (J. Urquhart and F. E. Yates, eds.), Vol. 2 of Alza Conference Series, Plenum, New York, 1973, pp. 107–127.
28. Soeldner, J. S., Chang, K. W., Aisenberg, S., and Hiebert, J. M., Progress towards an implantable glucose sensor and an artificial beta cell. In *Temporal Aspects of Therapeutics* (J. Urquhart and F. E. Yates, eds.), Vol. 2 of Alza Conference Series, Plenum, New York, 1973, pp. 181–207.
29. Robinson, J. R. and Eriksen, S. P., Theoretical formulation of sustained-release dosage forms. *J. Pharm. Sci.*, *55*:1254 (1966).

30. Fincher, J. H., Particle size of drugs and its relationship to absorption and activity. *J. Pharm. Sci.*, 57:1825 (1968).
31. Lee, V. H. and Robinson, J. R., Drug properties influencing the design of sustained or controlled release drug delivery systems. In *Sustained and Controlled Release Drug Delivery Systems* (J. R. Robinson, ed.), Marcel Dekker, New York, 1978.
32. Hansch, C. and Dunn, W. J., Linear relationships between lipophilic character and biological activity of drugs. *J. Pharm. Sci.*, *61*:1 (1972).
33. Fujita, T., Iwasa, J., and Hansch, C., A new substituent constant, derived from partition coefficients. *J. Am. Chem. Soc.*, *86*:5175 (1964).
34. Beerman, B., Hellstrom, K., and Rosen, A., Metabolism of propantheline in man. *Clin. Pharmacol. Ther.*, *13*:212 (1972).
35. Niebergall, P. J., Sugita, E. T., and Schnaare, R. L., Potential dangers of common drug dosing regimen. *Am. J. Hosp. Pharm.*, *31*: 53 (1974).
36. Brooke, D. and Washkuhn, R. J., Zero-order drug delivery system: Theory and preliminary testing. *J. Pharm. Sci.*, *66*:159 (1977).
37. Lipper, R. A. and Higuchi, W. I., Analysis of theoretical behavior of a proposed zero-order drug delivery system. *J. Pharm. Sci.*, *66*:163 (1977).
38. Cobby, J., Mayersohn, M., and Walker, G. C., Influence of shape factors on kinetics of drug release from matrix tablets. I: Theoretical. *J. Pharm. Sci.*, *63*:725 (1974).
39. Green, B. K., U.S. Patent 2,712,507 (1955), *Chem. Abstr. 50*:12479a (1956).
40. British Patent 490,001 (1938) through *Chem. Abstr.*, *33*:814 (1939).
41. Chang, T. M. S., *Science, 146*:524 (1964).
42. Chang, T. M. S., *Science J.*, *3*:63 (1967).
43. Deasy, P. B., *Microencapsulation and Related Drug Processes*, Marcel Dekker, New York, 1984, p. 120.
44. Asker, A. F. and Becker, C. H., *J. Pharm. Sci.*, 55:90−94 (1966).
45. Takenaka, H., Kawashima, Y., and Lin, S. Y., *J. Pharm. Sci.*, 69: 1388−1392 (1980).
46. Cusimano, A. G. and Becker, C. H., *J. Pharm. Sci.*, 5:1104−1112 (1968).
47. Hamid, I. S. and Becker, C. H., *J. Pharm. Sci.*, 59:511−514 (1970).
48. Pederson, A. M. et al., U.S. Patent 4,572,833, Feb. 25 (1986).
49. Colombo, P., Conte, U., Caramella, C., Gazzaniga, A., and LaManna, A., *J. Controlled Release*, 1:283−289 (1985).
50. U.S. Patent 3,400,185 (Sept. 3, 1968).
51. Jager, K. F. and Bauer, K. H., *Drugs Made in Germany*, 15:61−65 (1982).
52. Kawashima, Y., Ohno, H., and Takenaka, H., *J. Pharm. Sci.*, 70: 913−916 (1981).
53. U.S. Patent 4,401,456 (Aug. 30, 1983).
54. Roberts, A. G. and Shah, K. D., *Chem. Eng.*, 12:748−750 (1975).
55. Ghebre-Sellassie, I., Gordon, R. H., Fawzi, M. B., and Nesbitt, R. U., *Drug Dev. Ind. Pharm.*, 11:1523−1541 (1985).
56. Caldwell, H. C. and Rosen, E., *J. Pharm. Sci.*, 53:1387−1391 (1964).

57. U.S. Patent 4,083,949 (1978).
58. *Handbook of Avicel Spheres*, FMC Corp., Philadelphia, (1982).
59. Wan, L. S. L. and Jeyabalan, T., *Chem. Pharm. Bull.*, 33:5449–5457 (1985).
60. Conine, J. W. and Hadley, H. R., *Drug Cosmet. Ind.*, 106:38–44 (1970).
61. Jalal, I. M., Malinowski, H. J., and Smith, W. E., *J. Pharm. Sci.*, 6:1466 (1972).
62. Woodruff, C. W. and Nuessle, N. O., *J. Pharm. Sci.*, 61:787–790 (1972).
63. Malinowski, H. J. and Smith, W. E., *J. Pharm. Sci.*, 63:285–288 (1974).
64. O'Connor, R. E. and Schwartz, J. B., *Drug Dev. Ind. Pharm.*, 11:1837–1857 (1985).
65. Chien, T. Y. and Nuessle, N. O., *Pharm. Tech.*, 9(4):42–48 (1985).
66. Malinowski, H. J. and Smith, W. E., *J. Pharm. Sci.*, 64:1688–1692 (1975).
67. Scott, M. W., Robinson, M. J., Pauls, J. F., and Loritz, R. J., *J. Pharm. Sci.*, 53:670 (1964).
68. Osterwald, H. P., *Pharmaceut. Res.*, 2:14–18 (1985).
69. *Pharmaceutical Glazes Product Information Bulletin*, Somerset, New Jersey, William Zinsser & Company.
70. Stafford, J. W., *Drug Dev. Ind. Pharm.*, 8:513–530 (1982).
71. Bagaria, S. C. and Lordi, N. G., *Aqueous Dispersions of Waxes and Lipids for Pharmaceutical Coating*, Paper presented at the AAPS Second National Meeting, Boston, Massachusetts, (1987).
72. Bauer, K. H. and Osterwald, H., *Pharm. Ind.*, 41:1203–1209 (1979).
73. Pondell, R. E., *Drug Dev. Ind. Pharm.*, 10:191–202 (1984).
74. Banker, G. S. and Peck, G. E., *Pharm. Technol.*, 5(4):55–61 (1981).
75. Ghebre-Sellassie, I., Banker, G. S., and Peck, G. E., *Water-Based Controlled-Release Drug Delivery Systems*, Pharm. Tech. Conference 1982 Proceedings (Aster Publishing Corp., Springfield, Oregon, 1982), pp. 234–241.
76. Goodhart, F. W., Harris, M. R., and Nesbitt, R. W., *Pharm. Technol.* 8(4):64–71 (1984).
77. Lehman, K., *Acta Pharm. Fenn.*, 81(2):55–74 (1984).
78. Lehman, K., *Acta Pharm. Fenn.*, 91(4):225–238 (1982).
79. Lehman, K. and Dreher, D., *Int. J. Pharm. Tech. Prod. Mfr.*, 2(4):31–43 (1984).
80. Chang, R. K., Hsiao, C. H., and Robinson, J. R., *Pharm. Technol.*, 11(3):56–68 (1987).
81. Gurny, R., *Pharm. Acta Helv.*, 56(4–5):130–132 (1981).
82. Gurny, R., Peppas, N. A., Harrington, D. D., and Banker, G. S., *Drug Dev. Ind. Pharm.*, 7(1):1–25 (1981).
83. Willis, C. R. and Banker, G. S., *J. Pharm. Sci.*, 57:1598–1603 (1968).
84. Goodman, H. and Banker, G. S., *J. Pharm. Sci.*, 59:1131–1137 (1970).

85. Rhodes, C. T., Wai, K., and Banker, G. S., *J. Pharm. Sci.*, *59*: 1578–1581 (1970).
86. Rhodes, C. T., Wai, K., and Banker, G. S., *J. Pharm. Sci.*, *59*: 1581–1584 (1970).
87. Boylan, J. C. and Banker, G. S., *J. Pharm. Sci.*, *62*:1177–1183 (1973).
88. Larson, A. B. and Banker, G. S., *J. Pharm. Sci.*, *65*:838–843 (1976).
89. Garden, J. L., *High Polymers*, *29*:143–197 (1977).
90. Woods, M. E., Dodge, J. S., Krieger, I. M., and Pierce, P. E., *J. Paint. Technol.*, *40*(527):541–548 (1968).
91. Hansmann, J., *Adhaesian*, *20*(10):272–275 (1976).
92. Vanderhoff, J. W. et al., U.S. Patent 4,177,177 (Dec. 4, 1979).
93. Sanders, F. L. et al., U.S. Patent 3,652,676 (Feb. 15, 1972).
94. Burke, O. W., Jr., U.S. Patent 3,652,482 (1972).
95. Miller, A. L. et al., U.S. Patent 3,022,260 (1962).
96. Aelony, D. et al., U.S. Patent 2,899,397 (1959).
97. Burton, G. W. and O'Farrell, C. P., *Rubber Chem. Technol.*, *49*(2): 394 (1976).
98. Chang, R. K., Price, J. C., and Whitworth, C. W., *Pharm. Technol.*, *10*(10):24–33 (1986).
99. Chang, R. K., Price, J. C., and Whitworth, C. W., *Drug Dev. Ind. Pharm.*, *13*:1119–1135 (1987).
100. Chang, R. K., Price, J. C., and Whitworth, C. W., *Drug Dev. Ind. Pharm.*, *12*:2335, 2380 (1986).
101. Cooper, W., U.S. Patent 3,009,891 (1961).
102. Date, M. et al., Jpn. Patent 7306,619 (1973).
103. Warner, G. L. et al., U.S. Patent 4,123,403 (Oct. 31, 1978).
104. Leng, D. E. et al., U.S. Patent 4,502,888 (Mar. 5, 1985).
105. Judd, P., Brit. Patent 1,142,375 (1969).
106. Dieterich, D., Keberle, W., and Wuest, R., *J. Oil Col. Chem. Assoc.*, *53*(5):363–379 (1969).
107. Gurny, R., Bindschaedler, C., and Doelker, E., *Recent Advances in Latex Technology*, Proceedings Intern. Symp. Control. Rel. Bioact. Mater. 13, 1986 (Controlled Release Society, Inc., Lincolnshire, Illinois), pp. 130–131.
108. Li, L. C. and Peck, G. E., *Water Based Silicone Elastomer Dispersions as Controlled Release Tablet Coating (I) — Preliminary Evaluation of the Silicone Elastomer Dispersions*, Proceedings Intern. Symp. Control. Rel. Bioact. Mater., 14, 1987 (Controlled Release Society, Inc., Lincolnshire, Illinois), pp. 148–149.
109. Li, L. C. and Peck, G. E., *Water Based Silicone Elastomer Dispersions as Controlled Release Tablet Coating (II) — Formulation Considerations*, Proceedings Intern. Symp. Control. Rel. Bioact. Mater., 14, 1987 (Controlled Release Society, Inc., Lincolnshire, Illinois), pp. 150–151.
110. Mehta, A. M. and Jones, D. M., *Pharm. Technol.*, *9*(6):52–60 (1985).
111. *Sono-Tek Ultrasonic Nozzles*, Technical Information Bulletin, Poughkeepsi, New York, Sono-Tek Corporation, 1984.
112. Bindsschaedler, C., Gurny, R., and Doelker, E., *Labo-Pharma-Probl. Tech.*, *31/311*:389–394 (1983).

113. *Standard Test Method for Minimum Film Formation Temperature of Emulsion*, American Society for Testing and Materials, Designation D2354-81, pp. 407–409 (1981).

114. *Standard Test Method for Transition Temperature of Polymer by Thermal Analysis*, American Society for Testing and Materials, Designation D3418-75, pp. 840–843 (1976).

115. *Modern Plastics Encyclopedia*, McGraw-Hill, New York, 1984–1985, pp. 635–644.

116. U.K. patent Application GB 086725A.

117. Conte, U., Colombo, P., Caramella, C., and LaMonna, A., *Farmaco Ed. Pract.*, *39*:67 (1984).

118. Salomon, J. L., Doelker, E., and Buri, P., *Pharm. Ind.*, *41*:799 (1979).

119. Bludbaugh, F., Zapapas, J., and Sparks, M., *J. Am. Pharm. Assoc. (Sci. Ed.)*, *47*, *12*:857–870 (1958).

120. Decoursin, J. W., *Conference Proceedings of the Latest Developments in Drug Delivery Systems*, Aster Publishing Corp., 1985, pp. 29–32.

121. Sheth, P. R. and Tossounian, J., *Drug Dev. Ind. Pharm.*, *10*: 313–339 (1984).

122. Huber, H. F., Dale, L. B., and Christensen, G. L., *J. Pharm. Sci.*, *55*:974 (1966).

123. Kaplan, L. L., *J. Pharm. Sci.*, *54*:457 (1965).

124. Kornblum, S. S., *J. Pharm. Sci.*, *58*:125 (1969).

125. Lapidus, H. and Lordi, N. G., *J. Pharm. Sci.*, *55*:840 (1966).

126. Huber, H. F. and Christensen, G. L., *J. Pharm. Sci.*, *57*:164 (1968).

127. Baun, D. C. and Walker, G. C., *Pharm. Acta Helv.*, *46*:94 (1971).

128. Choalis, N. H. and Papadopoulos, H., *J. Pharm. Sci.*, *64*:1033 (1975).

129. Lapidus, H. and Lordi, N. G., *J. Pharm. Sci.*, *57*:1272 (1968).

130. Nystrom, C., Mazur, J., and Sjorgren, J., *Int. J. Pharm.*, *10*: 209–218 (1982).

131. Touiton, E. and Donbrow, M., *Int. J. Pharm.*, *11*:131–148 (1982).

132. Daly, P. B., Davis, S. S., and Kennerley, J. W., *Int. J. Pharm.*, *18*:201–205 (1984).

133. Buri, B. and Doelker, E., *Pharm. Acta Helv.*, *55*(7–8):189–197 (1980).

134. *Handbook on Methocel Cellulose Ester Products*, Dow Chemical Company, Midland, Michigan, 1984.

135. Raghunathan, Y. and Becker, C. H., *J. Pharm. Sci.*, *57*:1748 (1968).

136. Cusimano, A. G. and Becker, C. H., *J. Pharm. Sci.*, *57*:1104 (1968).

137. John, P. H. and Becker, C. H., *J. Pharm. Sci.*, *57*:584 (1968).

138. Robinson, M. J., Bondi, A., and Swintosky, J. V., *J. Am. Pharm. Assoc. Sci. Ed.*, *47*:874 (1958).

139. Kowarski, C. R., Volberger, B., Versanno, J., and Kowanski, A., *Am. J. Hosp. Pharm.*, *21*:409 (1964).

140. Yamamoto, R. and Baba, M., Jpn. Patent 1849,1960, through *Chem. Abstr.* 54,20100d, 1960.

141. Draper, E. B. and Becker, C. H., *J. Pharm. Sci.*, *55*:376 (1966).
142. Robinson, I. C. and Becker, C. H., *J. Pharm. Sci.*, *57*:49 (1968).
143. Lazarus, J., Pagliery, M., and Lachman, L., *J. Pharm. Sci.*, *53*: 798 (1964).
144. Sjogren, J. and Fryklof, L. E., *Pharm. Rev.*, *59*:171 (1960).
145. Rowe, R. C., *Manuf. Chem. Aerosol News*, *46*(3):23 (1975).
146. Desai, S. J., Simonelli, A. P., and Higuchi, W. I., *J. Pharm. Sci.*, *54*:1459 (1965).
147. Farhadien, B., Borodkin, S., and Buddenhagen, J. D., *J. Pharm. Sic.*, *60*:209 (1971).
148. Rowe, R. C., Elworthy, P. H., and Ganderton, D., *J. Pharm. Pharmacol.*, *24*(Suppl.):137P (1972).
149. Endicott, C. J., U.S. Patent 3,087,860 (1963).
150. Singh, P., Desai, S. J., Simonelli, A. P., and Higuchi, W. I., *J. Pharm. Sci.*, *56*:1542 (1967).
151. Farhadien, B., Borodkin, S., and Buddenhagen, J. P., *J. Pharm. Sci.*, *60*:212 (1971).
152. Rowe, R. C., Elworthy, P. H., and Ganderton, D., *J. Pharm. Pharmacol.*, *25*(Suppl.):112P (1973).
153. Rowe, R. C., Elworthy, P. H., and Ganderton, D., *J. Pharm. Pharmacol.*, *25*(Suppl.):12P (1973).
154. Desai, S. J., Singh, P., Simonelli, A. P., and Higuchi, W. I., *J. Pharm. Sci.*, *55*:1235 (1966).
155. Chang, R. C. and Price, J. C., *J. Biomater. Appl.*, *3*(1):80 (1988).
156. Jalsenjak, I., Nixon, J. R., Senjkovic, R., and Stivic, I., *J. Pharm. Pharmacol.*, *32*:678 (1984).
157. Jalsenjak, I., Nicolaidon, C. F., and Nixon, J. R., *J. Pharm. Pharmacol.*, *29*:169 (1977).
158. Nixon, J. R., Jalsenjak, I., Nicolaidon, C. F., and Harris, M., *Drug Dev. Ind. Pharm.*, *4*:117 (1978).
159. Nixon, J. R. and Agyilirah, G. A., *J. Pharm. Sci.*, *73*:52 (1984).
160. Chemtob, C., Chaumeil, J. C., and N'Dongo, M., *Int. J. Pharm.*, *29*:83 (1986).
161. Hasagawa, A., Nakagawa, H., and Sugimoto, I., *Yakugaku Zasshi*, *104*:889 (1984).
162. Walker, S. E., Ganley, J., and Eaves, T., *Tableting Properties of Potassium Chloride Microcapsules*. In F.I.P. Abstracts, 37th International Congress of Pharmaceutical Congress of Pharmaceutical Sciences, The Hague, Sept. 1977, p. 31.
163. Abdel Monem Sayed, H. and Price, J. C., *Drug Dev. Ind. Pharm.*, *12*:577 (1986).
164. Colbert, J. C., Controlled action drug forms. In *Chemical Technology Review*, No. 24, Noyes Data Corp., Park Ridge, New Jersey, 1974.
165. Johnson, J. C., Tablet manufacture. In *Chemical Technology Review*, No. 30, Noyes Data Corp., Park Ridge, New Jersey, 1974.
166. Green, M. A., One year's experience with sustained release antihistamine medication. *Ann. Allergy*, *12*:273 (1954).
167. Rogers, H. L., Treatment of allergic conditions with sustained release chlorpropenypyridamine maleate. *Ann. Allergy*, *12*:266 (1954).

168. Berkowitz, D., The effect of a long-acting preparation (Spansule) of belladonna alkaloids on gastric secretion of patients with peptide ulcer. *Gastroenterology, 30*:608 (1956).

169. Morrison, S., The use of a sustained release tranquilizer-anticholinergic combination in patients with disturbed digestive function. *Am. J. Gastroenterol., 29*:518 (1958).

170. Grahn, H. V., Antihypertensive effects of reserpine in sustained-release form: A comparative study. *J. Am. Geriatr. Soc., 6*:671 (1958).

171. Burness, S. H., Clinical evaluation of a sustained release belladonna preparation. *Am. J. Dig. Dis., 22*:111 (1955).

172. Heimlich, K. R., MacDonnell, D. R., Flanagan, T. L., and O'Brien, P. D., Evaluation of a sustained release form of phenylpropanolamine hydrochloride by urinary excretion studies. *J. Pharm. Sci., 50*:232 (1961).

173. Heimlich, K. R., MacDonnell, D. R., Polk, A., and Flanagan, T. L., Evaluation of an oral sustained release dosage form of trimeprazine as measured by urinary excretion. *J. Pharm. Sci., 50*: 213 (1961).

174. Vasconcellos, J. and Kurland, A. A., Use of sustained-release chlorpromazine in the management of hospitalized chronic psychotic patients. *Dis. Nerv. Sys., 19*:173 (1958).

175. Souder, J. C. and Ellenbogen, W. C., Laboratory control of dextroamphetamine sulfate sustained release capsules. *Drug Stand., 26*: 77 (1958).

176. Steigmann, F., Kaminski, L., and Nasatir, S., Clinical-experimental evaluation of a prolonged-acting antispasmodic-sedative. *Am. J. Dig. Dis., 4*:534 (1959).

177. Mellinger, T. J., Serum concentrations of thioridazine after different oral medication forms. *Am. J. Psychiatry, 121*:1119 (1965).

178. Hollister, L. E., Studies of prolonged-action medication. II: Two phenothiazine tranquilizers (thioridazine and chlorpromazine) administered as coated tablets and prolonged action preparations. *Curr. Ther. Res., 4*:471 (1962).

179. Mellinger, T. J., Mellinger, E. M., and Smith, W. T., Thioridazine blood levels in patients receiving different oral forms. *Clin. Pharmacol. Ther., 6*:486 (1965).

180. Vestre, N. D. and Schiele, B. C., An evaluation of slow-release and regular thioridazine and two medication schedules. *Curr. Ther. Res., 8*:585 (1966).

181. Swintosky, J. V., Design of oral sustained-action dosage forms. *Drug Cosmet. Ind., 87*:464 (1960).

182. Blythe, R. H., The formulation and evaluation of sustained release products. *Drug Stand., 26*:1 (1958).

183. Wagner, J. G., Carpenter, O. S., and Collins, E. J., Sustained action oral medication. I: A quantitative study of prednisolone in man, in the dog and in vitro. *J. Pharmacol. Exp. Ther., 129*:101 (1960).

184. Nash, J. F. and Crabtree, R. E., Absorption of tritiated d-desoxyephedrine in sustained-release dosage forms. *J. Pharm. Sci., 50*: 134 (1961).

185. Rosen, E. and Swintosky, J. V., Preparation of a ^{35}S labeled trimeprazine tartrate sustained action product for its evaluation in man. *J. Pharm. Pharmacol.*, *12*:237T (1960).

186. Hollister, L. E., Studies of delayed-action medication. I: Meprobamate administered as compressed tablets and as two delayed-action capsules. *N. Engl. J. Med.*, *266*:281 (1962).

187. Rosen, E., Tannenbaum, P., Ellison, T., Free, S. M., and Crosley, A. P., Absorption and excretion of radioactively tagged dextroamphetamine sulfate from a sustained-release preparation. *J.A.M.A.*, *194*:145 (1965).

188. Sugerman, A. A. and Rosen, E., Absorption efficiency and excretion profile of a prolonged-action form of chlorpromazine. *Clin. Pharmacol. Ther.*, *5*:561 (1964).

189. Rosen, E., Ellison, T., Tannenbaum, P., Free, S. M., and Crosley, A. P., Comparative study in man and dog of the absorption and excretion of dextroamphetamine-^{14}C sulfate in sustained-release and nonsustained-release dosage forms. *J. Pharm. Sci.*, *56*:365 (1967).

190. Rosen, E., Polk, A., Free, S. M., Tannenbaum, P. J., and Crosley, A. P., Comparative study in man of the absorption and excretion of amobarbital-^{14}C from sustained-release and nonsustained-release dosage forms. *J. Pharma. Sci.*, *56*:1285 (1967).

191. Khali, S. A. H. and Elgamal, S. S., In vitro release of aspirin from various wax-coated formulations. *J. Pharm. Pharmacol.*, *23*:72 (1971).

192. Royal, J., In vitro method for the determination of the rate of release of amphetamine sulfate from sustained release medication. *Drug Stand.*, *26*:41 (1958).

193. Royal, J., A comparison of in vitro rates of release of several brands of dextroamphetamine sulfate sustained release capsules. *Drug Stand.*, *27*:1 (1959).

194. Campbell, J. A., Nelson, E., and Chapman, D. G., Criteria for oral sustained release medication with particular reference to amphetamine. *Can. Med. Assoc. J.*, *81*:15 (1959).

195. Nash, R. A. and Marcus, A. D., An in vitro method for the evaluation of sustained release products. *Drug Stand.*, *28*:1 (1960).

196. Vliet, E. B., A suggested in vitro procedure for measuring the rate of drug release from timed release tablets and capsules. *Drug Stand.*, *27*:97 (1959).

197. Beckett, A. H. and Tucker, G. T., A method for the evaluation of some oral prolonged-release forms of dextroamphetamine in man, using urinary excretion data. *J. Pharm. Pharmacol.*, *18*:72S (1966).

198. Campbell, J. A., Evaluation of sustained-action release rates. *Drug Cosmet. Ind.*, *87*:620 (1960).

199. Ipsen, J., Mathematical relationship of in vitro release rates and biological availability of controlled-release nitroglycerin (Nitrong). *Curr. Ther. Res.*, *13*:193 (1971).

200. Feinblatt, T. M. and Ferguson, E. A., Timed-disintegration capsules. An in vivo roentgenographic study. *N. Engl. J. Med.*, *254*:940 (1956).

201. Feinblatt, T. M. and Ferguson, E. A., Timed-disintegration capsules (Tympcaps): A further study. An in vivo roentgenographic study,

blood level study and relief of anginal pain with pentaerythritol
tetranitrate. *N. Engl. J. Med.*, *256*:331 (1957).

202. Aming, Y. M. and Nagwekar, J. B., Rationale for apparent differences in pharmacokinetic aspects of model compounds determined
from blood level data and urinary excretion data in rats. *J. Pharm.
Sci.*, *65*:1341 (1976).

203. Henning, R. and Nyberg, G., Serum quinidine levels after administration of three different quinidine preparations. *Eur. J. Clin.
Pharmacol.*, *6*:239 (1973).

204. Green, D. M., Tablets of coated aspirin microspherules: A new
dosage form. *J. New Drugs*, *6*:294 (1966).

205. Magee, K. R. and Westerberg, M. R., Treatment of myasthenia
gravis with prolonged-action mestinon. *Neurology*, *9*:348 (1959).

206. Cass, L. J. and Frederik, W. S., Clinical comparison of a sustained-
and a regular-release aspirin. *Curr. Ther. Res.*, *7*:673 (1965).

207. Cass, L. J. and Frederik, W. S., A clinical evaluation of a sustained-release aspirin. *Curr. Ther. Res.*, *7*:683 (1965).

208. Sirine, G., Microencapsulation. *Drug Cosmet. Ind.*, *101*:56
(Sept. 1967).

209. Luzzi, L., Microencapsulation. *J. Pharm. Sci.*, *59*:1367 (1970).

210. Bakan, J. A. and Sloan, F. D., Microencapsulation of drugs. *Drug
Cosmet. Ind.*, *110*:34 (March 1972).

211. Nixon, J. R. and Walker, S. E., The in vitro evaluation of gelatin
coacervate microcapsules. *J. Pharm. Pharmacol.*, *23*:147S (1971).

212. Matthews, B. R. and Nixon, J. R., Surface characteristics of
gelatin microcapsules by scanning electron microscopy. *J. Pharm.
Pharmacol.*, *26*:383 (1974).

213. Tanaka, N., Takino, S., and Utsumi, I., A new oral gelatinized
sustained-release dosage form. *J. Pharm. Sci.*, *52*:664 (1963).

214. Phares, R. E. and Sperandio, G. J., Coating pharmaceuticals by
coacervation. *J. Pharm. Sci.*, *53*:515 (1964).

215. Madan, P. L., Luzzi, L. A., and Price, J. C., Microencapsulation
of a waxy solid: Wall thickness and surface appearance studies.
J. Pharm. Sci., *63*:280 (1974).

216. Madan, P. L., Luzzi, L. A., and Price, J. C., Factors influencing
microencapsulation of a waxy solid by complex coacervation.
J. Pharm. Sci., *61*:1586 (1972).

217. Luzzi, L. A. and Gerraughty, R. J., Effects of selected variables
on the microencapsulation of solids. *J. Pharm. Sci.*, *56*:634 (1967).

218. Merkle, H. P. and Speiser, P., Preparation and in vitro evaluation
of cellulose acetate phthalate coacervate microcapsules. *J. Pharm.
Sci.*, *62*:1444 (1973).

219. Luzzi, L. A. and Gerraughty, R. J., Effect of additives and formulation techniques on controlled release of drugs from microcapsules.
J. Pharm. Sci., *56*:1174 (1967).

220. Birrenbach, G. and Speiser, P. P., Polymerized micelles and their
use as adjuvants in immunology. *J. Pharm. Sci.*, *65*:1763 (1976).

221. McGinity, J. W., Cobs, A. B., and Martin, A. N., Improved method
for microencapsulation of soluble pharmaceuticals. *J. Pharm. Sci.*,
64:889 (1975).

222. Khanna, S. C., Jecklin, T., and Speiser, P., Bead polymerization technique for sustained-release dosage form. *J. Pharm. Sci.*, 59: 614 (1970).

223. Khanna, S. C. and Speiser, P., In vitro release of chloramphenicol from polymer beads of α-methacrylic acid and methylmethacrylate. *J. Pharm. Sci.*, 59:1398 (1970).

224. Seager, H. and Baker, P., The preparation of controlled release particles in the subsieve size range. *J. Pharm. Pharmacol.*, 24: 123P (1972).

225. Croswell, R. W. and Becker, C. H., Suspension polymerization for preparation of timed-release dosage forms. *J. Pharm. Sci.*, 63:440 (1974).

226. Willis, C. R. and Banker, G. S., Polymer-drug interacted systems in the physicochemical design of pharmaceutical dosage forms. I: Drug salts with PVM/MA and with a PVM/MA hemi-ester. *J. Pharm. Sci.*, 57:1598 (1968).

227. Goodman, H. and Banker, G. S., Molecular-scale drug entrapment as a precise method of controlled drug release. I: Entrapment of cationic drugs by polymeric flocculation. *J. Pharm. Sci.*, 59:1131 (1970).

228. Rhodes, C. T., Wai, K., and Banker, G. S., Molecular scale drug entrapment as a precise method of controlled drug release. II: Facilitated drug entrapment to polymeric colloidal dispersion. *J. Pharm. Sci.*, 59:1578 (1970).

229. Rhodes, C. T., Wai, K., and Banker, G. S., Molecular scale drug entrapment as a precise method of controlled drug release. III: In vitro and in vivo studies of drug release. *J. Pharm. Sci.*, 59:1581 (1970).

230. Boyland, J. C. and Banker, G. S., Molecular-scale drug entrapment as a precise method of controlled drug release. IV: Entrapment of anionic drugs by polymeric gelation. *J. Pharm. Sci.*, 62:1177 (1973).

231. Larson, A. B. and Banker, G. S., Attainment of highly uniform drug dispersions employing molecular scale drug entrapment in polymeric latices. *J. Pharm. Sci.*, 65:838 (1976).

232. Bell, S. A., Berdick, M., and Holliday, W. M., Drug blood levels as indices in evaluation of a sustained-release aspirin. *J. New Drugs*, 6:284 (1966).

233. Rotstein, J., Estrin, I., Cunningham, C., Gilbert, M., Jordan, A., Lamstein, J., Safrin, M., Wimer, E., and Silson, J., The use of a sustained-release aspirin preparation in the management of rheumatoid arthritis and osteoarthritis. *J. Clin. Pharmacol.*, 7:97 (1967).

234. Draper, E. B. and Becker, C. H., Some wax formulations of sulfaethylthiadiazole produced by aqueous dispersion for prolonged-release medication. *J. Pharm. Sci.*, 55:376 (1966).

235. Robinson, I. C. and Becker, C. H., Sulfaethylthiadiazole (SETD) release from synthetic wax prolonged-release particles. I: Effect of dispersant concentration. *J. Pharm. Sci.*, 57:49 (1968).

236. John, P. M. and Becker, C. H., Surfactant effects on spray-congealed formulations of sulfaethylthiadiazole-wax. *J. Pharm. Sci.*, 57:584 (1968).

237. Cusimano, A. G. and Becker, C. H., Spray-congealed formulations of sulfaethylthiadiazole (SETD) and waxes for prolonged-release medication. Effect of wax. *J. Pharm. Sci.*, 57:1104 (1968).

238. Raghuathan, Y. and Becker, C. H., Spray-congealed formulations of sulfaethylthiadiazole (SETD) and waxes for prolonged-release medication. Effect of modifiers. *J. Pharm. Sci.*, 57:1748 (1968).

239. Hamid, I. S. and Becker, C. H., Release study of sulfaethylthiadiazole (SETD) from a tablet dosage form prepared from spray-congealed formulations of SETD and wax. *J. Pharm. Sci.*, 59:511 (1970).

240. Wurster, D. E., U.S. Patent 2,648,609 (August 11, 1953).

241. Wurster, D. E., U.S. Patent 2,799,241 (July 16, 1957).

242. Doerr, D. W., Series, E. R., and Deardorff, D. L., Tablet coatings: Cellulosic high polymers. *J. Am. Pharm. Assoc., Sci. Ed.*, 43:433 (1954).

243. Gagnon, L. P., DeKay, H. G., and Lee, C. O., Coating of granules. *Drug Stand.*, 23:47 (1955).

244. Ahsan, S. S. and Blaug, S. M., A study of tablet coating using polyvinylpyrrolidone and acetylated monoglyceride. *Drug Stand.*, 26:29 (1958).

245. Wagner, J. G., Veldkamp, W., and Long, S., Enteric coatings. IV: In vivo testing of granules and tablets coated with styrene-maleic acid copolymer. *J. Am. Pharm. Assoc., Sci. Ed.*, 49:128 (1960).

246. Kleber, J. W., Nash, J. F., and Lee, C. C., Synthetic polymers as potential sustained-release coatings. *J. Pharm. Sci.*, 53:1519 (1964).

247. Asker, A. F. and Becker, C. H., Some spray-dried formulations of sulfaethylthiadiazole for prolonged-release medication. *J. Pharm. Sci.*, 55:90 (1966).

248. Lappas, L. C. and McKeehan, W., Polymeric pharmaceutical coating materials. II: In vivo evaluation as enteric coatings. *J. Pharm. Sci.*, 56:1257 (1967).

249. Seidler, W. M. K. and Rowe, E. J., Influence of certain factors on the coating of a medicinal agent on core tablets. *J. Pharm. Sci.*, 57:1007 (1968).

250. Powell, D. R. and Banker, G. S., Chemical modifications of polymeric film systems in the solid state. I: Anhydride acid conversion. *J. Pharm. Sci.*, 58:1335 (1969).

251. Tsevdos, T. J., Press-coated and multi-layer tablets. *Drug Cosmet. Ind.*, 78:38 (1956).

252. Windheuser, J. and Cooper, J., The pharmaceutics of coating tablets by compression. *J. Am. Pharm. Assoc., Sci. Ed.*, 45:542 (1956).

253. Cooper, J. and Pasquale, D., The present status of compression coating. *Pharm. J.*, 181:397 (1958).

254. Lachman, L., Speiser, P. P., and Sylwestrowicz, H. D., Compressed coated tablets. I: Measurement and factors influencing core concentration. *J. Pharm. Sci.*, 52:379 (1963).

255. Wurster, D. E., Air-suspension technique of coating drug particles. A preliminary report. *J. Am. Pharm. Assoc., Sci. Ed.*, 48:451 (1959).

256. Wurster, D. E., Preparation of compressed tablet granulations by the air-suspension technique. II. *J. Am. Pharm. Assoc., Sci. Ed., 49*:82 (1960).

257. Coletta, V. and Rubin, H., Wurster coated aspirin. I: Film-coating techniques. *J. Pharm. Sci., 53*:953 (1964).

258. Wood, J. H. and Syarto, J., Wurster coated aspirin. II: An in vitro and in vivo correlation of rate from sustained-release preparations. *J. Pharm. Sci., 53*:877 (1964).

259. Donbrow, M. and Friedman, M., Timed release from polymeric films containing drugs and kinetics of drug release. *J. Pharm. Sci., 64*: 76 (1975).

260. Higuchi, T., Mechanism of sustained-action medication. Theoretical analysis of rate of release of solid drugs dispersed in solid matrices. *J. Pharm. Sci., 52*:1145 (1963).

261. Borodkin, S. and Tucker, F. E., Drug release from hydroxypropyl cellulose-polyvinyl acetate films. *J. Pharm. Sci., 63*:1359 (1974).

262. Borodkin, S. and Tucker, F. E., Linear drug release from laminated hydroxypropyl cellulose-polyvinyl acetate films. *J. Pharm. Sci., 64*: 1289 (1975).

263. Bercher, P. R., Bevans, D. W., Gormley, J. D., Hubbard, R. E., Sullivan, D. D., Stevenson, C. R., Thomas, J. B., Goldman, R., and Silson, J. E., Sinusule: Timed-release therapy in allergic rhinitis, with human in vivo release rates and clinical statistics. *Curr. Ther. Res., 9*:379 (1967).

264. Sjogren, J. and Fryklof, L. W., Duretter: A new type of oral sustained action preparation. *Farm. Rev. (Stockh.), 59*:171 (1960).

265. Cooper, J., Lontab repeat action tablets. *Drug Cosmet. Ind., 81*: 312 (1957).

266. Sjogren, J. and Ostholm, I., Absorption studies with a sustained release tablet. *J. Pharm. Pharmacol., 13*:496 (1961).

267. Sjogren, J. and Ervik, M., A method for release rate determination from sustained-release tablets. *Acta Pharm. Suecica, 1*:219 (1964).

268. Collins, R. L. and Doglia, S., Theory of controlled release of biologically active substances. *Arch. Environ. Contam. Toxicol., 1*: 325 (1973).

269. El-Egakey, M. A., El-Khawas, F., El-Gindy, N. A., and Abdel-Khalik, M., Release study of some drugs from polymeric matrices. *Pharmazie, 29*:286 (1974).

270. Asker, A. F., Motawi, A. M., and Abdel-Khalek, M. M., A study of some factors affecting the in vitro release of drug from prolonged release granulations. I: Effect of method of preparations. *Pharmazie, 26*:170 (1971).

271. Asker, A. F., Motawi, A. M., and Abdel-Khalek, M. M., A study of some factors affecting the in vitro release of drug from prolonged release granulations. 2: Effect of dissolution retardent. *Pharmazie, 26*:213 (1971).

272. Asker, A. F., Motawi, A. M., and Abdel-Khalek, M. M., A study of some factors affecting the in vitro release of drug from prolonged release granulations. 3: Effects of particle size, enzymatic contents of pepsin and pancreatin, bile and ionic concentration. *Pharmazie, 26*:215 (1971).

273. Lapidus, H. and Lordi, N. G., Some factors affecting the release of a water-soluble drug from a compressed hydrophilic matrix. *J. Pharm. Sci.*, 55:840 (1966).

274. Huber, H. E., Dale, L. B., and Christenson, G. L., Utilization of hydrophilic gums for the control of drug release from tablet formulations. I: Disintegration and dissolution behavior. *J. Pharm. Sci.*, 55:974 (1966).

275. Javoid, K. A., Fincher, J. H., and Hartman, C. W., Timed-release tablets employing lipase-lipid-sulfamethiazole systems prepared by spray-congealing. *J. Pharm. Sci.*, 60:1709 (1971).

276. Javaid, K. A. and Hartman, C. W., Blood levels of sulfamethizole in dogs following administration of timed-release tablets employing lipase-lipid-drug systems. *J. Pharm. Sci.*, 61:900 (1972).

277. Farhadieh, B., Borodkin, S., and Buddenhagen, J. D., Drug release from methyl acrylate-methyl methacrylate copolymer matrix. II: Control of release rate by exposure to acetone vapor. *J. Pharm. Sci.*, 60:212 (1971).

278. Elbert, W. R., Morris, R. W., Rowles, S. G., Russell, H. T., Born, G. S., and Christian, J. E., In vivo evaluation of absorption and excretion of pentylenetetrazol-10-^{14}C from sustained-release and nonsustained-release tablets. *J. Pharm. Sci.*, 59:1409 (1970).

279. Farhadieh, B., Borodkin, S., and Buddenhagen, J. D., Drug release from methyl acrylate-methyl methacrylate copolymer matrix. I: Kinetics of release. *J. Pharm. Sci.*, 60:209 (1971).

280. Ritschel, W. A., Influence of formulating factors on drug safety of timed-release nitroglycerin tablets. *J. Pharm. Sci.*, 60:1683 (1971).

281. Sjuib, F., Simonelli, A. P., and Higuchi, W. I., Release rates of solid drug mixtures dispersed in inert matrices. III: Binary mixture of acid drugs released into alkaline media. *J. Pharm. Sci.*, 61:1374 (1973).

282. Sjuib, F., Simonelli, A. P., and Higuchi, W. I., Release rates of solid drug mixtures dispersed in inert matrices. IV: Binary mixture of amphoteric drugs released into reactive media. *J. Pharm. Sci.*, 61:1381 (1972).

283. Goodhart, F. W., McCoy, R. H., and Ninger, F. C., Release of a water-soluble drug from a wax matrix timed-release tablet. *J. Pharm. Sci.*, 63:1748 (1974).

284. Choulis, N. H. and Papadopoulos, H., Timed-release tablets containing quinine sulfate. *J. Pharm. Sci.*, 64:1033 (1975).

285. Chien, Y. W., Lambert, H. J., and Lin, T. K., Solution-solubility dependency of controlled release of drug from polymer matrix: Mathematical analysis. *J. Pharm. Sci.*, 64:1643 (1975).

286. Desai, S. J., Simonelli, A. P., and Higuchi, W. I., Investigation of factors influencing release of solid drug dispersed in inert matrices. *J. Pharm. Sci.*, 54:1459 (1965).

287. Desai, S. J., Singh, P., Simonelli, A. P., and Higuchi, W. I., Investigation of factors influencing release of solid drug dispersed in inert matrices. II: Quantitation of procedures. *J. Pharm. Sci.*, 55:1224 (1966).

288. Desai, S. J., Singh, P., Simonelli, A. P., and Higuchi, W. I., Investigation of factors influencing release of solid drug dispersed

in inert matrices. III. Quantitative studies involving the poly-ethylene plastic matrix. *J. Pharm. Sci.*, 55:1230 (1966).

289. Desai, S. J., Singh, P., Simonelli, A. P., and Higuchi, W. I., Investigation of factors influencing release of solid drug dispersed in inert matrices. IV: Some studies involving the polyvinyl chloride matrix. *J. Pharm. Sci.*, 55:1235 (1966).

290. Singh, P., Desai, S. J., Simonelli, A. P., and Higuchi, W. I., Release rates of solid drug mixtures dispersed in inert matrices. I: Noninteracting drug mixtures. *J. Pharm. Sci.*, 56:1542 (1967).

291. Singh, P., Desai, S. J., Simonelli, A. P., and Higuchi, W. I., Release rates of solid drug mixtures dispersed in inert matrices. II: Mutually interacting drug mixtures. *J. Pharm. Sci.*, 56:1548 (1967).

292. Singh, P., Desai, S. J., Simonelli, A. P., and Higuchi, W. I., Role of wetting on the rate of drug release from inert matrices. *J. Pharm. Sci.*, 57:217 (1968).

293. Schwartz, J. B., Simonelli, A. P., and Higuchi, W. I., Drug release from wax matrices. I: Analysis of data with first-order kinetics and with the diffusion-controlled model. *J. Pharm. Sci.*, 57:274 (1968).

294. Schwartz, J. B., Simonelli, A. P., and Higuchi, W. I., Drug release from wax matrices. II: Application of a mixture theory to the sulfanilamide-wax system. *J. Pharm. Sci.*, 57:278 (1968).

295. Levy, G. and Hollister, L. E., Dissolution rate limited absorption in man. Factors influencing drug absorption from prolonged-release dosage form. *J. Pharm. Sci.*, 54:1121 (1965).

296. Nicholson, A. E., Tucker, S. J., and Swintosky, J. V., Sulfaethyl-thiadiazole. VI: Blood and urine concentrations from sustained and immediate release tablets. *J. Am. Pharm. Assoc., Sci. Ed.*, 49:40 (1960).

297. Kaplan, L. L., Determination of in vivo and in vitro release of theophylline aminoisobutanol in a prolonged-action system. *J. Pharm. Sci.*, 54:457 (1965).

298. Lackenbacher, R. S., Chlortrimeton maleate repeat action tablets in the treatment of pruritic dermatoses. *Ann. Allergy*, 10:765 (1952).

299. Bancroft, C. M., Tripelenamine hydrochloride and chlorprophen-pyridamine maleate. A comparison of their efficacies in the treatment of hay fever. *Ann. Allergy*, 15:297 (1957).

300. Fuller, H. L. and Kassel, L. E., Sustained-release triethanolamine trinitrate biphosphate (Metamine) in angina pectoris. *Antibiot. Med.*, 3:322 (1956).

301. DeRitter, E., Evaluation of nicotinic alcohol Timespan tablets in humans by urinary excretion tests. *Drug Stand.*, 28:33 (1960).

302. Cass, L. J. and Frederik, W. S., Clinical evaluation of long-release and capsule forms of pentobarbital sodium. *Curr. Ther. Res.*, 4:263 (1962).

303. Webster, J. J., Treatment of iron deficiency anemia in patients with iron intolerance: Clinical evaluation of a controlled-release form of ferrous sulfate. *Curr. Ther. Res.*, 4:130 (1962).

304. Morrison, B. O., Tolerance to oral hematinic therapy: Controlled-release versus conventional ferrous sulfate. *J. Am. Geriatr. Soc.*, 14:757 (1966).

305. Crosland-Taylor, P. and Keeling, D. H., A trial of slow-release tablets of ferrous sulphate. *Curr. Ther. Res.*, 7:244 (1965).

306. Tarpley, E. L., Controlled-release potassium supplementation. *Curr. Ther. Res.*, *16*:734 (1974).

307. O'Reagan, T., Prolonged release aspirin. *Drug. Cosmet. Ind.*, *98*: 35 (April 1966).

308. Wiseman, E. H. and Federici, N. J., Development of a sustained-release aspirin tablet. *J. Pharm. Sci.*, 57:1535 (1968).

309. Wiseman, E. H., Plasma salicylate concentrations following chronic administration of aspirin as conventional and sustained-release tablets. *Curr. Ther. Res.*, *11*:681 (1969).

310. Harris, R. and Regalado, R. G., A clinical trial of a sustained-release aspirin in rheumatoid arthritis. *Ann. Phys. Med.*, 9:8 (1967).

311. Chandraesekaran, S. K., Benson, H., and Urquhart, J., Methods to achieve controlled drug delivery: The biomedical engineering approach, pp. 557—593. In *Sustained and Controlled Release Drug Delivery Systems* (J. R. Robinson, ed.), Marcel Dekker, New York, 1978.

5

The Pharmaceutical Pilot Plant

Charles I. Jarowski

St. John's University, Jamaica, New York

I. INTRODUCTION

A. Primary Functions of the Pharmaceutical Pilot Plant

The primary responsibility of the pilot plant staff is to ensure that the newly formulated tablets developed by product development personnel will prove to be efficiently, economically, and consistently reproducible on a production scale. Attention must be given to the cost of manufacture, since low production costs provide a competitive advantage. This is especially for tablets containing generic drugs. As a consequence, well-designed tablet formulas must be processed intelligently to insure that each unit operation is optimized. Thus, final compression conducted at a rapid rate is economically advantageous. However, some of this advantage will be lost if excessive production times are required and undesirable yield losses accrue during the blending, granulating, drying, and compression steps. Furthermore, excessive strain on the tablet presses can lead to the need for both more frequent press repair and resurfacing of the tablet punch faces.

The manufacturing instructions transferred to the production department should be clearly written, readily understood, and unambiguous. The widespread use of word processors makes standardization of such procedures desirable. Attention should be given to the use of in-house production equipment, unless sufficient data has been accumulated to support the economic advantage of purchasing new equipment. Alternate manufacturing equipment and procedures may also be required for international companies intending to manufacture pharmaceutical products at several sites.

The physical properties and specifications for the manufactured tablet formulation should match those established earlier by the product formulator, the pilot plant staff, and the quality control department. Therefore, the tablets manufactured on a production scale should possess the proper weight, thickness, and content uniformity. Tablet hardness, disintegration, and dissolution rates in simulated gastrointestinal media must be consistently attainable to ensure optimal bioavailability.

Additional responsibilities for pilot plant personnel include the evaluation of new processing equipment and aiding in finding causes and providing solutions for problems that occasionally arise during routine tablet manufacture. The manufacturer of quality tablets at a rate of 10,000 per minute attests to the competence of tablet technologists. Such achievements have been made possible by the interaction of skilled research, process development, and production personnel. Manufacturers of processing equipment have also played key roles by supplying excellent apparatus for improving unit operations, such as particle size reduction, mixing, drying, granulating, compressing, and coating.

II. SELECTED FACTORS TO BE CONSIDERED DURING DEVELOPMENT

The establishment of ideal formulations and procedures for plant manufacture must take into account a variety of factors.

A. Efficient Flow of Granules

The high speed of tablet manufacture currently attainable requires that the granule flow from hopper to die cavity be unimpeded. To accomplish such desired free flow, several parameters need study. First of all, the particle size distribution of the granules must be accurately defined. The addition of glidants such as talc, starch, and magnesium stearate may be indicated for the large-scale manufacture of the tablet formulas developed in the laboratory.

The efficiency of granule flow can be checked in the pilot plant by conducting experiments under extended running conditions at high speed. Tablets produced for at least 3 to 4 h will possess uniform weight and hardness if granule flow has been efficient. Granule flow may be judged to be satisfactory and still tablet weight and hardness may be unsatisfactory. Such deficiencies in many instances can be corrected by increasing the concentration of fines.

B. Ease of Compression, Speed of Manufacture, Yield of Finished Tablets

Tableting equipment, punches, and dies will require less maintenance if tablets are routinely easily compressed. Excessive compressional forces applied in the manufacture of tablets will lead to an increased frequency of maintenance and repair. Tablets that are produced under such conditions are apt to possess excessive hardness, and are apt to exhibit reduced dissolution rates and erratic bioavailability.

A high yield of finished tablets and the speed of their manufacture are obvious economic advantages that an ideal formulation should ensure.

C. Content Uniformity

The use of finely milled ingredients in tablet manufacture is advantageous. The oral absorption efficiency of poorly soluble neutral drugs is improved as their surface area in the intestinal tract is increased. Granulations prepared with such finely milled material and excipients possessing coarser particle size may lead to classification problems under high-speed, large-scale tablet manufacture. Particle size distribution and blending time must be well defined during the product development stage to avoid unacceptable variation in drug concentration between individual tablets.

D. Advantage of Accurately Defined Variables

Process development pharmacists must conduct well-controlled scale-up experiments on the tablet formulations developed in the laboratory. Such variables as drying time, residual moisture, granule particle size distribution, percentage of fines, and compressional force should be accurately defined within specified limits. Deleterious effects encountered outside these specified limits should also be recorded. Such detailed data developed during the pilot stage will become valuable as tableting problems arise in future production runs.

Reworking a production batch of tablets not meeting quality control standards has been complicated by recent rulings by the U.S. Food and Drug Administration (FDA). The reason for the poor content uniformity, the poor dissolution rate, or some discoloration, for example, must be discovered and explained before reworking of such batches can be considered. The value of a well-equipped pilot plant manned with a skilled staff will become increasingly apparent to managers of a pharmaceutical company whose volume and variety of tablets produced is increasing.

III. TYPES OF ORGANIZATIONAL STRUCTURES RESPONSIBLE FOR PILOT OPERATIONS

The types of organizational structures found in the drug-manufacturing industry depends upon a number of factors. In a small company, there may not be space allocated for pilot development of tablet formulations. The tablet formulator in the product development department may be responsible for the first few production batches of tablets. Most likely he or she would also be called upon to aid in the solution of problems encountered in future batches.

In a large organization, a pharmaceutical development team may be responsible for the transfer of new tablet formulations to production. A well-equipped space for conducting scale-up runs of new tablets will also be provided in such an organization. Such a developmental team may report administratively to the head of pharmaceutical research and development. In other instances, such a group will be a part of the production division.

The various types of organizational structures that can exist for pharmaceutical pilot development are mentioned below.

A. Research Pharmacist Responsible for Initial Scale-Up and Initial Production Runs

Figure 1 represents an example of an organizational structure wherein no direct responsibility exists administratively for the pilot operation. This abbreviated structure is concerned only with administrative responsibility for the research and production of tablet dosage forms. The solid lines connecting the boxes represent administrative lines of authority and responsibility. The broken lines represent lines of communication.

In such an organizational structure, direct responsibility rests with the director of pharmaceutical research and development and the manager of solid-dosage form research. The tablet formulators, who report administratively to the manager, are responsible for the scale-up and initial production runs of their tablet formulations.

There are advantages that can be cited for such an arrangement. Thus, the tablet formulators who know the most about their new tablet are directly involved with the manager and section head in the production division, who will be responsible for the routine manufacture of their tablet. Communicating such information as stability data, physical properties, and the reasons for the procedure adopted is best conveyed by the tablet formulator, who alone is aware of the variations in formulation that were investigated. Several batches of the preferred tablet formula had to be

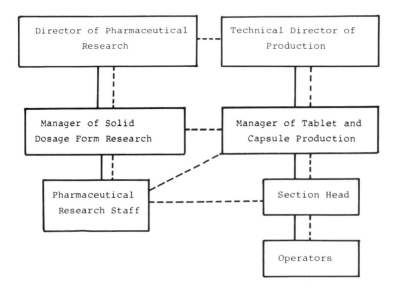

Figure 1   Abbreviated organizational diagram of a pharmaceutical company where no direct responsibility exists administratively for the pilot operation.

prepared for accelerated and long-term stability testing. In addition, many clinical batches may also have been prepared by the tablet formulator.

The advantage that accrues to the production division is that individuals with the most technical information concerning the new tablet are directly involved in the initial production runs of the new formula. The tablet formulators from the research division will also gain from such an arrangement. They in turn gain valuable experience concerning the types of problems that can arise during the large-scale manufacture of their tablets. Such experience will serve to improve their competence in developing future tablet products.

There are disadvantages that can be cited for such a working relationship. Assigning the research division the responsibility for the first three to five production batches means a significant commitment of research time. The research pharmacist may strive to develop formulations and procedures which are preferred by the production division in order to avoid complaints. Thus, for example, resistance to a direct-compression or double-compression procedure might be encountered. The heavy investment in equipment suitable for wet granulation methodology by the production division will naturally result in their continuing support for such procedures.

A person not thoroughly familiar with the production division's equipment, materials, etc., could cause unnecessary expense in urging the acquisition of new manufacturing equipment. Furthermore, a product development pharmacist is not as familiar with the plant operations as a pilot plant person whose job responsibility necessitates knowing the production division's personnel and facilities.

In a small company — where equipment and personnel are limited — the tablet formulator can more readily introduce a formula due to the limitations of facilities and personnel. In a big company, the pilot laboratory is called upon to bridge the gap between the production and research divisions. Manufacturing problems can arise with different lots of bulk materials. Efficient problem solving will be favored if the troubleshooter is familiar with the production division's facilities and has a good working relationship with research and production personnel.

The objective of the research pharmacist is to develop practical tablet formulas that cause minimal manufacturing problems. However, he or she must not become complacent. A less practical, more expensive procedure may produce a tablet exhibiting superior bioavailability. Such a formula modification may be difficult to promote within an organization while patent protection exists for the drug in the less-efficient tablet. The alert and capable tablet formulator will not wait for generic competition to initiate such an improvement in oral absorption through the use of a new manufacturing procedure.

Formulations that are manufactured very efficiently can still be improved by using less-expensive excipients. Automated procedures can significantly reduce manufacturing costs. Such improvements can only be made after an investment of time and effort. Frequent interruptions in research effort result when the research pharmacist is called upon to search for the solution to a problem that has arisen during the manufacture of a tablet formulation developed by him or her. Such interruptions are unfortunate because they are distracting and disruptive to long-term research.

B. Pharmaceutical Pilot Plant Controlled
    by Pharmaceutical Research

The abbreviated organizational diagram depicting such an administrative
structure is shown in Figure 2. There are a number of advantages in this
type of organizational structure. Thus, newly hired research pharmacists
can include service in the pharmaceutical pilot plant in their orientation
program. The scheduling of scale-up runs is under the research division's
control. Clinical supplies of a new drug in a tablet dosage form should be
controlled by the research division when it is prepared in the pilot plant.
If any scale-up problems are encountered in the preparation of clinical
lots, corrective measures, such as dosage formulation modification, can be
made immediately. Such corrective measures should be made as rapidly as
possible to ensure that the formulation being clinically evaluated will be
the one ultimately marketed and that it will prove to be practical to manufacture.

The pharmaceutical research and development division is dedicated to
developing dosage forms of new drugs and to search for more economical
manufacturing procedures and formulations. Thus, it is expected that in a
pilot plant under research control, new processing equipment, automated
procedures, and alternate excipients will be actively investigated. Ideally,
the pharmaceutical pilot plant facility should be located close to the manufacturing unit. With such proximity several advantages accrue:

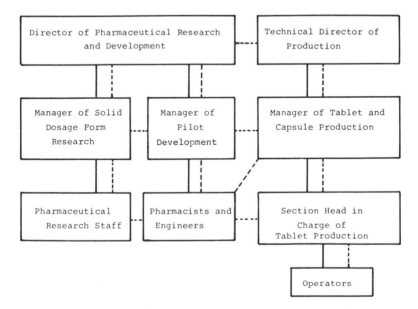

Figure 2   Abbreviated organizational diagram of a pharmaceutical company
where direct responsibility for the pilot plant is under the research
division.

1. Scale-up runs can be readily observed by members of the production and quality control divisions.
2. Supplies of excipients and drugs, cleared by the quality control division, can be drawn from the more spacious areas provided to the production division.
3. Supplies of packaging material will be easily accessible.
4. Access to engineering department personnel is provided for equipment installation, maintenance, and repair.
5. Subdivision and packaging of clinical supplies will be expidited by temporarily borrowing personnel from the production division.

The principal disadvantage that can arise from such an organizational structure is that inadequate time may be provided to solving production problems when they arise. The fact that such problems arise unpredictably makes it difficult to justify maintaining an adequately staffed troubleshooting team in the production division. An experienced pilot plant development team is technically trained to solve such problems. Its frequent interaction with both research and production personnel provides this team with an excellent base of diverse information which is of value in troubleshooting. All that would seem to be needed to surmount this possible disadvantage is the assignment of priorities by closely cooperating heads of production and research.

C. Pharmaceutical Pilot Plant Controlled by the Production Division

Pilot development of tablet formulations from the research division under such an organizational structure would be carried out by personnel reporting administratively to the production division. The abbreviated organizational diagram depicting this is shown in Figure 3.

In such an organization, the responsibility of the tablet formulator is to establish the practicality of his or her formula and manufacturing procedure in pilot plant equipment. Such equipment is most likely to be similar to that used in the production division. This similarity is advantageous because a successful scale-up in the pilot plant augers well for future success in large-scale manufacturing equipment.

The frequency of direct interaction of the tablet formulator with production personnel in the manufacturing area will be reduced under this organizational structure. The presence of a pilot plant team will make it likely that manufacturing problems will be directed to their own pilot plant personnel. High priority can be assigned because the pilot plant is under the control of the production division. Thus, any troubleshooting that is required will be initiated expeditiously. Having competent individuals in the pilot plant will serve to reduce interruptions on the research effort by the production division.

On the other hand, initiation of a developmental project that may require pilot plant equipment not representative of production models is likely to meet resistance. The pressures of manufacturing a line of products on schedule is bound to make the pilot group ever sensitive to production priorities. As a consequence, a sustained commitment on the development of new manufacturing procedures is likely to be assigned a lower priority.

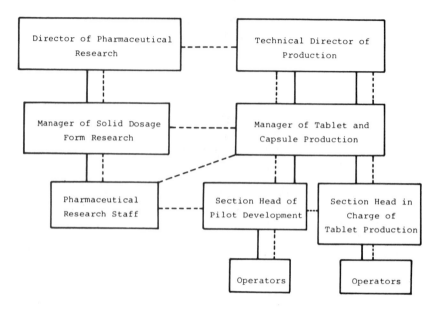

Figure 3   Abbreviated organizational diagram of a pharmaceutical company where direct responsibility for the pilot operation is under the production division.

IV. EDUCATIONAL BACKGROUNDS OF PILOT PLANT PERSONNEL

Pilot plant staff members concerned with the development of tablets should understand the functions of the ingredients used, the various unit operations involved, and the general methods of preparing tablets. They should possess knowledge of the physicochemical factors which could adversely affect the bioavailability of the drug component from a tablet dosage form. In addition, good communication skills, both oral and written, are essential because these individuals must frequently interact with members of the pharmaceutical research and production divisions.

An individual with graduate training in industrial pharmacy is well qualified for such a responsibility. Industrial pharmacy core curricula and electives usually include the following courses: product formulation (lecture and laboratory), manufacturing pharmacy (lecture and laboratory), industrial pharmacy, biopharmaceutics, homogeneous systems, pharmaceutical engineering, evaluation of pharmaceutical dosage forms, pharmaceutical materials, regulatory aspects of drug production and distribution, principles of quality assurance, reaction kinetics, and physical chemistry of macromolecules.

Tablet production operations are by no means static. The following technological trends attest to anticipated production complexity: (1) preparing tablets by continuous processing, (2) aqueous film coating, (3) direct compression of tablets, and (4) use of fluid-bed technology in granulating powder blends and in coating tablets. The addition of mechanical and chemical engineers would be advantageous in the selection of new equipment offerings being considered for such operations as well as in the organization of the most economical sequence of unit operations.

Whatever the technological trend, once the goals are defined, the best combination of trained personnel can be determined for the pilot plant.

V.   PILOT PLANT DESIGN FOR TABLET DEVELOPMENT

The 1979 amendments of Current Good Manufacturing Practices of the Food and Drug Act are fairly comprehensive with respect to the design, maintenance, and cleanliness of a production facility used in the manufacture of drugs and their various dosage forms. One of the paragraphs of the regulations on Current Good Manufacturing Practices reads as follows:

> Buildings shall be maintained in a clean and orderly manner and shall be of suitable size, construction and location to facilitate adequate cleaning, maintenance and proper operations in the manufacturing, processing, packaging, labelling or holdings of a drug.

Thus, a drug shall be deemed to be adulterated if the methods used for its manufacture, processing, packaging, or holding are not operated in conformity with good manufacturing practice. The above regulations apply to the pilot plant area as well, since it serves as the site for the preparation of clinical supplies of drugs in various dosage forms.

The design and construction of the pharmaceutical pilot plant for tablet development should incorporate features necessary to facilitate maintenance and cleanliness. If possible, it should be located on the ground floor to expedite the delivery and shipment of supplies. Extraneous and microbiological contamination must be guarded against by incorporating the following features in the pilot plant design:

1. Fluorescent lighting fixtures should be the ceiling flush type.
2. The various operating areas should have floor drains to simplify cleaning.
3. The area should be air conditioned and humidity controlled (75°F and 50% relative humidity). The ability to maintain a much lower relative humidity in a confined area may be desired if special processing conditions are required, such as the development of effervescent tablets. In other areas, only clean but not conditioned air is needed, such as in the site where the fluid-bed dryer is installed.
4. High-density concrete floors should be installed in all areas where there is heavy traffic or materials handling.
5. The walls in the processing and packaging areas should be enamel cement finish on concrete masonry for ease of maintenance and cleanliness.
6. Equipment in the pharmaceutical pilot plant should be similar to that used by the production division in the manufacture of tablets. The diversity of equipment on hand should enable the developmental team to conduct unit operations in a variety of ways. Space should be provided for evaluating new pieces of equipment.

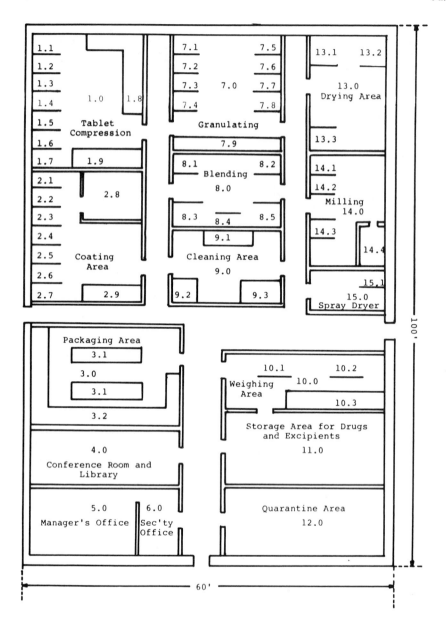

Figure 4   Floor plan for tablet development.

A typical floor plan is shown in Figure 4; the floor plan reference is shown in Table 1. A typical floor plan for a small pilot plant is shown in Figure 5, and its reference is shown in Table 2. The variety of equipment installed must be narrow because of space limitations. However, efficient use of such limited space can be made by borrowing from the production division, as needed, portable tablet presses, mills, and coating pans.

Table 1   Floor Plan Reference for the Tablet Development Area (Fig. 4)

1.0 Tablet compression room	2.8 Area for preparing syrups, solutions, and suspensions for sugar or film coating
1.1 Heavy-duty tablet press for dry granulation	
1.2 Rotary tablet press, 54 stations	2.9 Bench top with wall cabinets
	3.0 Packaging area
1.3 Rotary tablet press, 16 stations	3.1 Work tables
1.4 Compression-coating tablet press	3.2 Storage cabinets containing packaging supplies
1.5 Single-punch tablet press	4.0 Conference room and library
1.6 Tablet deduster	5.0 Manager's office
1.7 Storage cabinet for the punches and dies	6.0 Secretarial office
	7.0 Granulating area
1.8 Bench top with wall cabinets	7.1 Comminuting mill
Ancillary equipment: balances, friabilator, disintegration-testing apparatus, dissolution-testing apparatus, hardness tester	7.2 Sigma blade mixer
	7.3 Planetary-type mixer
	7.4 Tornado mill
	7.5 Fluidized bed spray granulator
1.9 Bench top with wall cabinets	7.6 Comminuting equipment
Ancillary supplies: tools, vacuum cleaner	7.7 Extructor
	7.8 Chilsonator
2.0 Coating area	7.9 Bench top with wall cabinets
2.1 Coating pan, 36-in diameter	8.0 Blending area
2.2 Coating pan, 30-in diameter	8.1 V shaped blender with intensifier bar, 1 ft^3 capacity
2.3 Coating pan, 20-in diameter	
2.4 Perforated coating pan, 24-in diameter	8.2 V shaped blender with intensifier bar, 5 ft^3 capacity
2.5 Polishing pan	8.3 V shaped blender with intensifier bar, 20 ft^3 capacity
2.6 Fluidized bed coating apparatus	
	8.4 Ribbon blender
2.7 Airless spray equipment	8.5 Lodige blender

Table 1 (Continued)

9.0 Cleaning area	13.0 Drying area
9.1 Sink	13.1 Tray and truck dryer
9.2 Ultrasonic cleaner	13.2 Fluidized bed dryer
9.3 Bench top with wall cabinets	13.3 Freeze dryer
10.0 Weighing area	14.0 Milling area
10.1 Scale	14.1 Hammer mill
10.2 Scale	14.2 Ball mill
10.3 Bench top with wall cabinets	14.3 Muller
Small scales and balances positioned on bench top	14.4 Fluid energy mill (micronizer), 2 in diameter
11.0 Storage area for drugs and excipients	15.0 Spray-drying area
12.0 Quarantine area	15.1 Spray-dryer

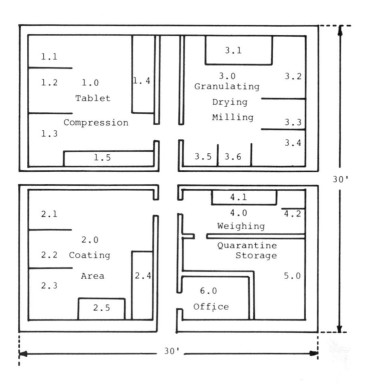

Figure 5   Floor plan for a small pilot plant for tablet development.

Table 2 Floor Plan Reference for the Small Pilot Plant (Fig. 5)

1.0 Tablet compression room	2.4 Area for preparing syrups, solutions, and suspensions for sugar or film coating
1.1 Tablet press, single-punch	
1.2 Rotary tablet press, 16 stations	2.5 Sink
1.3 Tablet deduster	3.0 Granulating, drying, and milling area
1.4 Bench top with wall cabinets	3.1 Tray and truck dryer
Ancillary equipment: balances, friabilator, disintegration-testing apparatus, dissolution-testing apparatus, hardness tester	3.2 Hobart mixer
	3.3 Comminuting mill
	3.4 Hammer mill
1.5 Bench top with wall cabinets	3.5 Fluidized bed dryer
Ancillary supplies: tools, vacuum cleaner	3.6 V-shaped blender with intensifier bar
2.0 Coating area	4.0 Weighing area
2.1 Polishing pan, 36-in diameter	4.1 Bench top with wall cabinets
2.2 Coating pan, 36-in diameter	4.2 Scale
2.3 Airless spray equipment	5.0 Quarantine and storage area
	6.0 Office

VI. PAPER FLOW BETWEEN RESEARCH, QUALITY CONTROL, AND PRODUCTION

When the tablet formulation has reached the pilot developmental stage it becomes the responsibility of the tablet formulator to issue clearly written instructions for its manufacture. In addition, analytical specifications for the ingredients must be thoroughly delineated. Thus, for example, the use of micronized drug may be specified. The in-process steps describing the milling conditions to be followed must be spelled out. In addition, particle size characterization of the micronized material must be included. In other instances, the latter characterization would be included as a quality control responsibility for purchased micronized bulk drug. The tablet formulator is well aware of the need to use micronized material on the basis of dissolution studies conducted during the early stages of formula development. When bulk drug specifications are being established, such information is related to members of the quality control and production divisions. A raw material (RM) number is designated for the micronized bulk drug along with any physical or chemical information deemed significant. Melting point is not only an important indication of the purity of a compound, it also serves as an additional checkpoint for the desired polymorphic form on a crystalline compound. A stringently low trace metal content may be specified in some instances if improved drug stability dictates it.

Specification Number RM 1000		Product Description
Specification Classification Release and Purchase		Ascorbic Acid, USP, FCC Empirical Formula $C_6H_8O_6$ Molecular Weight 176.13
Specification Effective Date 7/11/80	Supersedes 10/10/79	
Page 1 of 1	Grade Tablet	
Label Claim if Applicable Description		white, practically odorous, crystalline powder with a pleasantly tart taste
Specific Rotation at 25°C		+20.5 to 21.5°C
Heavy Metals		Maximum 20 ppm
Lead		Maximum 10 ppm
Arsenic		Maximum 3 ppm
Residue on Ignition		Maximum 0.1%
Assay		Minimum 99%
Mesh Size		100% through a No. 20 U.S. Std sieve
		Maximum 60% through a No. 80 sieve
		Maximum 8% through a No. 200 sieve

Figure 6   Example of a specification sheet for a bulk vitamin.

    A typical specification sheet for ascorbic acid is shown in Figure 6. As there may be several grades or particle sizes of ascorbic acid within the company, it is important to remember to specify the desired grade (in this example, RM-1000).

    Figures 7−9 illustrate manufacturing instructions for tablets containing 50 mg of hydrochlorothiazide. On the first sheet (Fig. 7) are listed the ingredients, the amounts per tablet, and the amounts of each required for the batch size. At the top of the figure there appears the words "product code number." Such a designation will help to avoid confusion by the various departments involved in the manufacture and release of the finished tablets. There may be hydrochlorothiazide tablet potencies other than 50 mg also being manufactured in the company. When a new drug is to be marketed in a tablet dosage form, a new product code number is assigned and subsequently used.

    There are columns headed by the words "compounded by" and "checked by." When each ingredient is weighed the individual who made the weighing puts his or her initials along side the ingredient weight; the observer

Product and Potency Hydrochlorthiazide Tablets, 50 mg		Product Code Number	Lot Number		Page 1 of 3		
		Batch Size 5,000,000	Date Started	Date Completed			
		Prepared By	Production Approval	Quality Control Approval			
Number	Ingredient	Grade	Grams/Tablet	Grams/Batch	Compounded By	Checked By	RM #	Lot #
1	Hydrochlorthiazide	U.S.P.	0.050	250,000				
2	Microcrystalline Cellulose (PH 101)	N.F.	0.050	250,000				
3	Dicalcium phosphate, dihydrate	N.F.	0.099	495,000				
4	Magnesium Stearate	N.F.	0.001	5,000				
	Total		0.200	1,000,000				

Figure 7   List of ingredients used in manufacturing hydrochlorothiazide tablets (50 mg) as they would appear in a set of manufacturing instructions.

Product and Potency Hydrochlorthiazide Tablets, 50 mg	Product Code Number	Lot Number	Page 2 of 3	
Steps	Manufacturing Instructions		Compounded By	Checked By
1	Pass items 1, 2 and 3 through a #16 screen using a comminuting mill to break up any lumps.			
2	Blend the three ingredients in a V shaped blender for 1 hour.			
3	Add the magnesium stearate and continue blending for 15 minutes.			
4	Subdivide the blended material into polyethylene-lined drums. Submit representative samples to the Quality Control division to determine if the blend is homogeneous.			
5	Upon receipt of clearance from Quality Control, tablet the blend with 5/16" standard, round concave punches on the 54 station, rotary tablet machine.			
6	Submit representative samples of the finished tablets to the Quality Control division for final release.			

Figure 8   An example of manufacturing instructions for the preparation of tablets.

Product and Potency Hydrochlorthiazide Tablets, 50 mg	Product Code Number	Lot Number	Page 3 of 3

Tablet Specifications

Weight of Tablet	0.200 g
Weight Range	0.190 - 0.210 g
Potency	50 mg/tablet
Range in Potency	46.25 - 53.75 g /tablet
Hardness Range	7 - 9 (Strong-Cobb units)
Disintegration Time	Less than 5 minutes (U S P method)
Dissolution Rate	60% of the labeled potency shall dissolve within 30 minutes (U S P method)
Color of Tablet	White

Figure 9 An example of a tablet specification form which is attached to the manufacturing instructions.

of the operation also places his or her initials as a double check on the accuracy of the weighing operation. A similar procedure should be followed for each step in the compounding operation. Such double checking is required by the Food and Drug Administration for all new drug application-type products. However, even if it were not required, such a double-checking procedure should be followed to ensure that there are no weighing or compounding errors.

The lot number of each ingredient used must be recorded. Such recordings become of special importance when one is attempting to trace the history of a particular batch of tablets. Troubleshooting will be simplified in some instances by tracing the source of a raw material. A typical problem that may arise can be due to a particular lot number of a substandard excipient that could have been inadvertently used.

On the second sheet of the proposed manufacturing instructions (see Fig. 7) the stepwise procedure to be followed is described. The words chosen should be readily understood by the variety of individuals who will be reading these instructions. Thus, quality control personnel considering the establishment of in-process controls and pilot and production operators who will be following the procedure for the first time should not be confused by cryptic phrases containing technical words not easily understood. The tablet formulator should keep in mind that his or her manufacturing procedure may also be circulated to foreign manufacturing plants. Manufacturing instructions that are clearly written are advantageous because they avoid confusion which may lead to errors.

Figure 9 illustrates a list of specifications for the finished tablets. As can be seen in Figures 7–9, spaces for the product code and lot number are provided at the top of the form. The three forms become a part of the file for the lot number of the batch of tablets prepared. These three sheets serve as a historical record. Attachments that are included, for example, would be the clearance data from the quality control division and a record of the physicians receiving the material for clinical study.

VII.   USE OF THE PILOT PLANT SCALE-UP TO SELECT THE OPTIMAL PROCEDURE FOR THE PREPARATION OF DEXAMETHASONE TABLETS

A company was planning to expand its tablet-manufacturing facility. The company's tablet products in greatest demand were potent corticoids and cardiovascular drugs. These water-insoluble, neutral drugs were to be used in concentrations ranging from 0.1 to 5.0 mg per tablet.

The presence of 0.1 mg of drug in a tablet weighing 200 mg represents a drug dilution with tablet excipients of 1:2000. Maintaining content uniformity could be a problem in the routine manufacture of such tablets. In addition to content uniformity, the dissolution rates of such water-insoluble drugs can be a problem. Such drugs as the corticoids and the cardiac glycosides, on occasion, have been recalled by the Food and Drug Administration because of a lack of bioequivalency.

The company's top management requested the pharmaceutical research and development department to determine which tablet-manufacturing procedure should be adopted for this line of tablet products. Their 0.25-mg dexamethasone tablets were considered to be representative of the several drugs whose production volume were to be expanded.

One of four tablet-manufacturing procedures were to be considered: (1) wet granulation, (2) microgranulation, (3) direct compression, and (4) double compression. Each of these procedures had been used successfully by the pharmaceutical research department in the development of the 0.25-mg dexamethasone tablets. The responsibility now rested with the pilot plant personnel to scale-up each of the four procedures. The basis for selection of the optimal procedure would take into consideration the following: (1) simplicity of manufacture, (2) physical properties of the finished tablets, (3) content uniformity, (4) dissolution rate of the dexamethasone from the tablets, and (5) cost of manufacture. On the basis of the procedure selected decisions could be made about new equipment purchases for the expanded manufacturing facility. The tablet formulations are listed in Table 3 [1–3].

Dexamethasone was chosen as the drug in this study because it is a water-insoluble, neutral compound whose bioavailability can be adversely

Table 3   Formulations of Experimental Dexamethasone Granules and Tablets[a]

Ingredients (mg/tablet)	Wet granulation	Micro-granulation	Direct compression	Slugging
Dexamethasone	0.25	0.25	0.25	0.25
Starch, dry	10.00	11.00	15.00	11.00
Acacia, powdered	2.60	3.00	3.00	3.00
Lactose	130.75	130.25	–	126.75
Lactose, direct compression[b]	–	–	127.75	–
Starch[c]	1.00	–	–	–
Acacia, powdered[c]	0.40	–	–	–
Purified water	18.60	8.00	–	–
Starch, dry[d]	4.00	4.00	–	4.00
Magnesium stearate	1.00	1.00	2.00	1.00
Talcum, powdered	–	0.50	2.00	3.00
Magnesium stearate[e]	–	–	–	1.00
Total	150.00	150.00	150.00	150.00

[a]Batch size for each method was 10,000 tablets.

[b]Directly compressible lactose.

[c]Used as starch/acacia paste.

[d]Added to the dry granules.

[e]Added for the final compression.

Source: From Refs. 1–3.

affected by a poor tablet formulation. In each procedure the micronized dexamethasone was mixed with the excipients by using a geometric dilution procedure in a V-shaped blender of 3 kg capacity. The four procedures followed are summarized below.

A. Wet Granulation

Homogeneous blends of the dexamethasone and excipients were granulated with starch/acacia in a planetary mixer. The wet mass was passed through an oscillating granulator equipped with a No. 8 screen and oven dried overnight at 45°C. After dry screening through a No. 16 screen, the granulations were blended with the remaining dry starch, lubricated, and compressed.

B. Microgranulation

Microgranulates were prepared by a procedure first described by de Jong [4]. An advantage cited for this procedure is that a blend of finely powdered drug and excipients can be converted into compressible granules with only minor changes in particle size. Thus, microgranulation is differentiated from conventional wet granulation by the absence of large agglomerates. A relatively small quantity of granulating liquid is used in the process of forming microgranulates. As a consequence, the blended powder particles become coated by a thin film of binder which reduces interparticular attraction and yields a free-flowing powder which can be compressed to form a tablet. Hydrophobic powders coated in such a manner are rendered less hydrophobic, and thus more readily dispersible in water. Since such microgranulations are devoid of large agglomerates, powder blends granulated in this manner exhibit excellent content uniformity, rapid dissolution, and excellent bioavailability.

   In the preparation of dexamethasone microgranulates a homogeneous blend of micronized drug, powdered acacia, starch, and lactose was placed in a planetary mixer and uniformly moistened with a minimal quantity of purified water. The uniform distribution of water is a critical step. Failure to distribute the water uniformly will mean that portions of the blend will have been inadequately granulated. As a result excessive capping will result during the compression stage. The addition of excessive water during the granulating step will result in the formation of macrogranules.

   The uniformly moistened granules were passed through a No. 16 sieve and tray dried at 45°C overnight. The dried granules were passed through a No. 16 sieve. Additional starch and magnesium stearate were added to the sieved microgranules and the blend was compressed into tablets.

C. Double Compression

Slugs were made using a heavy-duty press with 1-in diameter punches. The slugs were granulated through an oscillating granulator fitted with a No. 16 sieve. Additional lubricant was added to the granules and, after additional blending, the granules were compressed into tablets.

D. Direct Compression

The dexamethasone, binder, disintegrant, and anhydrous lactose were blended by geometric dilution. The homogeneous blend was lubricated and compressed.

The granules prepared by the three granulation procedures and the directly compressible blend were compressed on a 16-station tablet machine in which only 4 stations were used. Flat punches measuring 5/16 in in diameter were employed. Particle size analyses were performed on samples of the powder blend before granulation, after granulation, and after compaction and disintegration by using a nest of sieves and an electromagnetic sieving machine. The particle size distribution of the granules after compaction and disintegration was determined by the method of Khan and Rhodes [5].

These authors prepared compacts by means of a hydraulic press. To effect disintegration of the compacts without agitation, which might cause granule fracture, a particularly effective disintegrant was included in the compacts. In the case of compacts prepared from insoluble materials, such as dicalcium phosphate, distilled water was used as the disintegration vehicle; for other systems appropriately saturated solutions were used. Particle size determinations of the disintegrated compacts were made using a particle size counter or an air-jet sieve.

The dexamethasone tablets were allowed to disintegrate into particles and granules by soaking them in absolute ethanol saturated with the drug. Aqueous media were avoided because of the presence of water-soluble lactose. The particles and granules were separated by filtration and dried at 40°C for 16 h. The dried particles and granules were then gently brushed through a 16-mesh screen. The screened particles and granules were then subjected to a particle size analysis using a nest of sieves and an electromagnetic sieving machine.

Representation of Particle Size Distribution Data

In Table 4 are shown the weight percentages and cumulative weight percentages of particles on each of the sieves for the following: (1) the dexamethasone powder blend, (2) dried granules prepared by wet granulation before compaction, and (3) dried granules after compaction and disintegration.

Inspection of the data in Table 4 reveals that 100% of the particles in the dexamethasone powder blend have a particle size of less than 251 μm, since all the particles passed through the 60-mesh sieve. Approximately 50% of the material should have diameters of less than 152 μm and greater than 75 μm. This follows, since 13% of the material was collected on the 120-mesh sieve and 43% was collected on the 200-mesh sieve. The aperture for the 100-mesh sieve is 152 μm and the aperture for the 200-mesh sieve is 75 μm.

A method of representing the particle size data to obtain a rough estimate of the average diameter is to plot the cumulative percentage over or under a particular size versus particle size. This is shown in Figure 10, using the cumulative percentage oversize for the data in Table 4.

As an example, the points on the dexamethasone powder blend curve were generated as follows. All of the particles of the dexamethasone

Table 4 Fractional and Cumulative Weight Percentages Collected on a Nest of Sieves for Dexamethasone Powder Blend, Dried Granules Prepared by Wet Granulation, and Dried Granules After Compaction and Disintegration

Sieve mesh no. (ASTM)	Aperture (μm)	Dexamethasone powder blend Fractional	Dexamethasone powder blend Cumulative	Granules (wet granulation) Fractional	Granules (wet granulation) Cumulative	Granules after compaction Fractional	Granules after compaction Cumulative
30	598	0	0	20	20	15	15
40	424	0	0	20	40	16	31
50	296	0	0	17	57	14	45
60	251	0	0	5	62	5	50
80	178	1	1	12	74	8	58
100	152	8	9	10	84	5	63
120	124	13	22	11	95	5	68
200	75	43	65	0	95	21	89
325	44	35	100	0	95	10	99
Receiver	—	0	100	5	100	1	100

Column group header: Weight percentages

Source: From Refs. 1–3.

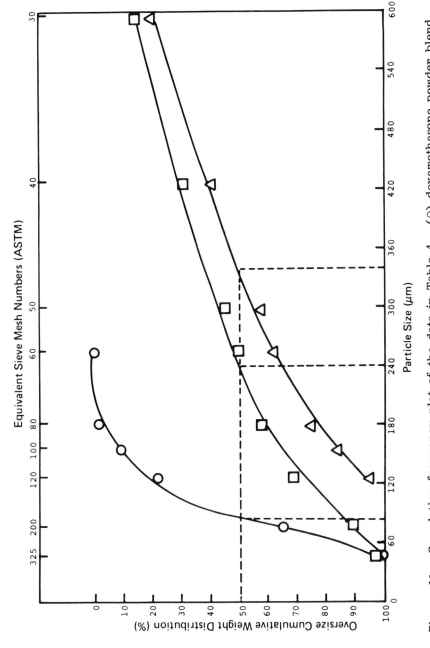

Figure 10 Cumulative frequency plot of the data in Table 4. (○) dexamethasone powder blend, (△) dried granules prepared by wet granulation before compaction, (□) dried granules after compaction and disintegration. (From Refs. 1–3.)

powder blend passed through the 60-mesh sieve, therefore 0% are greater than 251 μm (sieve aperture diameter). Only 1% of the particles that passed through the 60-mesh sieve were retained on the 80-mesh sieve. Hence, only 1% of the particles are greater than 178 μm. Of the particles that passed through the 80-mesh sieve, 8% were retained on the 100-mesh sieve. As a consequence, 9% of the particles have diameters greater than 152 μm (1 plus 8%). The remaining points on the dexamethasone powder blend curve as well as the curves for the dried granules before compaction and after compaction and disintegration were plotted in a similar fashion.

The curves shown in Figure 10 can be used to estimate the average particle size of the particles. This is determined by drawing a line parallel to the abscissa which meets the ordinate at the 50% point. Perpendicular lines are drawn at the points where the horizontal line intersects each curve. The average particle size diameter is read on the abscissa.

A rough estimate of the average diameter of the particles can be obtained from the sigmoid curves in Figure 10. A perpendicular to the abscissa is drawn from the point where the 50% point on the ordinate meets the curves. By this method, the dexamethasone powder blend has an average diameter of 84 μm. The dried granules obtained after wet granulation have an average diameter of 339 μm; the dried granules obtained after compaction and disintegration have an average diameter of 237 μm.

Extrapolation of data from sigmoidal curves as shown in Figure 10 is not recommended. A linear relationship is preferred for greater accuracy. When the weight of particles lying within a certain size range is plotted against the size range or average particle size a frequency-distribution curve is obtained. Such plots are valuable because they give a visible representation of the particle size distribution. Thus, it is apparent from a frequency-distribution curve which particle size occurs most frequently within the sample. Hence, it is desirable to determine if the data will yield a normal frequency-distribution curve.

A normal frequency-distribution curve is symmetrical around the mean. The standard deviation is an indication of the distribution about the mean. In a normal frequency-distribution curve, 68% of the particles lie ±1 standard deviation from the mean, 95.5% of the particles lie within the mean ±2 standard deviations, and 99.7% lie within the mean ±3 standard deviations.

Unfortunately, a normal frequency-distribution curve is not commonly found in pharmaceutical powders. Pharmaceutical powders tend to have an unsymmetrical, or skewed, distribution. However, when the data are plotted as frequency versus the logarithm of the particle diameter, then frequently a typical bell-shaped curve is obtained. A size distribution fitting this pattern is referred to as a log-normal distribution.

A log-normal distribution has several properties of interest. When the logarithm of the particle diameter is plotted against the cumulative percentage frequency on a probability scale a linear relationship is observed. Selected data from Table 4 is plotted in this manner as shown in Figure 11.

On the basis of the linear relationship of the data shown in Figure 11, one can determine the geometric mean diameters and the slopes of the lines. The geometric mean diameter is the logarithm of the particle size equivalent to 50% of the weight of the sample on the probability scale.

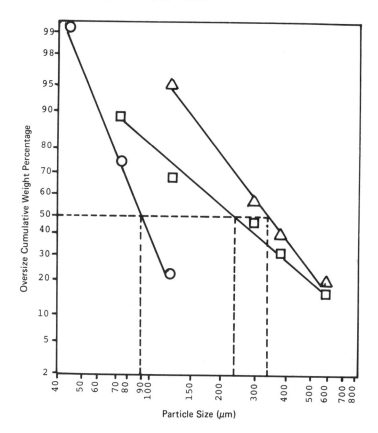

Figure 11 A plot of oversize cumulative weight percentage versus particle size. (○) dexamethasone powder blend, (△) dried granules prepared by wet granulation, (□) dried granules after compaction and disintegration. (From Refs. 1–3.)

The values for the geometric mean diameters as shown in Figure 11 are (1) 88 μm for the dexamethasone powder blend, (2) 322 μm for the dried granules prepared by wet granulation, and (3) 250 μm for the dried granule granules obtained after compaction and disintegration.

The slopes of the lines are given by the geometric standard deviations, which are the quotients of any one of the following ratios:

$$\frac{84\% \text{ undersize}}{\text{geometric mean diameter}} \qquad \frac{16\% \text{ oversize}}{\text{geometric mean diameter}}$$

$$\frac{\text{geometric mean diameter}}{84\% \text{ oversize}} \qquad \frac{\text{geometric mean diameter}}{16\% \text{ undersize}}$$

Knowing the two parameters, slope and geometric mean diameter, one can determine the particle size distribution at various fractional weights of the sample from the graph and reconstruct a log-normal distribution curve. Mention should be made of the origin of the numbers 84 and 16%. In a

normal or log-normal distribution curve, 68% of the particles will lie less than one standard deviation away from the mean or geometric mean diameter. To put it another way, 34% of the particles will be larger than the
mean or geometric mean (34 + 50 = 84) and 34% of the particles will be smaller than the mean or geometric mean (50 − 34 = 16).

In Figure 11, the ordinate data are spaced logarithmically. Equally good linear data are obtained if semilog plots are used; that is, one plots oversize cumulative weight percentage versus the logarithm of the particle size. A comparison of the average particle size of granules obtained from log-probability and semilog plots is shown in Table 5. In the table, the average particle size data tabulated attest to the close agreement of the two procedures. Semilog plots were adopted for the presentation of all particle size data (Figs. 12−15). The average particle diameters determined from the figures are summarized in Table 6.

Slugging produced the widest particle size distribution and the largest average particle diameter (Fig. 14). Forty percent of the weight of the sample had particle diameters greater than 596 μm. Furthermore, only 91% of the sample was collected on the nest of sieves, and thus 9% of the sample possessed particle diameters less than 44 μm. The original dexamethasone powder blend was completely collected on sieves ranging from 80 to 325 mesh. After compaction and disintegration, the granules with the largest particle diameter amounted to only 7%. Fifteen percent of the sample after compaction and disintegration passed through the 325-mesh screen. Such data are indicative of size reduction occurring during the two compressional stages. Such size reduction was not found to be deleterious, since the granulations prepared by slugging yielded satisfactory tablets. If the concentration of particles with diameters less than 44 μm had exceeded 25 to 30%, irregular granule flow and capped tablets could have been obtained.

Table 5   A Comparison of Average Particle Sizes of Granules Prepared by Three Granulating Methods and a Direct-Compression Powder Blend[a]

Granulating method	Average particle size (μm)	
	Log probability plot	Semilog plot
Wet granulation	322	315
Microgranulation	100	100
Slugging	410	400
Direct compression	122	120

[a]The average particle sizes were obtained from log probability and semilog plots.

Table 6 Average Particle Diameters of Dexamethasone Powder Blends and Granules Prepared by Wet Granulation, Microgranulation, and Slugging[a]

Processing stage	Average particular diameter (μm)			
	Wet granulation	Micro- granulation	Slugging	Direct compression
Powder blend	88	88	88	120
Granules	315	100	400	–
Disintegrated tablets	235	90	120	120

[a]Also included are dried granules obtained after compaction and disintegration and tablets prepared by direct compression.

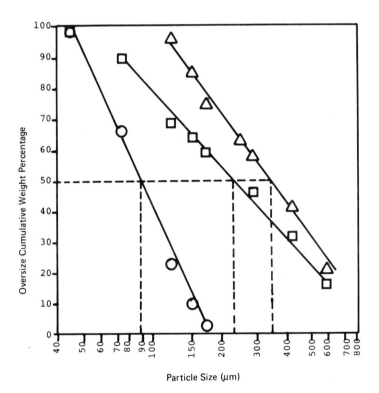

Figure 12 Effect of wet granulation on the particle size distribution of a dexamethasone powder blend before and after compaction and disintegration. (○) dexamethasone powder blend, (△) dried granules before compaction, (□) dried granules after compaction and disintegration. (From Refs. 1–3.)

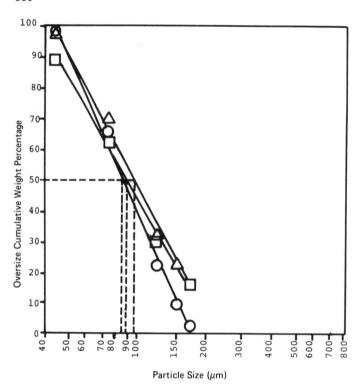

Figure 13 Effect of microgranulation on the particle size distribution of a dexamethasone powder blend before and after compaction and disintegration. (○) dexamethasone powder blend, (△) dried granules before compaction, (□) dried granules after compaction and disintegration. (From Refs. 1–3.)

Microgranulation brought about the least change in particle size distribution (see Fig. 13). The slopes of the three lines are similar. The amounts of material passing through the 325 mesh screen were 0% (dexamethasone powder blend), 2% (before compaction), and 10% (after compaction and disintegration). Such increases in fine particles are not significant.

Granules prepared by wet granulation were much larger than the original powder blend (see Fig. 12). Ninety-five percent of the sample was collected on 30- to 120-mesh sieves. Only 5% of the sample passed through the 325-mesh sieve. After compaction and disintegration a significant size reduction occurred. The 200-mesh sieve collected 21% of the granules and the 325-mesh sieve retained 10% of the sample. Prior to compaction and disintegration none of the granules had been retained by either of these sieves.

Direct compression produced the least change in particle size before and after compaction and disintegration (see Fig. 15). The slopes of the two lines are practically identical. Ninety-seven percent of the particles

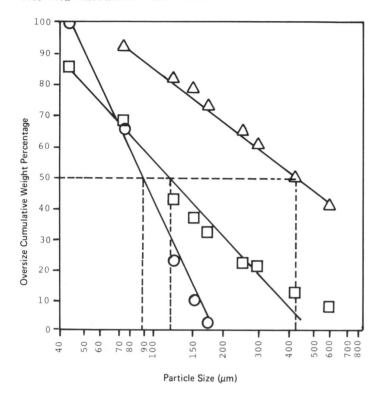

Figure 14 Effect of slugging on the particle size distribution of a dexamethasone powder blend before and after compaction and disintegration. (○) dexamethasone powder blend, (△) granules prepared by slugging, (□) dried granules after compaction and disintegration. (From Refs. 1–3.)

in the directly compressible blend were collected on 50- to 325-mesh sieves, whereas 92% of the particles after compaction and disintegration were collected on such sieves. The fines which were collected in the receiver (3 and 8%, respectively) are of concern in this instance, since micronized dexamethasone accounts for only 0.16% of the sample weight. As a consequence, classification and poor content uniformity might be anticipated. None of the original dexamethasone powder blend passed through the 325-mesh sieve. Hence, compressed tablets prepared from granules obtained by the three granulating procedures could be expected to exhibit differences in content uniformity and weight uniformity.

Dexamethasone Homogeneity in the
Granules and Tablets

The relative homogeneity of dexamethasone in the granules prepared by the four procedures is shown in Table 7. Microgranulation produced the best dispersion of dexamethasone. The fine granule size most likely accounts for the homogeneity of drug distribution in the microgranulate.

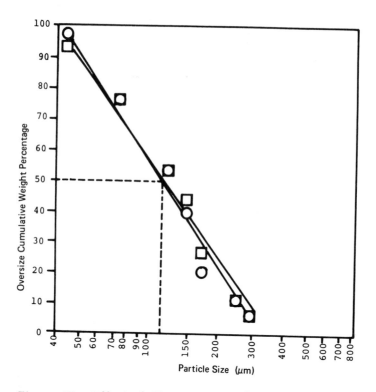

Figure 15 Effect of direct compression on the particle size distribution of a dexamethasone powder blend before and after compaction and disintegration. (○) direct compression powder blend, (□) dried granules after compaction and disintegration. (From Refs. 1–3.)

Table 7 Homogeneity of Dexamethasone Distribution in Granules Prepared by Four Different Methods

Granulating method	Average content (mg)	Maximum content (mg)	Minimum content (mg)	Coefficient of variation (%)
Wet granulation	0.240	0.265	0.222	5.97
Microgranulation	0.251	0.253	0.247	0.99
Direct compression	0.249	0.267	0.238	3.90
Slugging	0.247	0.252	0.243	1.43

Source: From Refs. 1–3.

On the other hand, wet granulation exhibited the poorest homogeneity. This is attributable to the larger particle size and the wider distribution of particle size of the granules before and after compaction. The slugging method was found to be the second best granulating procedure for producing homogeneous granules. In the slugging method, dexamethasone was dispersed in powdered lactose in a suitable blender. After the addition of a portion of the starch and acacia the blend was lubricated with magnesium stearate and slugged under high pressure. Unlike wet granulation, the slugging method did not call for so many processing steps, such as wetting, wet screening, drying, dry screening, lubricating, and compressing. Moreover, bonding of drug excipient had occurred during the slugging operation. Subsequent granulation did not result in segregation of dexamethasone because of such bonding. Thus, the homogeneity of drug distribution in granules is not only dependent on granule size distribution and/or drug particle size, but also is dependent on the granulation method. The coefficient of variation is also high for the blend prepared for direct compression. This is attributable to the great difference in particle size between the active ingredient and the excipients. The dexamethasone was micronized (size range 1−5 μm); the directly compressible lactose had an average particle diameter of 120 μm.

Control charts for the weight variations of dexamethasone tablets are shown in Figures 16−19. The control chart is a useful measure for process control. It is based on standard deviation or range (R).

Each of the circled points in Figures 16−19 represent the average weight of five tablets ($\bar{X}$) taken at 5-min intervals up to 40 min. Thus, a total of 40 tablets were individually weighed. The highest and lowest weight of each time interval are also shown in the four figures. The average for the 40 tablets ($\bar{\bar{X}}$) is represented by the solid horizontal line. The horizontal broken lines above and below the solid line represent 3 standard deviations from the mean. For a normal curve distribution of

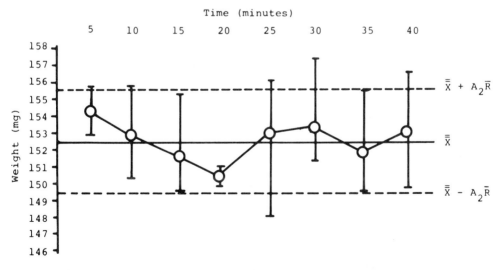

Figure 16   Control chart for the weight variation of dexamethasone tablets prepared by the wet granulation method. (From Refs. 1−3.)

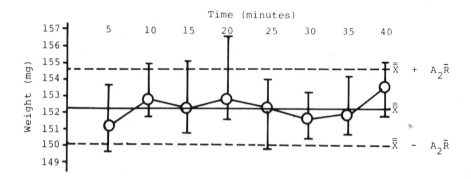

Figure 17 Control chart for the weight variation of dexamethasone tablets prepared by microgranulation. (From Refs. 1–3.)

weights, this means that 99.73% of the tablets in the batch will weigh within the range represented by the upper and lower limits; for a skewed curve distribution, 95% or more of the tablets will weigh within the upper and lower limits represented by the horizontal broken lines.

The standard deviation is used as the measure of spread for almost all industrial frequency distributions. It is the root mean square deviation of

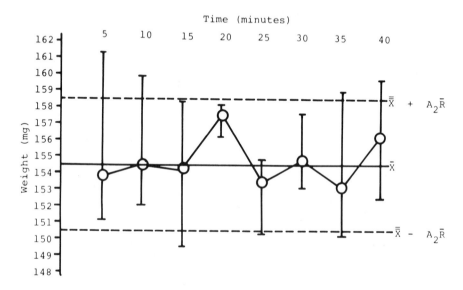

Figure 18 Control chart for the weight variation of dexamethasone tablets prepared by slugging. (From Refs. 1–3.)

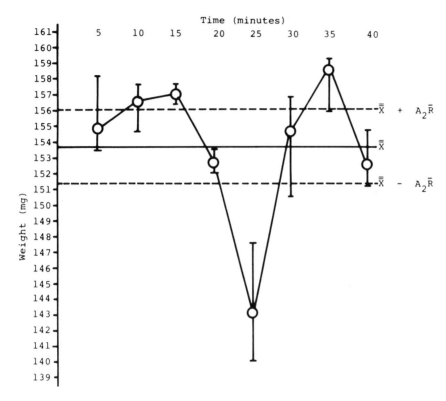

Figure 19 Control chart for the weight variation of dexamethasone tablets prepared by the wet granulation method. (From Refs. 1—3.)

the readings in a series from their average. The sample standard deviation is obtained by extracting the square root of the sums of the squares of the series from the average, divided by the number of readings. This is represented symbolically as follows:

$$\text{Standard deviation} = \sqrt{\frac{(X_1 - \overline{X})^2 + (X_2 - \overline{X})^2 + (X_3 - \overline{X})^2 + \cdots + (X_n - \overline{X})^2}{n}}$$

where $X_1, X_2, X_3 \cdots X_n$ = value of each reading

$\overline{X}$ = average value of the series

n = number of readings

The standard deviation of the data presented in Figure 16 is calculated as follows: X, the average weight for the 40 tablets = 152.4 mg

Time (min)

5		10		15	
$(X - \bar{\bar{X}})$	$(X - \bar{\bar{X}})^2$	$(X - \bar{\bar{X}})$	$(X - \bar{\bar{X}})^2$	$(X - \bar{\bar{X}})$	$(X - \bar{\bar{X}})^2$
+2.8	7.84	−0.4	0.16	+2.8	7.84
+1.6	2.56	+3.3	10.89	−1.6	2.56
+3.2	10.24	+0.1	0.01	−2.6	6.76
+1.2	1.44	−2.1	4.41	−3.1	9.61
+0.4	0.16	+0.2	0.04	−0.2	0.04

Time (min)

20		25		30	
$(X - \bar{\bar{X}})$	$(X - \bar{\bar{X}})^2$	$(X - \bar{\bar{X}})$	$(X - \bar{\bar{X}})^2$	$(X - \bar{\bar{X}})$	$(X - \bar{\bar{X}})^2$
−2.4	5.76	+2.8	7.84	−0.2	0.04
−1.8	3.24	−4.5	20.25	+5.1	26.01
−2.3	5.29	−1.2	1.44	−1.0	1.00
−2.6	6.76	+0.6	0.36	−1.0	1.00
−1.5	2.25	+3.6	12.96	+1.0	1.00

Time (min)

35		40	
$(X - \bar{\bar{X}})$	$(X - \bar{\bar{X}}^2)$	$(X - \bar{\bar{X}})$	$(X - \bar{\bar{X}}^2)$
−1.2	1.44	+0.1	0.01
+3.1	9.61	+4.2	17.64
−2.9	8.41	−2.8	7.84
+1.6	2.56	−1.8	3.24
−3.0	9.00	+2.6	6.76

$$\text{Standard deviation} = \sqrt{\frac{226.27}{40}} = \sqrt{5.657} = \pm 2.38$$

$$\frac{\text{Standard deviation of}}{\text{the sample average}} = \frac{\text{standard deviation of the lot}}{\sqrt{n}}$$

$$= \frac{2.38}{\sqrt{5}} = \frac{2.38}{2.24} = 1.06$$

Three standard deviations of the sample average = 3 × 1.06 = ±3.18

From the calculations shown, the upper line of the control chart (see Fig. 16) is set at 152.4 = 3.18 = 155.58; the lower line of the control chart is set at 152.4 + 3.18 = 149.22.

Obviously, it would be tedious to gather a series of samples of small size, determine the values for central tendency and spread for each of these samples, and then go through the laborious calculations that are involved. However, statisticians have simplified the calculations by preparing a table of constants (Table 8) [6].

Through the use of the following equation the control limits can be calculated much more easily ($\overline{R}$ = average of the range values):

Upper broken line (Fig. 16) = $\overline{\overline{X}} + A_2\overline{R}$

Lower broken line (Fig. 16) = $\overline{\overline{X}} - A_2\overline{R}$

Thus, for samples consisting of five units at each time interval the value for A_2 has been calculated to be 0.577 (see Table 8). Substitution of the factor into the above equations is shown at the bottom of Figure 16. Note the close agreement of the limit values derived by either method of calculation.

Table 8 Factors for Computing
Control Limits When Range is Used
as a Measure of Spread

Number of observations in sample (n)	Factor for control limits (A_2)
2	1.880
3	1.023
4	0.729
5	0.577
6	0.483
7	0.419
8	0.373
9	0.337
10	0.308
11	0.285
12	0.266
13	0.249
14	0.235
15	0.223

Source: From Refs. 1–3.

Examination of Figures 16–19 reveals that the tablets prepared by the microgranulation procedure were most uniform in weight (Fig. 17). This conclusion can be drawn from the following considerations: (1) the average range value, 3.85, is the smallest for the four granulation procedures; (2) the average value for the five tablets at each time interval always fell between the upper and lower limits; and (3) the weight spread between the 40 tablets was least for the microgranulation procedure (156.6 − 150 = 6.6 mg).

An interesting correlation can be seen between the average range values $\bar{R}$ from the four control charts (see Figs. 16–19) and the average particle size of the granules used in preparing the tablets (see Table 5). On the basis of the data in Table 5, one can conclude that the lower the average particle size of the granules the lower the average range value. Thus, the four granulating procedures rank in the following order with respect to increase in average particle size and $\bar{R}$ value: microgranulation, 100 μ, 3.85 mg; direct compress., 120 μ, 3.9 mg; wet gran., 315 μ, 5.35 mg; and slugging, 400 μ, 6.6 mg. Thus weight variation is a function of the average particle size of the granules.

Content uniformity was determined for the tablets prepared by the four manufacturing procedures. Assay data collected on 40 tablets were treated in a fashion similar to that shown in Figure 16. Control charts for content variation of dexamethasone tablets are shown in Figures 20–23. Each point on these figures represents the average spectrophotometric absorbance (at 239 nm) for five tablets individually assayed at 5-min intervals up to 40 min.

Microgranulation and slugging can be seen to be the best procedures for preparing dexamethasone tablets possessing good content uniformity (see Figs. 21 and 22). Their average range values of 0.017 and 0.016, respectively, were much lower than those values for the wet granulation and direct-compression procedures.

Confirmation of these conclusions was derived from assays performed on 50 individual tablets selected at random from each batch of tablets. The coefficients of variation (standard deviation/average) were significantly lower for tablets prepared by the microgranulation and slugging procedures (Table 9).

Table 9   Coefficient of Content Variation for Dexamethasone Tablets Prepared by the Four Manufacturing Procedures[a]

Manufacturing procedure	Number of assays	Average absorbance	Standard deviation	Coefficient of variation (%)
Wet granulation	50	0.430	0.0248	5.77
Microgranulation	50	0.452	0.0092	2.04
Direct compression	50	0.450	0.0182	4.04
Slugging	50	0.455	0.0129	2.84

[a]Contents expressed in terms of absorbance.
Source: From Refs. 1–3.

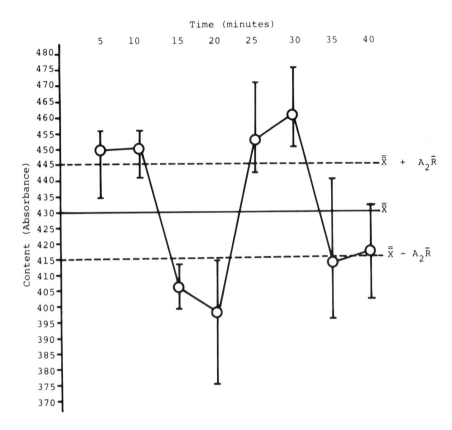

Figure 20 Control chart for the content variation of dexamethasone tablets prepared by the wet granulation method. (From Refs. 1–3.)

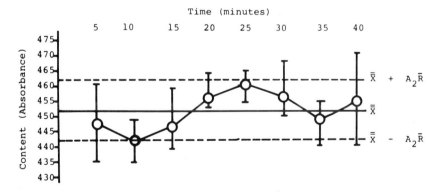

Figure 21 Control chart for the content variation of dexamethasone tablets prepared by microgranulation. (From Refs. 1–3.)

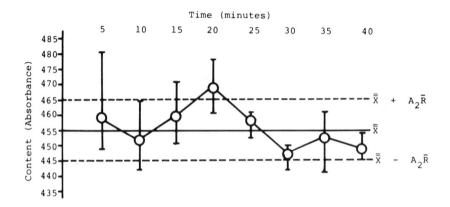

Figure 22   Control chart for the content variation of dexamethasone tablets prepared by slugging. (From Refs. 1–3.)

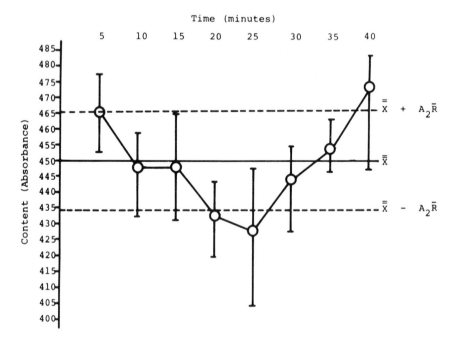

Figure 23   Control chart for the content variation of dexamethasone tablets prepared by direct compression. (From Refs. 1–3.)

Additional Properties of the Granulations and
Compressed Dexamethasone Tablets

Additional properties of the granulations that were studied are (1) loss on drying, (2) tapped, bulk, and true density, (3) compressibility, (4) porosity, (5) angle of repose, (6) flow rate, (7) mean granule diameter. Properties of the compressed tablets that were studied are (1) average weight, (2) hardness, (3) disintegration time. These properties are summarized in Table 10.

LOSS ON DRYING. Residual moisture in the granules was determined with a moisture determination balance on duplicate samples. The samples were kept at 70°C for 30 min. The loss in weight was expressed in percentage units.

TAPPED, BULK, AND TRUE DENSITY. Tapped (packed) density was measured by using a granulated cylinder and a motorized tapping device set to operate 200 cycles/5min. Volumes of the tapped granules (5-gm samples) were read in the granulated cylinder after the device was run for 10 min. The results in Table 9 are the average of three determinations.

Bulk densities were determined by measuring the volumes of 5-gm samples of granules placed in graduated cylinders. True densities of the

Table 10   Properties of Dexamethasone Granules and Tablets Prepared by Four Different Methods

Property	Wet granulation	Micro-granulation	Direct compression	Slugging
Loss on drying (%)	2.0	1.60	1.70	1.90
Density (gm/ml)				
Tapped	0.754	0.798	0.872	0.961
Bulk	0.691	0.646	0.683	0.820
True	1.511	1.511	1.562	1.511
Compressibility (%)	8.35	19.04	21.67	14.67
Porosity (%)	54.27	57.25	56.25	45.74
Angle of repose (%)	27.4	37.2	44.5	39.2
Flow rate (sec)	2.53	8.91	20.18	2.66
Flow (rotary press)	Very good	Very good	Good	Very good
Mean granule diameter (μm)	315	100	120	400
Average weight (mg)	152.5	152.3	153.5	154.6
Hardness (kg)	3.6	3.9	3.4	3.9
Disintegration (min)	2.5–3.8	1.1–1.5	3.7–4.7	1.4–1.7

Source: From Refs. 1–3.

powdered blends shown in Table 3 were determined with a pycnometer
using benzene as the immersion fluid.

COMPRESSIBILITY. Compressibility [7] was calculated by using the
following equation:

$$\text{Percent compressibility} = \frac{\text{packed density} - \text{bulk density} \times 100}{\text{packed density}}$$

POROSITY. Porosity [8] was calculated by dividing the bulk density
values by the true density values.

ANGLE OF REPOSE. The angles of repose [9,10] of the granules were
measured after the lubricant had been blended in. Sixty-gram samples
were poured into a 10-cm funnel having a stem diameter of 0.8 cm and
resting atop a rubber stopper having a diameter of 5.4 cm. The funnel
was then slowly raised a distance of 7 cm, allowing the granules to flow
out and form a conical heap. The angle of repose was calculated by using
the following equation:

$$\text{Tangent of the angle of repose} = \frac{\text{height of the cone}}{\text{radius of the cone}}$$

Thus, it is evident that the angle of repose is the base angle of the cone
formed when the granules fell freely on a flat surface from the funnel.
The values reported in Table 9 were obtained by referring to a table of
trigonometric functions.

The repose angle values listed in Table 9 are the averages obtained
from five determinations made on the various granulations and the directly
compressible powder blend. The angle of repose gives some indication of
the flow properties of granulations. Thus, granulations having repose
angles of less than 40° will flow freely through a hopper orifice. The repose angle depends on the nature of the powder and on variables which
include the shape and size distribution of the granules, presence of
moisture, density of the particles, and technique of measurement. The
relative humidity was kept constant during the determinations, and the
moisture content of the various granulations studied was less than 2%.

FLOW RATE. The flow rate was determined by passage of 50 gm of
granules through a stainless steel funnel with a 1-cm opening. The funnel was attached to a granule flow tester which recorded flow time
automatically.

The three factors of compressibility, angle of repose, and flow rate,
which give information on flow properties, predict that the granulations
prepared by the wet method will flow better. The lower the compressibility
factor and the smaller the angle of repose, the faster is the predicted flow
rate of the granules. Microgranulation was found to produce a blend
which had a high porosity, indicating bridging due to cohesive forces [9].
The porosity values of the granulations prepared by slugging were found
to be minimal, indicating little intraparticular void volume in the granules.
The disintegration rates of the dexamethasone tablets prepared by any of
the granulating procedures or by direct compression were all satisfactory.

DISSOLUTION RATE OF DEXAMETHASONE FROM GRANULES AND
TABLETS. The dissolution rates of dexamethasone from granules prepared
by the four granulation procedures (Fig. 24) were slower than the rates
of dissolution from their corresponding tablets (Fig. 25). A possible explanation for such increases in dissolution rates may be the compaction
behavior of the dexamethasone formulations. During compaction, particle
size of the granules was reduced and the distribution was narrowed. As
a result the specific surface area of the disintegrated granules was increased, thereby increasing the dissolution rate. Another reason may be
that dexamethasone was more rapidly wet by the dissolution medium when
introduced as tablets. It was noted that the tablets submerged and rapidly disintegrated, whereas when granules were introduced they settled beneath the dissolution medium more slowly. The dissolution rate of the tablets prepared by microgranulation proved to be the greatest; the poorest
dissolution rate was exhibited by those tablets prepared by the slugging
procedure.

All four tablet granulation procedures compressed equally well with regard to the rate of compression and the yield of finished tablets. The
content uniformity of tablets by all four procedures conformed to the

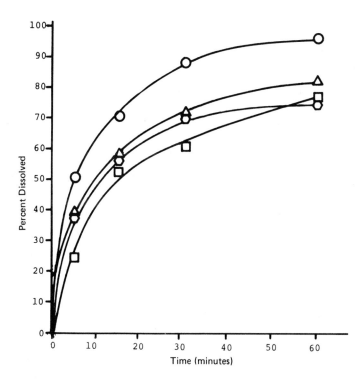

Figure 24 Dissolution rates of dexamethasone from granules prepared by
four procedures. (○) microgranulation, (△) wet granulation, (○)
slugging, (□) direct compression. (From Refs. 1–3.)

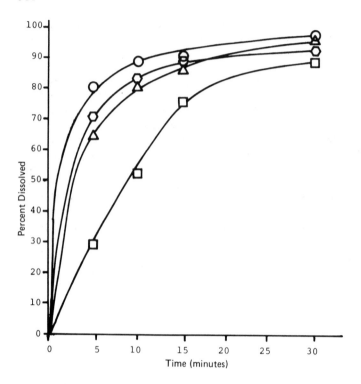

Figure 25 Dissolution rates of dexamethasone from tablets prepared by four procedures. (○) microgranulation, (△) wet granulation, (◇) slugging, (□) direct comprssion. (From Refs. 1–3.)

United States Pharmacopeia (USP) XIX limits of ±15%. On the basis of all the data collected, one must conclude that for dexamethasone tablets the optimal procedure with the excipients used is microgranulation. Microgranulation requires no special processing equipment. The average diameter of the granules obtained by microgranulation were the smallest before and after compaction and disintegration. Content uniformity of the granules and the finished tablets prepared by this procedure was best. This is not unexpected because of the lesser disparity between drug and excipient particle size. Finally, the dexamethasone tablets prepared by microgranulation had the greatest dissolution rates. Rapid dissolution would favor rapid release of the dexamethasone after oral administration of the tablets and thus favor reproducible absorption efficiency.

VIII. PROBLEM CAUSED BY A CHANGE IN EXCIPIENT SUPPLIER

Following is an experimental tablet formula for an oral hypoglycemic agent:

Chlorpropamide	250 mg
Kel acid	30 mg
Dicalcium phosphate	50 mg
Cornstarch	30 mg
Magnesium stearate	7 mg

Granules of the above blend of powders with half of the magnesium stearate requirement were prepared by slugging and passage of the slugs through an oscillating granulator. The granules were lubricated with the remainder of the magnesium stearate and compressed into tablets. Tablets prepared in this manner disintegrated in less than 15 min in simulated gastric fluid at 37°C. The physical properties of the tablets prepared on a pilot and production scale duplicated those specified by research. After several successful production size runs had been made a subsequent production run yielded tablets that did not disintegrate within the specified time limit. The pilot plant research pharmacist was asked to determine the cause of the poor disintegration.

At the outset the cause for such poor disintegration was difficult to determine. All the raw materials that had been used had been cleared for use by quality control. The manufacturing procedure had been followed exactly as written. Eventually a clue to the cause of the problem was found. A new lot of kel acid had been purchased and used in making the batch in question. This ingredient had been included in the tablet formula because of its disintegrant property. Discussions with the purchasing department revealed that this new lot of kel acid had been purchased from a new supplier. Microscopic inspection of the new supplier's kel acid revealed that it had been micronized. The original supplier's kel acid appeared as 10- to 20-μm fibers under the microscope. Thus, the cause of the problem was discovered. It is well known that when water-swelling gums are used as disintegrants, they are effective as relatively coarse particles because the swelling of coarse particles does not form a continuous film on the tablet surface as does a finely subdivided powder.

An attempt was made to rework the tablets in order to salvage them. The tablets were converted to granules by passage through a comminuting mill. Additional starch (5%) was added to the granules to ensure that the time limit for disintegration would be met. Additional magnesium stearate (1%) was added and the reworked blend compressed. The disintegration time for the reworked tablets was less than 15 min, but the dissolution rate of the chlorpropamide was unsatisfactory. A blood level study in dogs confirmed that the oral absorption of the chlorpropamide had been impaired. One might have anticipated that the release of chlorpropamide from the granules obtained after disintegration of the reworked tablets would be slow in vitro and in vivo because they contained the micronized kel acid. As a result of this experience, a particle size specification for the kel acid component was added by quality control.

IX. FRIABILITY RELATED TO PARTICLE SIZE DISTRIBUTION

Lantz et al. [11] described how the cause of a friability problem was discovered. After many days of production no problems had been encountered

Table 11   Acetophenetidin Particle Size Difference

Mesh size	Acceptable material (%)	Unacceptable material (%)
60	6.7	7.4
60–80	11.5	33.6
80–100	13.5	18.3
100–200	38.6	29.4
<200	29.8	8.3

Source: From Ref. 11.

with an acetophenetidin tablet formulation. With production apparently proceeding satisfactorily one day, on three successive lots of tablets the quality control and production departments reported that tablet friability was higher than usual. The statistics department ran an analysis on the friability data and concluded that a significant change had occurred. A check with the production operators revealed that nothing unusual had occurred. A check with the production operators revealed that nothing unusual had occurred during the production of these three lots of tablets.

A collaborative effort between the research, production, and quality control departments was initiated. A checking of the physical specifications on the raw materials used in the manufacture of these tablets revealed that the acetophenetidin was different in particle size distribution from previous lots (Table 11). The tablet blend containing the unacceptable material would not compress well. In the form of small particles it acted as a binder when compressed with the other tablet excipients. The quality control division did not use particle size distribution as a basis of accepting or rejecting acetophenetidin at the time this problem had arisen. Inclusion of a particle size specification for bulk acetophenetidin corrected the problem in subsequent production batches. The data in Table 11 clearly show that 30% of the acceptable bulk material passed through a 200-mesh sieve. Only 8.3% of the unacceptable acetophenetidin bulk passed through the 200-mesh sieve.

X. EFFECT OF DISINTEGRANT VISCOSITY ON DISINTEGRATION RATE

Sodium starch glycolate is an excellent disintegrating agent. It is formed by reacting starch with monochloracetic acid. It was being used as a disintegrating agent in a research tablet formula at a 3% concentration based on the weight of the tablet. Such tablets consistently disintegrate in less than 30 s in simulated gastric juice at 37°C. The first clinical batch of tablets prepared in the pilot plant exhibited disintegration times greater than 30 min. Discussions between research and pilot plant personnel revealed that a low viscosity grade had been used by research, whereas a regular grade had been used in the pilot plant. The two grades differ markedly in viscosity. Aqueous dispersions of the regular grade (3.3%) have viscosities ranging from 100 to 700 centipoise (cp). The low-viscosity grade (3.3%) in aqueous dispersion can range from 10 to 40 cp in viscosity. The establishment of a specification of <40 cp for an aqueous dispersion (3.3%) of the low-viscosity grade corrected the problem. All subsequent lots of tablets disintegrated within the time limits specified.

XI. INFLUENCE OF INGREDIENT MOISTURE CONTENT ON FRIABILITY

A multivitamin film-coated tablet containing a high concentration of ascorbic acid had been routinely manufactured by direct compression. The film coating was applied to the tablet cores in a fluidized-bed apparatus. In-house stability data had established that a moisture content above 2% in the finished tablets would not provide a 2-year shelf life. As a consequence, the moisture content of each of the components of the tablet formula were specified to be as low as possible. The moisture content of the purchased bulk ascorbic acid, for example, was specified to be less than 0.6%.

During an intensive production campaign, serious friability problems were encountered which led to a shutdown of the film-coating operation. A search for the cause of the friable cores ultimately led to an inspection of the quality control division's file samples and records of the raw materials used in the manufacture of the cores. Since ascorbic acid possessed the greatest percentage of the finished tablet weight, its file samples were scrutinized most thoroughly. Particle size distribution of file samples that had been used in making excellent batches of multivitamin tablets in the past were similar to the more recent material used in the friable cores.

The solution to the problem was finally found to be the low moisture content in the bulk ascorbic acid. When the bulk ascorbic acid had a moisture content of 0.5−0.6% firm cores were obtained which could be film coated with ease. However, if the bulk ascorbic acid had a moisture content of 0.2−0.3%, then the multivitamin tablet cores were apt to be friable and cause problems in the film-coating step. Additional studies were conducted to establish an ideal moisture content for the bulk ascorbic acid. Through the use of an instrument press it was established that a favorable compressibility/hardness ratio resulted when the bulk ascorbic moisture content was raised to 1.1%. Tablets prepared with such material produced cores which were efficiently film-coated. The moisture content of the finished tablets was less than 2%, and as a consequence shelf stability was assured.

XII. DRUG AND DYE MIGRATION IN WET GRANULATION

A. Drug Migration

Serious problems of content uniformity were being encountered in the manufacture of tablets containing small quantities of potent drugs. Wet granulation had been established as the method of choice for such tablets. The management of the firm was reluctant to invest in alternate granulating equipment, or in the purchase of more expensive direct-compression excipients. Additional problems of maintaining content uniformity could be anticipated because the company was planning to market several tablet formulas containing low concentrations of active ingredients. As a consequence, a development team from the pilot plant was asked to solve this problem.

Discussions with the pharmaceutical research formulators were not revealing. Poor content uniformity had not been encountered either during the development of the formulations or in the preparation of clinical batches ranging from 25,000 to 50,000 tablets. It was only during production campaigns to prepare several million tablets that such problems had arisen. The developmental team from the pilot plant focused their attention on the drying step. They realized that when water-soluble dyes are used in wet granulation tablet procedures dye migration can readily be noted both in the dried granulations and in the compressed tablets. The degree to which dye migration occurs is dependent upon (1) the water solubility of the colorant, (2) the rate of drying, (3) the thickness of the bed of wet granules, and (4) the granulating solvents used.

Chaudry and King [12] studied the extent of sodium warfarin migration in compressed tablets prepared by the wet granulation procedure. A dry blend of excipients and drug was proven to be uniform by assay. The blend was mixed with starch paste or acacia dispersion, passed through a No. 8 screen, and dried in a layer 1.27 cm thick at 65−70°C for 16−18 h in a shelf dryer. During the drying step migration of the sodium warfarin occurred. Higher concentrations of the drug were found in the outer layers, with a reduced amount toward the center. The dried material was passed through a No. 20 screen. The granules were blended with lubricant and tableted. Of the 50 tablets assayed only 12% fell within USP limits. Addition of 15% alginic acid to the blend of calcium phosphate and sodium warfarin prior to granulating with the acacia dispersion nullified drug migration during the drying step. As would be expected, content uniformity in the compressed tablets was significantly improved. The disintegration time was significantly increased by the addition of alginic acid. Thus, sodium warfarin tablets prepared with calcium phosphate and starch paste disintegrated in less than 12 s. On the other hand, tablets containing 15% alginic acid which had been granulated with an aqueous dispersion of acacia disintegrated in 16−18 min.

Warren and Price [13,14] reported on the effect of particle size of the major diluent, dispersion viscosity, and drying temperature on propoxyphene hydrochloride migration in wet granules during the drying step. Wet granulations of the drug were prepared using lactose as the major diluent and starch as the disintegrant. Particle size fractions of lactose ranging from 53 to 177 μm in diameter were employed. Determination of drug content at various depths in a dried granulation bed was accomplished by using a drying cell consisting of four layers. The cell was open on both ends of the cylinder formed by the layers. When used for migration studies the drying cell was placed on an oven tray lined with porous paper. Migration increased with decreasing particle size of the major diluent, lactose. The authors singled out two factors that could explain the results obtained: (1) increased entry suction due to decreased intragranular capillary size and (2) increased intergranular contact area. The drug concentrations were greatest at the top and bottom layers of granules. This was not unanticipated, since it was expected that the drug, solubilized in the water present, would be transported toward the evaporating surfaces by capillary action.

Binder solutions ranging in viscosity from 1 to 1000 cp were used to determine the effect of viscosity on drug migration. Binder solutions with viscosities greater than 90 cp produced granulations that exhibited insignificant drug migration during the drying step. Drying temperatures ranging from 40 to 80°C had little influence on the extent of drug migration.

Tablets prepared from a granulation in which drug migration was high showed a greater drug content variation than a granulation with lesser migration. This was so even though each dried granulation was blended before tableting.

On the basis of the published data reported above, the decision was made to prepare granules with more viscous binder solutions. As a further deterrent to drug migration, fluid-bed dryers were used in the interest of reducing drying time. An additional refinement was introduced in the form of an automatically controlled temperature profile. Temperature probes that recorded the air-in granules and air-exit temperatures were installed. The result of such refinements in the granulating and drying steps was that tablets containing small quantities of active ingredients were routinely produced which had excellent content uniformity.

B. Effect of Aged Simple Syrup on Dye Migration in Sugar-Coated Tablets

Soluble dyes, lake dyes, or insoluble pigments are added during the final stages in the sugar coating of tablets to facilitate identification and to enhance the esthetic appearance of the final product. There is an increasing tendency to use the lake dyes as tablet colorants.

Lake dyes are made by adsorbing a dye onto some inert substance surface such as aluminum hydroxide. The dye adsorbates are less sensitive to light degradation. Furthermore, when lakes are employed in the sugar-coating operation it is generally not necessary to use a variety of increasing concentrations of colorant to produce a uniform color. As a consequence, excellent results in tablet coloring are consistently being obtained by tablet coaters who use lake dyes in the regular and finishing coats.

A newly hired tablet coater was in the process of applying color coats to an established sugar-coated tablet. Dye migration and mottling were noted during the coating operation even though a lake dye was being used. Discussions with the tablet coater led to the solution of the problem. Although the proper lake dye had been used and the syrup contained the extender, calcium carbonate, their order of addition had been reversed. The simple syrup being used in the coating operation was slightly acidic. Adding the lake dye to the slightly acidic simple syrup resulted in partial solution of the dye from the surface of the aluminum hydroxide. Such partial dye solubilization was the cause of the dye migration and mottling observed. However, when the calcium carbonate was added to the syrup first any acidity in the latter was effectively neutralized because the calcium carbonate is alkaline.

A revised manufacturing procedure was issued which stressed the significance of adhering to the order of addition of the calcium carbonate and the lake dye. The dye migration and mottling problem was thereby effectively eradicated.

C. Effect of Acidic Salts on the Mottling of Tablets Containing Lake Dyes

A directly compressible tablet blend containing spray-dried lactose, starch, microcrystalline cellulose, magnesium stearate, and a lake dye showed signs of mottling on exposure to 50% relative humidity. The drug, a weakly basic compound, was present as the more soluble hydrochloride salt. A 5% aqueous solution of the salt had a pH of 4.2. The cause of the mottling problem was readily explained by the troubleshooter when these facts were presented. The close contact of the acidic salt, lake dye, and moisture led to elution and migration of the dye from the aluminum hydroxide surface. The mottling problem was readily overcome by inclusion of an alkaline buffer in the directly compressible tablet formula.

XIII. EFFECT OF AGED SIMPLE SYRUP ON SMOOTHING AND ROUNDING STEPS IN THE SUGAR COATING OF TABLETS

The steps involved in sugar coating of tablets may be subdivided into the following: (1) waterproofing and sealing, (2) subcoating, (3) smoothing or rounding, (4) coloring and finishing, and (5) polishing. Often the waterproofing and sealing steps are omitted. However, with sensitive drugs or vitamin mixtures they must be included. Subcoating involves alternately wetting the tablets with subcoating solution and partially dry sprinkling with dusting powder. This causes the tablets to be rapidly filled out. Rounding or smoothing involves applications of heavy syrup so that a hard, smooth surface is produced. Coloring and finishing involves the application of thinner, colored syrup in order to build up the tablet further and obtain the desired shade of color. Polishing involves rolling the tablets with wax or the application of a wax solution or suspension in order to give the finished tablets a high gloss.

During a routine sugar-coating operation on an established product, a drying problem was encountered during the smoothing and rounding step. Ordinarily, when subcoated tablets are revolving in the coating pan, a sufficient quantity of warm simple syrup is added to cover the tablets. The quantity of syrup is sufficient to loosen previous applications, so that the tablets will tend to cluster or adhere to the pan. However, stirring should be maintained to prevent clustering. When the tablets are rolling freely, air is blown on them until they are dry. The problem that arose during this routine coating operation was that the tablets showed no tendency to stick to the coating pan. The tablets slid rather than rolled. Drying was exceedingly slow. The dried tablets had a wrinkled, orange peel appearance.

Once the tablet surface becomes rough during this smoothing stage, recovery is difficult. Roughness can be created by (1) excess dust that remains after the dusting process. Such residual dust deposits on tablets as agglomerates when the next application of syrup is applied. (2) The tablets may be allowed to roll too long after the dusting power has been applied. (3) Insufficient syrup may have been added, so that incomplete wetting of the tablets resulted.

After extensive discussions with production division personnel, no plausible explanation could be found for the roughness encountered. Attention was then given to the possible implication of the simple syrup used. Production records revealed that the simple syrup had been on hand for several weeks. Furthermore, it had been heated, as required, on three previous occasions. Such heating of simple syrup favors the formation of invert sugar by the partial hydrolysis of sucrose. An analysis of the suspected syrup showed that 9% invert sugar was present. Thus, the cause of the drying problem was discovered. As is well known, invert sugar is frequently added to syrupy dosage forms to obviate the crystallization of sucrose beneath threaded bottle caps. Such sucrose deposition results in freezing of the caps. After establishment of tight specifications for invert sugar content in the coating syrup, the drying problem encountered during the smoothing operation disappeared.

XIV. EFFECT OF FILM-FORMER VISCOSITY ON DISINTEGRATION RATE

Developmental work had been initiated to film coat a tablet dosage form of a bitter-tasting drug. A 9:1 weight ratio of hydroxypropylmethylcellulose/ethylcellulose was found to be satisfactory because it masked the bitter taste.

Hydroxypropylmethylcellulose is a popular film former because of its solubility in organic solvents and its facile dispersibility in gastrointestinal juices. Such solubility and dispersibility characteristics permit its use in usual amounts without interfering with tablet disintegration and drug availability. Ethylcellulose was included in the film because its presence imparts film strength and elasticity. It cannot be used alone or in too high a concentration as it is completely insoluble in water.

Several lots prepared in research and in the pilot plant had disintegration times of less than 5 min in simulated gastric juice at 37°C. The uncoated cores consistently disintegrated within 2 min. A subsequent pilot batch of tablets did not disintegrate within the time limits specified. Discussions between research and pilot plant personnel were initiated to ascertain the cause of the slow disintegration.

The weights of the film-coated tablets were within specification limits. Check weight records and inventory supplies confirmed that the intended 9:1 weight ratio had been used. Nothing unusual had been noted by the pilot plant operators who had prepared the film-coated tablets. As a consequence, the decision was made to check the viscosities of the various lots of hydroxypropylmethylcellulose and ethylcellulose used in preparing the various batches of tablets. An interesting relationship between viscosity limits and tablet disintegration was found. The viscosity of a 2% aqueous dispersion of hydroxypropylmethylcellulose must be lss than 15 cp and the viscosity of ethylcellulose in toluene/ethanol must be less than 10 cp. The poorly disintegrating film-coated tablets had been coated with hydroxypropylmethylcellulose exhibiting a viscosity of 50 cp for a 2% aqueous dispersion. The ethylcellulose used in the poorly disintegrating tablets was type 10 cp. Viscosity specification limits were set in collaboration with quality control to obviate recurrence of the problem.

XV. TABLET BINDING

When tablets adhere, seize, or tear in the die the cause is usually inadequate lubrication. A film is formed in the die and ejection of the tablet is difficult. Such tablets have rough or vertically scratched sides. The surface of the tablets lacks a smooth or glossy finish, and they are often cracked on the top edge. Additional lubricant or substitution of a more effective one will usually correct this problem. The method of adding the lubricant can sometimes be the cause of binding in the die. Some formulators recommend introducing the lubricant by sifting through a 100-mesh silk screen.

Binding may be caused by attempting to compress granules that are too dry, too moist, too coarse, too hard, or too abrasive. Granules that are too dry could be regranulated. However, an in-process control specification on moisture content would effectively guard against overly dried granules. Granules that are too moist will likewise be prevented by an accurately defined in-process moisture specification. Granules that are too coarse are apt to cause lubricant failure. Corrective measures that can be considered are (1) reduce the size of the granules, and (2) increase the amount of lubricant. In the event the granules are too hard or too abrasive, modification of the granule formula should be considered.

After the compressional stage some tablets expand excessively. In such instances tapered dies should be considered as a practical corrective measure. When binding in the die occurs in one or two stations of a rotary tablet press, the tooling should be checked. Replacement or polishing of those punches and dies that are poorly finished or rough from abrasion would solve the problem.

XVI. PICKING AND STICKING

The term *picking* is used to describe the removal of material from the surface of the tablet and its adherence to the face of the punch. Specifically, this term refers to monograms, lettering, or numbering. Letters such as A, B, P, and R, which possess small, enclosed areas, are apt to cause picking. Letters such as M, N, W, and Z, which have sharp angles, are also troublesome. All such areas and angles are difficult for the engraver to cut cleanly and for the toolmaker to polish smoothly. Picking is usually due to moist granules when plain punches are used.

The term *sticking* may also refer to the build up of material on the punch faces. However, the term is more often used to describe the adhesion of granulation to the die wall. Sticking is usually due to improperly dried or improperly lubricated granulations. Sticking or picking is more apt to occur if excessive binder is used, if the humidity is high, or if a low-melting component such as stearic acid is present.

When lettered punches are to be used, the letters should be made as large as possible. This is especially useful on punches with small diameters. Increasing the diameter and weight of the tablet will be useful from two standpoints. Not only would the enlargement permit larger letters to be used, but a low-melting drug component could be diluted further to minimize the picking and sticking tendency. Others have found it beneficial to include colloidal silica in the tablet formula. The colloidal silica acts as a polishing agent and makes the punch face smooth, and thus deters the adhesion of the granulation. Additional lubricant should be added when colloidal silica is present, since the latter's frictional nature may deter easy ejection of the tablet from the die.

XVII. SELECTED TABLET PROBLEMS; SUGGESTED SOLUTIONS

In the interest of conserving space, a partial listing of several tablet problems that can arise and suggested solutions to such problems is given in Table 12.

Table 12   Selected Tablet Problems and Suggested Solutions

Tablet problem	Suggested solution
1. Tablets exhibit good dissolution rate but poor disintegration time	1. Use a less water-soluble excipient, lower the concentration of binder
2. Granule flow too slow for high-speed press	2. Reduce percent of fines; add glidant
3. Press-coated tablet core crumbling	3. Increase hardness of core (good range to shoot for 3−7 kg)
4. Separation of multilayer tablet layers	4. Keep lubricant concentration as low as practical to ensure better adhesion of layers
5. Excessive lamination of slugs	5. Reduce the depth of fill, speed, and tool size and increase the clearance by tapering
6. "Dead" effervescent tablets	6. Carry out the compression of dry ingredients in a dry atmosphere (less than 10% RH) kept at a temperature higher than ambient temperature
7. Excessive capping of tablets	7. Reduce concentration of fines, reassess lubricant concentration as it may be too high or too low, reassess moisture content in the granulation as it may be too high or too low

Source: From Refs. 1−3.

XVIII. SELECTED PROCESS DEVELOPMENT
PROJECTS OF CURRENT INTEREST

Pilot plant personnel must ever be alert to significant new equipment offerings that can reduce manufacturing costs. In addition, process modifications should be evaluated that appear to offer economic advantages over existing procedures and which do not sacrifice product quality. Selected pilot plant developmental projects of current interest are briefly summarized below.

A. High-Volume Granulation Operation

Increasing the size of batches of granules is economically advantageous because it reduces assay costs as there would be fewer batches. Furthermore, the cost of blending would be reduced because it requires little additional time to prepare a much larger batch.

The Lodige mixer [15] can be used to blend as well as to granulate tablet components. A 90 ft^3 Lodige mixer with air-sealed bearings, equipped with chopper blades, has a capacity for approximately 3000 kg of granulation. A higher degree of uniformity in distribution of tablet components has been reported to occur within 3 min as compared with 30 min in a double-cone blender. Depending on the weight of the final tablet, the capacity of granulation is sufficient for $3-5$ million tablets.

Recently, equipment based on the fluidized-bed principle has been introduced which can mix, granulate, and dry the granules formed in the same bowl. Obvious advantages of adopting such a mixer$-$dryer$-$granulator [16$-$20] are (1) less dusty plant operation, (2) reduction in granulating time, (3) drug exposed to less heat, and (4) better control of moisture content in the finished granulation.

Granulation by preliminary compression has been used for several years. Heavy-duty tablet presses were used to prepare the initial "slugs." More recent equipment introductions to prepare granulates by preliminary compression aim at increasing production capacity. The Chilsonator [21], a roll compactor, produces agglomerates by squeezing the tablet components.

Continuous processing should be considered when the volume of tablets manufactured is sufficiently large. The significant reduction achievable in manufacturing costs is well worth the investment in equipment and developmental time [22]. The purchase of such equipment and its ultimate adoption by the production division must have been preceded by a thorough pilot plant developmental study. Existing tablet formulas may have to be modified radically in order to ensure optimal performance and adherence to quality.

B. Tablet-Coating Innovations

A modification of the normal pear-shaped or subglobular coating pan which has been adopted by several companies is the side-vented coating pan [23]. Such pans have the advantage of a one-way flow of air through the tablet bed and the perforations in the pan. The increased popularity of such pans is due to the increased coating efficiency resulting from their use.

Delivery of the coating solutions manually by ladling is being replaced
by spraying with and without the aid of an air jet. Two general sprays
are available. Airless spraying relies on hydraulic pressure to produce a
spray when material is forced through a nozzle. Atomization of the spray
is achieved by the introduction of turbulent jets of air. The airless or
atomized spray of coating material can be applied to tablets contained in
the conventional pan, the side-vented pan, or in equipment based on the
fluidized-bed principle developed by Wurster [24].

A concerted effort is being made by several companies to replace organic solvent solutions of film formers with aqueous dispersions. The obvious advantage of reduced cost and reduction in environmental contamination by the solvents are compelling reasons. The perfection of coating
tablets with aqueous dispersions of film-forming materials requires lengthy
and thorough developmental efforts. The use of heated, less porous,
highly compressed tablets have been found to be promising. Various gums
and gum combinations are being evaluated. Here again, existing tablet
formulas may have to be radically modified in order to perfect coating with
aqueous dispersions of film formers.

XIX. ADDITIONAL PILOT PLANT RESPONSIBILITIES

A. Clinical Supplies, Validation and Revalidation

The large number of patients that must be treated in the evaluation of new
drugs to be given chronically means that clinical batches of tablet will be
large. The preparation of several clinical batches in the pilot plant provides its personnel with the opportunity to perfect and validate the
process.

Papariello [25] has suggested that validation of tablet dosage forms of
not only new drugs, but also those already being marketed should be conducted in the pharmaceutical pilot plant. He states that pharmaceutical
research and its development division have developed the formulas and
manufacturing processes for the tablet dosage forms. Hence, the history
and experiences gained in the development of the manufacturing process
are most familiar to the research and pilot plant personnel. This knowledge will prove to be most helpful during the validation process. Such
validation conducted on a pilot scale should simplify production scale
validation.

Reworking a clinical batch of tablets that did not meet established
specifications followed by revalidation will prove to be of future value during the production operation. Chambliss and Hendrick [26] pointed out
that if an FDA-approved reprocessing instruction exists for a particular
combination of product and problem, the manufacturer may release and distribute the product without notifying the FDA. Lack of such approved
reprocessing instructions will necessitate submission of New Drug Application (NDA) supplement in which the reprocessing and revalidating are
described. After receiving FDA approval, the reworked batch can then
be distributed. An extensive delay in obtaining approval could lead to
the sacrifice of the reprocessed batch.

Desirable goals to aim for are zero defects and zero batch rejections.
Confidence in attaining such goals according to Berry [27] can be
achieved and verified by process validation. Exhaustive finished testing

of product is not a substitute for in-process controls and process validation.

B. Bulk Drug Variation and Alternate Excipient Suppliers

During the clinical evaluation phase chemical processing modifications may be considered in the interest of improving the yield of the new compound. Solvents used for the final crystallization step during the early stages in synthesizing the new compound may be replaced by less costly ones. Slower cooling cycles encountered on scale-up could lead to large crystals differing in shape from those prepared on a small scale. The preferred larger crystals would be more rapidly filtered or centrifuged and washed. Size reduction by milling could lead to drug batches differing in particle size distribution, bulk density, dissolution rate, and static charges from earlier batches. Hence, another responsibility for the pharmaceutical pilot plant personnel is to validate the use of new batches of drug in the tablet formula under clinical study.

In many instances, the drug may be purchased by a drug company as are the purchase of excipients. Using alternate suppliers for such materials makes it less likely that supply problems may arise. Furthermore, competitive pricing will be assured. Such drug and excipient supplies should be carefully characterized. Tablets prepared with the excipients and drugs obtained from alternate suppliers should be compared with the tablets being evaluated clinically. The various physical properties of the standard formula such as hardness, disintegration time, dissolution rate, and friability as well as tability should all be matched by the tablets containing the supplies from each alternate source of materials.

Chowhan [28] described the significant differences that were encountered with a water-soluble drug that had been crystallized from different solvents. The tablets under consideration contained 64% of drug. Tablets containing bulk compound crystallized from denatured ethanol (Source B) instead of methanol (Source A) developed a serious tendency toward capping during the aqueous film-coating procedure. Additional comparisons were made with three batches of bulk drug from Source B plus one from Source A. The Source B bulks were crystallized from methanol, ethanol, or isopropanol. Significantly different wetting characteristics were noted during the granulation of these batches. Although the volume of the granulating solution, the rate of addition, and the mixing-granulating time were the same for each batch, finer granules were obtained from the methanol-crystallized drug (Source A) than from the isopropanol-crystallized drug (Source B). The two batches with coarser granules had significantly higher bulk densities than did the two batches that contained finer granules. The drug crystallized from ethanol was the least compressible. Tablets containing isopropanol-crystallized drug exhibited greater friability than those obtained from methanol.

Dissolution studies on tablets containing the differently crystallized drug revealed that more rapid rates were observed with tablets made with methanol-procesed drug from Source A than the isopropanol-treated drug from Source B. The results of this study demonstrated that the drug itself can cause major differences in the pharmaceutical scale-up process, and therefore should be thoroughly characterized. The final crystallization and isolation step for the drug can significantly affect the powder, granulation, compression, and tableting operation.

C. Processing Equipment Selection and Selected New Technology

The establishment of ideal procedures for plant manufacture must take into account a variety of factors. The small-scale equipment used by the research pharmacist in developing the original tablet formulation is too simplistic for direct scale-up to production-size batches. The pilot plant function is to conduct scale-up runs and recommend the pieces of equipment required for the large-scale manufacture of the particular tablet dosage form. The size of these pilot batches should be large enough to assure that the results obtained can be duplicated in production lot-size runs with a minimum of procedural modifications. The equipment selected should be cost effective, simple to operate, easy to clean and capable of producing high yields of quality tablets which consistently meet established specifications.

Blending

Initial blending time of the tablet ingredients in a V- or double-cone blender according to Sweitzer [29] is a function of the void space in the blender. The following relationship was established for the double-cone blender. At the 80% fill level, the blend was not completely uniform even after lengthier blending. Since all solids pick up surface charges owing to mechanical work, blending time cycles should be kept at a minimum to prevent too much static buildup. Excessive static buildup will cause a balling tendency which will make blend uniformity more difficult to attain.

A ribbon mixer could have been selected instead of the double-cone or V-blender. However, the latter two blenders will consume relatively small horsepower, since they are just lifting and folding the material, whereas the action in a ribbon mixer is largely frictional. Lower horsepower consumption is more cost effective.

Table 13 Blending Time Required in a Double-Cone Blender at Various Fill Levels

Fill level (%)	Test blend time required (min)	Approximate blend time for large production units (min)
50	3	10
65	4.2	14
70	5.4	18
75	7.2	24
80	12.0	40

Granulation

Harder and Van Buskirk [30] have stated that the most common reasons to justify granulation are: (1) to impart good flow properties to the material so that the tablet presses can be properly fed and a uniform tablet weight maintained, (2) to increase the apparent density of the powders, (3) to alter the particle size distribution so that the binding properties on compaction can be improved, and (4) to disperse potent active ingredients by solvent deposition.

In addition to the traditional sigma blade or planetary mixer, the double-cone or V-blender equipped with agitators and a liquid feed mechanism could be used to carry out the granulation step. In the interest of achieving greater efficiency and reduced cost, the Littleford Lodige Multifunctional Processor (Littleford Brothers, Florence, Kentucky) can be used. In such equipment, dry blending, wet granulation, drying, sizing, and lubrication can be conducted in a continuous process. Chowhan [28] has pointed out that the volume of granulating fluid is perhaps the most important factor that affects the granulation and tablet properties when such a continuous processor is used.

To evaluate the effects of small variations in the volume of granulation fluid, three 175-kg batches of granulation were prepared in a 22-ft^3 Littleford Lodige apparatus under identical mixing and granulating conditions. The volume of granulating solution was varied slightly in order to optimize the fluid volume for the mixer. In general, the granules were finer when a small amount of fluid was used in the granulation process. As the volume of granulating fluid was increased, the bulk and tapped densities increased correspondingly. At a granulation moisture content of 3.9%, all three granulations were equally compressible. At lower levels of moisture content, the differences in compressibility that were caused by the fluid volume used in the granulation step became evident. The granules that were made using lower fluid volumes were more compressible than the granules made with the higher fluid volumes.

At a granulation moisture content of 3.9%, the various volumes of granulating fluid did not affect the friability of the tablets. At lower moisture of the granulation such as 3.4% and 2.7%, tablets that were compressed from granulations made with the lower volumes of granulating fluid were slightly more friable than those tablets that were compressed with the higher volumes of granulating fluid.

A significant difference was observed for the in-vitro dissolution rate when the volume of granulating fluid was altered. The magnitude of this effect depends on the moisture content of the granulation and the hardness of the tablet. In general, a high volume of granulating fluid yields harder tablets exhibiting a low rate of drug dissolution and vice versa.

Fluid-Bed Granulation

The fluid-bed process has been shown to be superior to high-shear mixing with regard to processing time and yield of product. Rowley [31] has described scale-up factors that should be considered in converting from a conventional high-shear granulating process to a fluid-bed granulator. The unit operational steps for the former process include: (1) wet massing (Littleford Lodige mixer); (2) wet milling (Fitzmill, Fitzpatrick Company, Elmhurst, Illinois); (3) remilling (Fitzmill); (4) drying (Dryer/ Granulator); (5) dry milling (Tornado Mill, Stokes, Division of Pennwalt

Table 14 Major Test Parameters Used to Granulate a Sample Product in a
Fluid-Bed Granulator

| | Trial number | | | | |
Parameter	1	2	3	4	5
Bowl charge (kg)	15.0	15.0	15.0	15.0	15.0
Mix cycle (min)	5.0	5.0	5.0	5.0	5.0
Spray cycle					
Total solution (kg)	2.0	2.0	2.0	2.0	2.0
Spray rate (ml/min)	200.0	300.0	400.0	300.0	300.0
Atomizing air (bar)	2.0	2.0	2.0	2.0	2.0
Inlet-air temperature (°C)	40.0	40.0	40.0	40.0	40.0
Total cycle time (min)	12.0	10.0	8.0	10.0	10.0
Wet bulb LOD (%)	10.0	19.5	19.3	19.3	19.2
Dry cycle					
Inlet-air temperature (°C)	50.0	55.0	55.0	60.0	60.0
Total cycle time (min)	17.0	16.0	18.0	16.0	16.0
Final loss-on-drying (%)	3.0	2.9	2.9	2.9	2.8
Total run time (min)	34.0	31.0	31.0	31.0	31.0

Corp., Warminster, Pennsylvania); and (6) final blending (PK Blender,
Patterson Kelley Co., East Stroudsburg, Pennsylvania, 18301). The dryer/
granulator can be used for the mixing, wetting, and drying steps. The
dry milling and final blending steps can be conducted as previously stated
in steps (5) and (6). Rowley recommends that a dryer/granulator with a
15- to 20-kg capacity be used in feasibility studies. The investigator can
determine whether the fluid-bed granulator can be incorporated into the
process after inspection of the experimental data from five 15-kg lots. The
major test parameters Rowley employed in his pilot studies are summarized
in Table 14 [31].

The formulation consisted of drug, povidone, starch, lactose, and magnesium stearate. The content uniformity of the blend was determined after
the 5-min mix cycle. Time for mixing was added or subtracted as indicated
by the data. The spray rate of 200 ml/min was increased during the
feasibility studies, since the total moisture content of the wet mass after
spraying was less than 85% (w/w) of the granulating solution introduced.

The final granulation from trial 1 produced soft tablets that exhibited
some tendency to cap. The granulation from trial 2 produced tablets that
exhibited good weight control and a hardness that ranged from 9−12 SCU;
furthermore, no capping was evident. Trial 3 produced tablets that had

excellent weight control, a hardness from 12–13 SCU, and no capping.
The tablets from trials 2 and 3 passed current process specifications.
Trial 4 was used to verify the results obtained in trial 2. The granulation
from trial 4 had the same compression characteristics as the one from
trial 2, and it also produced excellent tablets. Trial 5 served as the final
third batch to complete the validation package and to support the process
change.

Recently, an excellent review article on wet granulation of a pharmaceutical product in fluidized beds and high shear mixers was published
[32]. The fundamentals of granule growth, granulation variables, scale-up,
and endpoint control are thoroughly covered.

*Drug Granules Prepared by Precompression, Wet
Granulation, Fluidized-Bed Granulation, and
Spray Drying*

Seager [33] compared the following methods of producing paracetamol granulations: precompression, wet massing, fluidized-bed granulation, and
spray drying. Precompressed granules containing 1–7% of hydrolyzed
gelatin were compared by roller compaction. Such granules consist of compressed drug and binder particles welded together through bonds formed
during the compaction process; for example, varying melting points in the
same treated batch and differences in brittleness or plastic deformation.
The granules are dense and may contain an uneven distribution of binder
particles. However, the binder makes little contribution to the granulation
process, since it was added as dry particles.

Wet-massed granules were obtained by mixing the drug in a planetary
mixer with an aqueous solution of hydrolyzed gelatin. The wet mass was
then forced through a sieve and dried. The granules obtained consisted
of more porous aggregates having drug particles held together in a sponge-
like network of binder. The drug particles are entrapped within the binder matrix and are partially bonded through crystalline bridges of drug and
binder which form during the granulation process.

The fluidized-bed granules were prepared by spraying a hydrolyzed
gelatin solution onto a bed of paracetamol being fluidized in the warm air
stream of a fluidized-bed dryer. The fluidized-bed granules were similar
to granules prepared by the wet-massing process. The intragranular porosity was greater, however, and the surface of the granules contained an
uneven distribution of binding agent.

The granules prepared in an industrial spray dryer by spray drying
a suspension of the drug in an aqueous solution of hydrolyzed gelatin consisted of spherical particles composed of an outer shell of binder with an
inner core of drug powder. The granules retained their integrity through
encapsulation by the binder and through the crystalline bridges which
formed between the drug particles during the spray-drying process. The
granules were porous, and the core contained vacuoles of encapsulated
air.

Tablets were prepared by mixing and then compressing the four types
of paracetamol granules with 10% microcrystalline cellulose, and 1% each of
Explotab and magnesium stearate. At all binder concentrations the tablets
prepared with spray-dried granules were the hardest and exhibited dissolution rates equal to or greater than softer tablets prepared with wet-
massed granules. Roller-compacted granules yielded tablets which were
soft at all compaction pressures. The dissolution rate of paracetamol

from tablets containing roller-compacted granules was slower compared to tablets containing wet-massed drug granules. Similar results were found for the tablets prepared from the larger granules manufactured by the fluidized-bed and wet-massing processes. Both the disintegration time and the dissolution rate of the more porous fluidized-bed product were superior to those of the wet-massed tablets for compacts of the same tensile strength even though in the case of the fluidized product, lower forces of compaction were used.

Seager [33] concluded that the binder distribution affects the compression characteristics of the granules. Furthermore, tablet strength is proportional to the concentration of binder at the granule surfaces and compact strength increases through intergranular bonding when the granules are prepared by precompression, wet massing, fluidization and spray drying, respectively. Finally, dissoluton rates are related to the degree of intergranular bonding and to the compact porosities, which in turn are governed by the nature and position of the binder within the granule structure of the tablet.

Carrier Granulation and Moisture-Activated Dry Granulation

Whenever new and significant granulation techniques are described in the literature, alert pharmaceutical research and development personnel will ascertain if their adoption might be advantageous. In many instances, the pharmaceutical pilot plant may be the most suitable area in which to evaluate such new procedures. Thus, as an example, Michoel et al. [34] have described the advantages of carrier granulation as a method that should be considered for the production of low-dosage-type tablets.

Carrier granulation is a one-step production process that greatly decreases the potential for segregation of drug particles encountered in some instances with conventional direct-compression operations. Furthermore, the carrier technique yields granulations that exhibit improved flow and compressibility. Content uniformity in tablets containing a small amount of drug is of concern when direct-compression procedures are employed. To favor content uniformity finely milled drug is used. The drug is blended with a directly compressible excipient, such as, spray-dried lactose. The finely milled drug may differ significantly in particle size with the directly compressible excipient. As a consequence, drug classification may occur during the blending operation.

In the carrier granulation technique, a portion of excipient is moistened with a small amount of solution containing a binder. The finely milled drug and additional excipient are mixed with the excipient moistened with binder solution. Granules obtained in this manner are less apt to classify.

The carrier granulation procedure was carried out on a laboratory scale as well as on an industrial scale using a Topo Granulator (Machines Collette, Wommelgem, Belgium). The Topo Granulator is a double-jacketed, cylindrical vessel that can be operated under vacuum conditions. Mixing is performed by a helical mixing arm that can rotate at variable speeds in both directions.

The following tablet excipients were employed in the article cited [34]: (1) filler, 200-mesh hydrous lactose in which a minimum of 90% of the particles were less than 100 µm in diameter; (2) carrier, hydrous lactose in which 20% of the particles were less than 63 µm and a minimum of 80% of the particles were less than 200 µm in diameter; (3) adhering material, anhydrous lactose in which 90% of the particles were less than 45 μm in diameter; (4) binder, microcrystalline cellulose and povidone; (5) disintegrants, starch, and sodium starch glycolate; and (6) lubricant, magnesium stearate.

In a typical pilot run 4 kg of hydrous lactose, carrier grade, was moistened with 175 ml of aqueous solution containing 100 gm of povidone. After mixing at 60°C for 15 min, 200 gm of drug and 600 gm of 450-mesh lactose were introduced. After 10 more minutes of mixing, the mixture was dried under a 5-kPa vacuum and then sized through a 1000-μ sieve. The carrier granulations possessed smaller geometric diameters and exhibited superior flowability than those granulations produced by conventional direct-compression or conventional wet-granulation procedures. The 175-ml of solution containing 100 gm of povidone represented 3.5% of the total weight of the granulation. In the conventional wet-granulation procedure, the volume of povidone solution introduced represented 15% of the total weight of the granulation.

After adding the disintegrants and lubricant, then blending and compressing, the carrier-granulation process yielded tablets which exhibited excellent hardness and better content uniformity than those prepared by direct compression. Tablets prepared by conventional wet granulation were slightly harder than those containing carrier granulation; however, the dissolution rate of drug from the latter was more rapid. As was mentioned earlier, carrier granulation is a one-step process that requires a low demand on resources, such as, time, room space, and personnel. Since the process limits the amount of water added to effect granulation, energy for removal of the water is considerably reduced.

Avoidance of the costly drying step in the preparation of granules can be achieved by following a modified wet process that has been referred to as moisture-activated dry granulation (MADG) by Ullah et al. [35]. Agglomeration and moisture distribution are the two basic steps of the MADG process. In the agglomeration step, 30−60% of the final formula weight is blended with a dry binder. The binder must become tacky when moistened and should be uniformly distributed throughout the powder that is intended for agglomeration. Since only a small amount of water is to be added, this moisture must also be uniformly distributed.

During blending, a small quantity of moisture that is equal to 1−4% of the final formula weight is added in the form of fine droplets or spray. With the addition of moisture, the dry binder is activated and agglomeration takes place. If the dry binder and the moisture are equally dispersed throughout the powder, the process does not require the usual large amount of shear to cause agglomeration; the shear generated by conventional wet-granulating equipment is adequate.

As blending continues, the balance of the drug or excipients, or both, is added to the agglomerated mass. During this step, the least absorbent material is added first and the most absorbent last; this sequence facilitates the uniform distribution of the moisture. A highly absorbent material, such as microcrystalline cellulose, is added last to absorb any remaining free water. At this stage, the granules can be sieved, if necessary, to obtain a more uniform particle size distribution or to further distribute the moisture throughout the granulation. The addition of a disintegrant and a lubricant completes the formulation. The type and amount of dry binder and excipients that are used as well as the amount of moisture that is added all control the agglomeration operation and determine the characteristics of the final granule and ultimately the tablet. The purpose of the agglomeration step in the MADG process is to eliminate fines.

To understand the mechanism involved in the MADG process, one can consider the amount of powder used for agglomeration representing 30% of the final formula weight. If an amount of moisture that is equivalent to 3% of the final weight is added to the powder, this would create a 10% moisture level at the agglomeration stage. This amount of moisture is often sufficient for agglomeration. For any particular formulation, the amount of starting material as well as the quantity of moisture to be added to effect agglomeration must be determined experimentally.

Ullah et al. [35] prepared acetaminophen tablets using MADG granulations and compared their properties to tablets made by wet-granulation and direct-compression methods. The excipients for the three types of tablets were similar except that the water added in the MADG process was not removed. Each tablet prepared by the MADG process contained (in milligrams):

Acetaminophen, USP	325
Povidone, USP	20
Purified water, USP	15
Microcrystalline cellulose, NF	179.5
Sodium starch glycolate, NF	7.5
Magnesium stearate, NF	3

The acetaminophen and povidone were blended for 10 min in a twin-shell blender and then passed through a 30-mesh screen. The screened blend was placed in a planetary mixer and agglomerated with water, which was added as a fine stream. While continually stirring, the microcrystalline cellulose was incorporated. After additional stirring for 5 min, the granulation was again passed through a 30-mesh screen and then blended with sodium starch glycolate and magnesium stearate by mixing for 10 min in a twin-shell blender. This granulation was compressed without difficulties into highly satisfactory tablets.

This study illustrated that the MADG process combined the ease and speed of a dry-blending process with the homogeneous distribution of drug and tablet hardness achieved by wet granulation. The MADG process was capable of reducing fines, improving powder flow, and reducing the compressional force required to produce tablets with appropriate hardness. Of particular significance, the MADG process does not require any special granulating equipment. Finally, since the water added to effect granulation is not removed, the MADG process is cost effective by eliminating the customary drying operation. However, water-sensitive drugs cannot be used in this tableting process.

Instrumented Tablet Presses

The benefit of having instrumented tablet presses in pharmaceutical research and development as well as in production has been described in an excellent review article [36]. A Stokes Model F single-punch press instrumented with piezoelectric transducers is used by the Pharmaceutical Development Laboratory at Merck Sharp & Dohme [37]. This instrumented tablet press is interfaced with a PDP-11 Laboratory Computer (Digital Equipment Corporation, Marlboro, Massachusetts). The computer was selected because it (1) allowed for rapid collection of data concerning a large number of tablets, (2) increased the accuracy of force versus time readings, and (3) facilitated the determination of peak height (compressional force) and other compression parameters.

The objectives in building the system were twofold. First, to generate compression profiles of currently marketed products or those in the final stages of development in order to provide a baseline for future comparisons. Second, to provide a tool for use in the development of future tablet formulations. Thus, for example, one could study the effects on tablet compression characteristics with changes in excipients. Third, compression profiles for excipients or only active ingredients may aid in future formulation studies.

According to Schwartz [38], the first of the above cited objectives provides a basis for comparison that can be most useful once the formulation is in production. Processing concerns, such as (1) initial scale-up runs; (2) changes in location of manufacture; (3) changes in equipment; (4) changes in batch size; (5) excipient-supplier changes; (6) active-ingredient changes, such as a change in solvent used in the crystallization step; (7) formulation changes; and (8) generation of validation data, may each be accommodated much more efficiently through proper use of the baseline data made available by the basic compression data generated by the instrumented press. Furthermore, such an instrumented tablet press will be a valuable aid for investigating the behavior of various formulations when they are subjected to a range of different compaction forces or when they are compressed at different rates. Such a system will allow each batch of granulation to be checked before it is compressed in order to establish the normal compression profile for a particular formulation and to check future batches for the same compression properties.

The rapid development of computer-integrated systems makes possible fully automatic, unattended tablet production feasible. Weight monitoring and control systems for tablet production have been in use for several years. Ideally, the weight of every single tablet should be checked. Some modern presses are capable of producing 125 tablets/s. This speed is beyond the capability of any currently available weighing system. Rather than use direct weight data from a small statistical sample, the majority of systems have employed compaction force for each and every tablet as an indirectly measured variable. The assumption is that for a given tablet thickness there is a fixed relationship between compaction force and weight deviations. This is only valid if variations in granule consistency, humidity, temperature, or compaction in the hopper for the feed chute do not adversely affect feeding. Routine weight checks on sample tablets need to be made and machines adjusted from time-to-time. This is done by automatic weight control systems available today.

With both direct and indirect systems, compression force and fill depth are the variables. Weight, however, is not the only parameter of importance. Change in compaction force can result in considerable variation in tablet thickness and hardness, the latter of which may alter dissolution properties so that they are outside allowable limits.

Huddlestone [39] described the Kilian-developed automatic system for tablet production designated as CIT by the developer. Kilian, a German-based tablet press manufacturer, utilizes compaction force as the primary control on every individual tablet, which in turn is routinely monitored and regulated using actual weight, thickness, and hardness data generated by an integrated test module. The real advance made by Kilian has been the introduction of an electromechanical quality control unit to establish quality parameters and to integrate signaled data into the adaptive control system.

The quality assurance module in the CIT system takes a predetermined number of sample tablets and performs individual weight, thickness, and hardness measurements. After integration of this data, signals are sent to the control processor. This controller is capable of adjusting each of these parameters. For example, if the actual weight of the sampled tablets falls outside the preset range, the compaction fill set point for the primary control will be adjusted. This in turn affects the weight of the tablet.

The actual weight data can only be used over a limited range as the compaction variation affects hardness and dissolution. In its full form, CIT introduces tablet hardness as another control variable. Hardness changes caused by compaction force variation are compensated by altering tablet thickness.

The total Kilian process management system, CIT, consists of three controls operating synchronously: (1) compaction force/fill depth; (2) actual weight with constant compaction force, varying fill and tablet thickness; and (3) hardness control with constant fill, varying compaction force set value and thickness.

Pharmaceutical Pilot Operation in
Small and Large Companies

The instrumented tablet presses described in the preceding section are very expensive. The small manufacturer not only is unable to provide such sophisticated equipment, the company may not even be able to afford pilot plant space or personnel. In such instances, the pharmaceutical development personnel will be responsible for conducting scale-up runs and to validate the manufacturing procedures on production presses. The accumulated in-house experience should be taken advantage of when pilot runs are scheduled between production runs. Agreement should be sought with production and quality assurance personnel on the in-process controls recommended. Close cooperation, frequent communication, and unambiguous written procedures are essential if the established specifications for the newly developed tablet formulation are to be consistently and competently matched by the production department personnel.

The large manufacturer can provide well-equipped pilot plant space and personnel. More numerous newly developed tablet formulations can be readied for transfer to the production department without causing frequent scheduling interruptions. Such well-equipped areas can more efficiently evaluate and incorporate new tablet technology for the financial benefit of the company. Here again, the same desirable spirit of cooperation, communication, and unambiguous written procedures between the various difisions of the company should prevail.

REFERENCES

1. Das, S. and Jarowski, C. I., Effect of granulating method on particle size distribution of granules and disintegrated tablets. *Drug Dev. Ind. Pharm.*, 5(5):479–488 (1979).
2. Das, S. and Jarowski, C. I., Effect of granulating method on content uniformity and other physical properties of granules and their

corresponding tablets. II. *Drug Dev. Ind. Pharm.*, 5(5):489−500 (1979).

3. Das, S. and Jarowski, C. I., Effect of granulating method on dissolution rate of compressed tablets. III. *Drug Dev. Ind. Pharm.*, 5(5): 501−505 (1979).

4. de Jong, E. J., The preparation of microgranulations, an improved tableting technique. *Pharm. Week Blad.*, *104* (1979).

5. Khan, K. A. and Rhodes, C. T., Effect of compaction on particle size. *J. Pharm. Sci.*, *64*:444−446 (1979).

6. Feigenbaum, A. V., *Total Quality Control Engineering and Management*. McGraw-Hill, New York, 1961, p. 265.

7. Schwartz, J. B., Martin, E. T., and Dehner, E. J., Intragranular starch: Comparison of starch USP and modified corn starch. *J. Pharm. Sci.*, *64*:329 (1975).

8. Martin, A. N., Swarbrick, J., and Cammarata, A., *Physical Pharmacy*, 2nd ed. Lea & Febiger, Philadelphia, 1969, pp. 485−490.

9. Jones, T. M. and Pilpel, N., The flow properties of granular magnesia. *J. Pharm. Pharmacol.*, *18*:81 (1966).

10. Martin, A. N., Swarbrick, J., and Cammarata, A., *Physical Pharmacy*, 2nd ed. Lea & Febiger, Philadelphia, 1969, pp. 491−492.

11. Lantz, R. J., Jr., Daruwala, J., and Lachman, L., The importance of interdisciplinary cooperation in pharmaceutical production trouble shooting. *Drug Dev. Commun.*, *1*(4):349−368 (1975).

12. Chaudry, I. A. and King, R. E., Migration of potent drugs in wet granulations. *J. Pharm. Sci.*, *61*:1121−1125 (1972).

13. Warren, J. W., Jr. and Price, J. C., Drug migration during drying of tablet granulations. I: Effect of particle size of the major diluent. *J. Pharm. Sci.*, *66*:1406−1409 (1977).

14. Warren, J. W., Jr. and Price, J. C., Drug migration during drying of tablet granulations. II: Effect of binder solution viscosity and drying temperature. *J. Pharm. Sci.*, *66*:1409−1412 (1977).

15. *Technical Evaluation of the Littleford Horizontal Mixer.* Littleford Brothers, Florence, Kentucky.

16. Schaefer, T. and Worts, O., Control of fluidized bed granulation. I: Effects of spray angle, nozzle height and starting materials on granule size and size distribution. *Arch. Pharm. Chem.*, *5*:51−60 (1977).

17. Schaefer, T. and Worts, O., Control of fluidized bed granulation. II: Estimation of droplet size of atomized binder solution. *Arch. Pharm. Chem.*, *5*:178−193 (1977).

18. Schaefer, T. and Worts, O., Control of fluidized bed granulation. III: Effects of inlet air temperature and liquid flow rate on granule size and size distribution. Control of moisture content of granules in the drying phase. *Arch. Pharm. Chem.*, *6*:1−13 (1978).

19. Schaefer, T. and Worts, O., Control of fluidized bed granulation. IV: Effects of binder solution and atomization on granule size and size distribution. *Arch. Pharm. Chem.*, *6*:14−25 (1978).

20. Schaefer, T. and Worts, O., Control of fluidized bed granulation. V: Factors affecting granule growth. *Arch. Pharm. Chem.*, *6*: 69−82 (1978).

21. *Technical Bulletin on the Evaluation of the Chilsonator.* Fitzpatrick Co., Chicago.

22. *Continuous Liquid–Solids Blender Processor.* Patterson-Kelley Co., East Stroudsburg, Pennsylvania.
23. *Survey Bulletin on the Operation of the Accela-Cota.* Thomas Engineering, Hoffman Estates, Illinois.
24. Wurster, D. E., *Fluidized Bed Technique for Research and Development.* Glatt Air Techniques, New York.
25. Papariello, G. J., *Organizing for Validation-Process Development (R&D Division)*, Proceedings of the PMA Seminar Program on validation of solid dosage form processes (May), 31–35, 1980.
26. Chambliss, W. G. and Hendrick, M. G., One approach to reprocessing, *Pharm. Tech.*, 12:37–43 (1986).
27. Berry, I. R., Practical process validation of pharmaceutical products, *Drug Cosmet. Ind.*, 10:36–46 (1986).
28. Chowhan, Z. T., Aspects of granulation scale-up in high shear mixers, *Pharm. Technol.*, 2:26–44 (1988).
29. Sweitzer, G. R., Blending and drying efficiency; Double cone vs V-shape, Internal publication of the General Machine Co. of New Jersey, Middlesex, New Jersey.
30. Harder, S. and Van Buskirk, G., Pilot plant scale-up techniques. In *The Theory and Practice of Industrial Pharmacy*, 3rd Ed. (L. Lachman, H. A. Lieberman, and J. L. Kanig, eds.), Lea & Febiger, Philadelphia, 1986, p. 687.
31. Rowley, F. A., Scale-up factors in adapting a conventional granulating process to a fluid-bed granulator, *Pharm. Technol.*, 9:76–79 (1987).
32. Kristensen, H. G. and Schaefer, T., A review on pharmaceutical wet-granulation, *Drug Dev. Ind. Pharm.*, 4,5:803–872 (1987).
33. Seager, H., Relationship between the process of manufacture and the structure and properties of granules and tablets, Paper presented at the Pharm. Tech. conference in New York, 1982.
34. Michoel, A., Verlinden, W., Rombaut, P., Kinget, R., and De Smet, P., Carrier granulation: A new procedure for the production of low-dosage forms, *Pharm. Technol.*, 6:66–82 (1988).
35. Ullah, I., Carrao, R. G., Wiley, G. J., and Lipper, R. A., Moisture-activated dry granulation: A general process, *Pharm. Technol.*, 9:48–54 (1987).
36. Schwartz, J. B., The instrumented tablet press: Uses in research and production, *Pharm. Technol.*, 9:102–132 (1981).
37. Rosenberg, A. S., Faini, G. J., Allegretti, J. E., and Schwartz, J. B., Development of an instrumented press-computer system. Presented to the IPT Section of the Academy of Pharmaceutical Sciences meeting, San Antonio Texas, November 1980.
38. Schwartz, J. B., Dehner, E. J., and Allegretti, J. E., Formulation and process monitoring by computerized instrumented press. Presented to the IPT Section of the Academy of Pharmaceutical Sciences meeting, San Antonio, Texas, November 1980.
39. Huddlestone, K., New developments for automatic tabletting, *Manuf. Chem.*, 12:45–48 (1987).

6

Tablet Production

Robert J. Connolly and Frank A. Berstler

Superpharm Corporation, Central Islip, New York

David Coffin-Beach

Schering-Plough, Inc., Kenilworth, New Jersey

I. INTRODUCTION

Over the last decade the science of tablet production has changed as at no
other time in recent history. There are many factors that have contributed to this. In the authors' opinion, the two dominant reasons are:
(1) the manufacturers' realization for the need to improve their compet-
itiveness owing to the increase of both foreign and domestic competition,
and (2) the growth of the generic industry that mandates a less labor-
intensive environment and that by nature has greater numbers of products and normally shorter runs than the manufacturer of the brand name
products.

   With the realization that tablet production is an evolving technology-
based science, wherever possible, an attempt has been made to provide
not only "current practice" but also emerging trends in this area. In so
doing, the goal of this chapter is to provide the readership with information which will serve today's needs as well as, hopefully, some of to-
morrow's needs. With these objectives the following information is provided.

II. FOUR BASIC REQUIREMENTS FOR SUCCESSFUL
TABLET PRODUCTION

A. Design

The formulation and the ease with which that formulation can be processed
is basic to productivity. The "equipment package" ultimately used to
prepare the dosage form is primarily determined during the formulation
development stages of the product. The efficient transfer of a product to
production is predicated on a close working relationship between research

and production personnel to assure that research initiatives can be addressed when the product is commercialized. The importance of this close working relationship cannot be overemphasized, as typically the majority of production calamities can be traced back to initial formulation development. Formulation development, which centers on equipment or technology which the production organization neither possesses nor recognizes the need for, typically results in significant delays and/or changes when the formulation is transferred to production. This detail becomes particularly important when new technologies are introduced.

Organizationally, a committee with appropriate representation from research, production, management, marketing, and quality assurance is typically utilized as a facilitator for the transfer of products from research to production. Active planning and participation in the development and implementation of an integrated plan for product development and introduction by this group is essential.

B. Equipment

The selection of equipment, the proper maintenance of the equipment, adequate training in its use and care, and a review of the types of equipment available for each phase of the tablet-manufacturing process are as important as the initial design of the product in determining the success of a tablet-production facility.

C. Facility

A comprehensive understanding of the current good manufacturing practices (CGMPs) is essential for determining the facility requirements such as adequate space for separation of operations, construction materials that are not absorptive, additive, or reactive, and allow for proper cleaning and housekeeping. Both dust control that will preclude airborne cross contamination and material flow that progresses with a minimum of material crossover are also musts.

D. Personnel

There can be no substitute for properly trained personnel at all levels of the production flow. A review of the type and intensity of training required for each individual involved in the manufacturing and support functions will be addressed later in this chapter.

A thorough review and understanding of each section cf CGMPs are absolute requirements for all personnel involved in the design, construction, and operations of a tablet-manufacturing facility.

III. OVERVIEW OF THE PROCESS

A. Ordering

The manufacturing process begins with a work order or supply plan and the required materials are put on order from an approved bill of materials (master batch card and master packaging order card). In order for any production planning/inventory control function to operate efficiently with a minimum of errors and/or delays, the accuracy of the bills of materials must be at a 99.5% level and the accuracy of the inventory at any given time must be greater than 95%. An active vendor approval program will generate significant savings from a reduction in rejected materials and labor losses due to work stoppages and nonstandard processing. Ideally, the supplier of raw materials and packaging components should have a close working relationship with the purchasing department to fine tune their product specifications to more closely fit the manufacturer's requirements. This obviously becomes more difficult if there are multiple vendors of the same components. Whatever efforts are expended toward this end will be rewarded with consistency and quality during the entire production process.

B. Receiving

A centralized warehousing function should be responsible for the receipt and storage of components in whatever stage of the process they are in. There must be adequate space for the receiving process. The initial step is to identify the materials being received against the component code and name, the purchase order number, and the vendor lot number. A receiving number is then assigned that will be traceable throughout the manufacturing cycle. These numbers are clearly marked on all receipts according to CGMPs and company policy.

C. Sampling

The quality assurance group should have a separate area central to the receiving area to take the required samples. Timely notification of receipt and expeditious sampling of materials will greatly reduce the space required and minimize confusion and clutter in the warehouse, assuring better material control.

D. Warehouse

The clearly marked quarantined materials are stored in a separate and identified storage area until released by quality control personnel. The materials are then labeled as released and moved into a separate and identified area for released material. Conversely, rejected material must be immediately labeled as such and moved to a remote and clearly identified reject storage area for ultimate disposition. As the components are physically moved through each of the aforementioned stages they must also be traceable by inventory controllers so the availability of the inventory is known at all times. This is being accomplished, to an ever increasing extent, by computer tracking systems such as Material Requirements Planning (MRP) or all inclusive Manufacturing Resource Planning (MRP II). Obviously, it is as important to know the status of your inventory as it is to have adequate inventory on hand.

E. Dispensing

Once adequate released materials are on hand, the processing of a manufacturing order may begin. There are many ways to design a weighing
area; however, it must be designed so as to minimize the generation of
dust. By having adequate dust-collection equipment placed strategically,
material may be prevented from becoming airborne and from unnecessarily
settling on table and floor surfaces. This will greatly reduce the time required to clean each area after the specific weighing is accomplished.

Before weighing commences, the area must be inspected and certified
as clean and any raw material containers being brought into the area must
be inspected and certified as clean.

The weighing must be performed on calibrated weighing devices that
are sufficiently sensitive to the quantity of materials being weighed. Each
raw material must be weighed by one operator and checked by a second
operator. A weigh ticket must be generated for each material weighed
and an identifying label placed on each container of material weighed.
Many companies have label printers interfaced with their weighing devices
to perform this task. Many have also integrated this process further by
employing automated dispensing and weighing equipment, label printing,
and interfacing with their MRP or MRP II systems to automatically record
the withdrawal and instantly update the inventory. A running inventory
must be kept on materials used for each manufacturing lot and the balance
returned to stock. At the end of each raw material lot, a reconciliation
must be performed and any significant discrepancies thoroughly investigated.

F. Granulating

Each manufacturing order as received from the weigh room must be checked
against the master formula and the weigh tickets as received in the batch
folder. This check must consist of identifying each component by its label,
checking the correctness of the weights, and a visual inspection of the
containers and material contained therein.

The size of the area in which this is accomplished must be adequate to
prevent any crossover of batches being processed, and it must also have
been inspected and certified as clean. The mixing and granulating areas
must be designed with adequate space for ease of cleaning and safety of
employees. Each operation must be separated from any other activities to
ensure that no crossover of materials can occur. All containers must be
clean and identified as well as the equipment being used.

With each manufacturing order a specific quantity of equipment and
container identification labels are issued to the operators in a master batch
record folder. This folder must be kept with the batch at all stages.
As each ingredient is added to the processing equipment and each step of
the production process is performed, one operator must sign that the ad-
ditions took place and the step was completed and the second operator
must verify it with his/her signature.

At the completion of each major step of the process (i.e., after drying
and sizing or after final mixing), a reconciliation of yield is performed
and verified and any discrepancies outside the norm are immediately investigated. The blend is staged while the final check of the master production record is performed and a blend analysis is completed if required.

Four major processing techniques are employed in the manufacture of oral, solid-dosage forms today. These include direct compression, dry granulation (slugging/roll compacting), wet granulation, and combination processing (a modification of one of the cited methods). Details of each of these processing techniques are to be found elsewhere in this text, but, from a manufacturing/processing perspective, the following considerations should be emphasized.

Direct Compression

The direct-compression processing technique offers simplicity, economy, and the potential for high-volume output. Equipment considerations are minimal, since typically only mixing and compression equipment are required. Facilities designed exclusively for this type of processing can concentrate on efficient methods for bulk granulation processing and transfer to dosage-form production. Batch sizes are limited typically only by the capacity of the mixing equipment utilized, and operator handling of the granulation is, in a well-designed facility, minimal. Mindful of the limitations which this type of processing possesses, from a production perspective it still represents the ideal methodology for dosage-form manufacture. In addition, with the continuing trend toward low-dose therapeutic entities, and with stability in the supply, functionality, and uniformity of direct-compressing excipients, many of the historical objections to this type of processing are no longer valid.

Dry Granulation

The dry-granulation technique offers an alternative to direct-compression processing with many of the same advantages. Slugging is a technique which has existed as long as tableting. Newer roll-compaction equipment has greatly improved potential granulation throughput rates and provided a justifiable economic basis for the adoption of this technology over traditional slugging. As with direct-compression processing, equipment requirements for this type of processing are minimal. Essentially, the addition of only a roll compactor to the equipment package for direct-compression processing is required. Similar to direct-compression processing, dry-granulation processing has benefited from the changes cited in actives as well as excipients. Today it constitutes one of the manufacturing methods of choice for antibiotics and moisture-sensitive active ingredients.

Wet Granulation

The traditional wet-granulation technique has benefited from the introduction of processing equipment which improves its historic economic liabilities. The introduction of the fluid-bed dryer, and later the dryer/granulator (Fig. 1) and also the adaptation of the high-shear granulator to the pharmaceutical processing environment have both contributed significantly to the maintenance of this technique for granulation processing.

The significant investment both in facilities and required equipment to perform this type of processing has already been made by most companies. Consequently, this technique is often employed in lieu of dry granulation where additional expenditures may be required. Perhaps, more significantly, the wet-granulation technique represents the tried and true, and many of today's marketed products were developed utilizing this methodology.

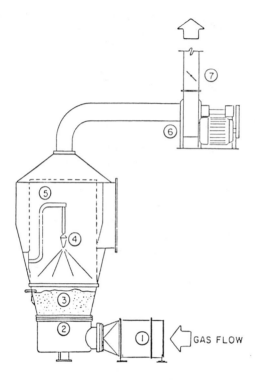

GAS FLOW

Figure 1   Fluid-bed dryer/granulator. (1) Inlet gas conditioning,
(2) entrance plenum, (3) product container with bottom screen and product, (4) granulator spray head in filter chamber, (5) filter bag, (6) fan,
and (7) damper. (Courtesy of Fluid Air, Inc.)

The economic justification for conversion to a newer, perhaps just as acceptable processing technique cannot be made for many of these "mature"
products. Obviously, of the granulation processing techniques thus far
described, wet granulation requires the largest amount of facility space,
equipment, and processing time.

Combination Processing

The category of combination processing is included in this discussion for
sake of completeness. It represents processing techniques which employ
more than one of the methods just described. Obviously, combination
processing typically results in high labor costs due to the large amount of
material handling, but in some instances, it may be the only means by
which a granulation can be manufactured. As most pharmaceutical manufacturers have equipment to perform the traditional granulating techniques,
this modality of granulation processing typically can be performed without
additional equipment expenditure. It should be noted that an emerging
trend in equipment design has resulted in the market introduction of
machines capable of complete granulation processing. Typically, a high-
intensity mixing environment is combined with a heat source/transfer

mechanism (Fig. 2). This type of equipment allows for high-speed mixing in the case of direct-compression formulations, but wet granulation with drying can also be accomplished in the same equipment. From a facilities/ equipment use perspective, the processor-type equipment represents a highly efficient and flexible method of granulation preparation.

G. Tablet Compression

In the United States, tablets are the preferred vehicle for delivering medication to the patient. The advantages include convenience of administration, precision of dosage, efficiency of manufacturing and packaging, and the ability to withstand extended storage.

There are several factors that must be taken into consideration when selecting the final manufacturing equipment for a specific tablet formulation. The size of the tablet, quality of batch, ease of compressibility (is precompression required), and abrasiveness of product are factors that will not only determine the type of tablet press used (large die, small die, single sided, or double sided), but also the type of tooling needed (standard steel, premium steel, or chromium plated). Tooling manufacturers are usually experts in determining the type of steel required for the size, shape, and abrasiveness of a product. Another factor that should be considered is the size of the run. Generally, it would not be economical on relatively short runs to have to set up a high-speed multitooled tablet press.

The tablet-compression area should be designed with separate booths or rooms that are large enough to accommodate all equipment, materials, and personnel required for the batch. The rooms must be designed with adequate dust removal and containment. The materials of construction must be those that are easily cleanable but also have sound-absorbing qualities. The aisles should be of sufficient size to allow for the free movement of materials in and out of the compression rooms and for the personnel required to operate, repair, or monitor the process.

The control of dust is of utmost importance when designing a tablet-compression area. Each room should be serviced by a centralized dust-collection system for the dust pickup stations on the tablet press, the tablet deduster, and at the feeding points unless the method of feeding precludes the escape of any product dust. In some cases, such as in the compression of control substances, there are advantages in placing cyclone collectors between the dust pickups and the central dust collector. A cyclone collector traps and contains particles drawn into the dust collector without reducing the airflow. The trapped material can then be easily removed for reconciliation.

When locating in-process test equipment, consideration should be given to centrally locating this equipment outside of the compression rooms. The advantages include the elimination of the duplication of expensive test equipment, and if no product is ever returned to the compression rooms, another potential source of product crossover is eliminated. A typical in-process test station should consist of a balance, hardness tester, friability tester, and thickness gauge. There is equipment on the market to perform all of these tests automatically and to give a computer-generated statistical profile of each batch (Fig. 3). Batch records may also be held in the centralized area for ease of reference by supervision and for

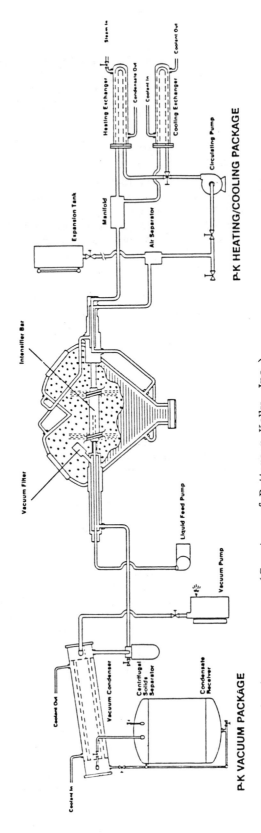

Figure 2   Combination processor.   (Courtesy of Patterson-Kelly, Inc.)

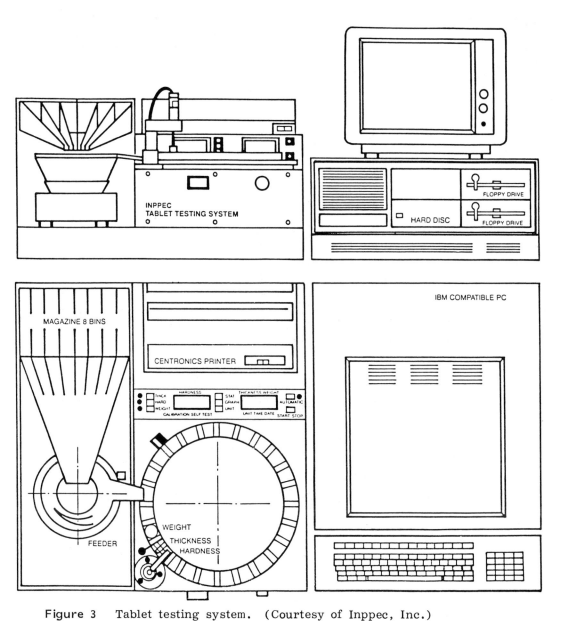

Figure 3 Tablet testing system. (Courtesy of Inppec, Inc.)

Superpharm Corporation
IN – PROCESS WEIGHT CHECK

PRODUCT:	CODE NO:	LOT NO:

DESCRIPTION:_____

	MINIMUM	TARGET	MAXIMUM
WEIGHT OF 10 TABLETS	_____		_____
INDIVIDUAL HARDNESS	_____		_____
INDIVIDUAL THICKNESS	_____		_____

NO	DATE	TIME	BOX NO	WEIGHT (mg)	HARDNESS (Kp)	THICKNESS INCHES	BY	NO	DATE	TIME	BOX NO	WEIGHT (mg)	HARDNESS (Kp)	THICKNESS INCHES	BY
1								17							
2								18							
3								19							
4								20							
5								21							
6								22							
7								23							
8								24							
9								25							
10								26							
11								27							
12								28							
13								29							
14								30							
15								31							
16								32							

WEIGHT   CONTROL CHART

1 2 3 4 5 6 7 8 9 10 11 12 13 14 15 16 17 18 19 20 21 22 23 24 25 26 27 28 29 30 31 32

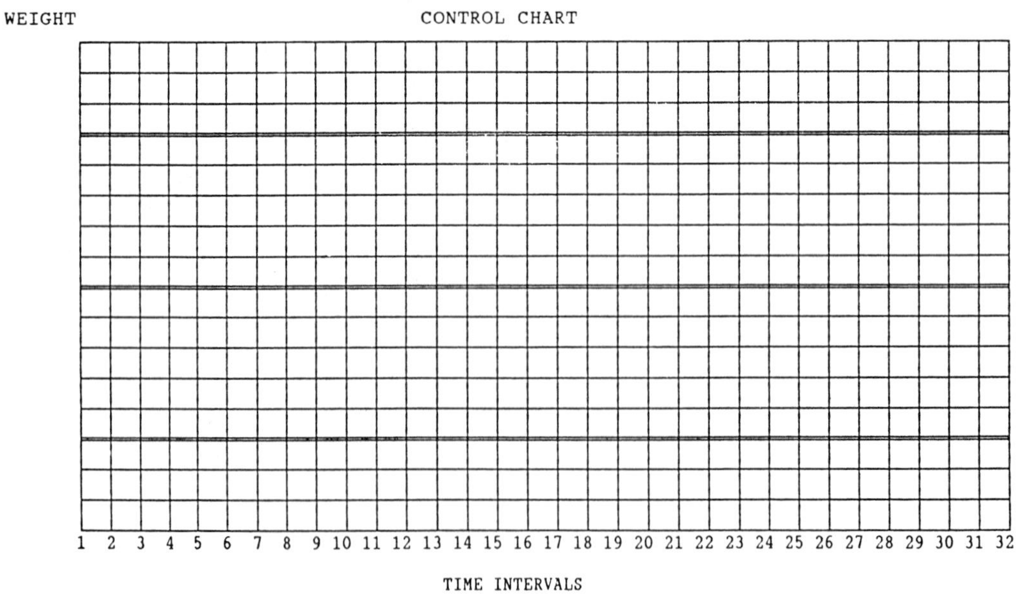

TIME INTERVALS

Figure 4   In-process weight sheet with control chart.

consistency of control over these important documents. A running control chart of tablet weights should be kept at each work station so that a trained operator can recognize a potential problem before an out-of-control situation occurs (Fig. 4).

When a batch is selected for compression, a precise series of steps may then start.

1. The machine, room, and any ancillary equipment being used are thoroughly inspected for proper cleaning and to make sure all logs are completed. These steps are then verified by a second individual.
2. The required tooling is withdrawn from the tool room and the accompanying records are inspected for accuracy and completeness. The tooling is brought to the compression machine and individually checked by a second person.
3. After the press is set up, a final review of proper alignment and lubrication is done along with another cleanliness check before granulation is introduced to the machine.
4. Once the set-up operator is satisfied that the tablets are of the proper weight, hardness, and thickness, a sample of these tablets is given to the Quality Assurance Department for a verification of all tablet specifications. This is performed and recorded as approved or rejected.
5. If all is in order, the compression of the batch may start.
6. During the compression run the tablet press operator monitors all quality aspects at predetermined intervals: Usually weight checks are performed at 15-min intervals, visual inspection more often, and hardness and friability at least once an hour. Quality assurance personnel will also periodically check and verify that all specifications are being met.
7. After the completion of the batch, the weight of the final product is recorded on the master production record and the yield is calculated. An investigation is undertaken immediately if the yield is outside the norm for this product.
8. A thorough review of the master batch record is performed and the batch is staged as quarantined in-process material until a final release to package is obtained.

H. Tablet Coating

The process of tablet coating has evolved over the years from the gold (literally) coating once applied to hand-rolled pills to the automated batch process of today. Where once sugar coating was the only option available, the development of water-soluble polymers and the combined pressures of environmentalists and concerns over worker safety have ushered in the aqueous-coating era. Although some specialty coating processes still require the use of solvents, the current trend within the pharmaceutical industry is to limit and whenever possible eliminate the use of all organic solvents in the coating process.

Three separate processing modalities are currently used to apply coating materials to "core" tablets or pellets. In addition, compression coating is sometimes employed as a processing technique, but really has very little in common with applied coating techniques. Each of the classic techniques employs equipment which functions to not only provide mechanical agitation to the dosage forms (coating substrate), but also creates a drying environment in which the excess solvent, whether water or other, can be evaporated during the coating cycle. Logically, each technique offers certain advantages and disadvantages which may be summarized as follows.

Conventional Pan

The conventional pan technique is arguably the oldest, but still finds widespread use throughout the industry, although the popularity of the conventional pan coating is waning. This technique involves the use of a solid-wall coating pan (Fig. 5) which revolves at approximately 10−15 revolutions per minute. The pan is supplied with both a warm-air inlet and an exhaust duct through the opening for loading and unloading tablets. Excess air is commonly supplied to the pan to compensate for the poor thermal energy transfer provided by the equipment. The coating solution is either poured onto the agitated tablet bed, or it can be atomized and sprayed onto the tablets. This design has several severe limitations, including poor agitation of the tablet bed, poor heat transfer to cause evaporation, and relatively long process times, which typically push the cost to coat by this modality out of consideration. Sugar coating represents the main use of this type equipment today and, in many instances, even that process has changed to the use of more modern perforated pans.

Perforated Pan

The perforated pan design of coating equipment evolved to address the technical problems which existed with the conventional pan. These systems (Fig. 6) are designed to allow airflow through the tablet bed by providing warmed drying air through a plenum to the enclosed pan with the exhaust air being drawn through perforations in the wall of the pan. This design obviously allows for much more precise control of drying conditions and consequently shorter processing times. In addition, the coating solution is atomized through spray guns situated within the pan, which also

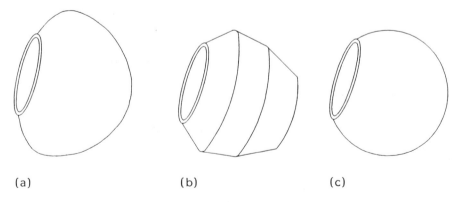

(a)   (b)   (c)

Figure 5   Conventional coating pans. (a) Pear shaped, (b) hexagonal, and (c) spherical.

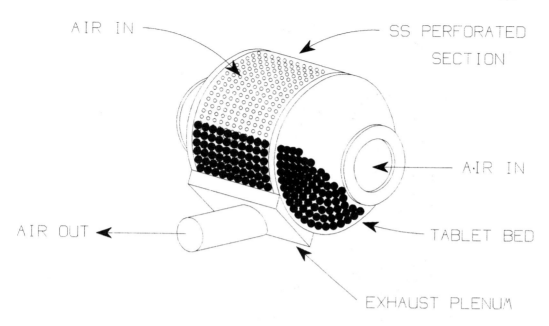

Figure 6 Perforated coating pan.

results in much more uniform application of the coating solution. These
systems are available for purchase today with the capability to perform
sugar, solvent, and aqueous coating with equal facility, and it is for this
reason this technique enjoys such widespread and growing popularity in
the industry today. Several other advantages of the perforated pan over
conventional pans include the capacity to coat substantial quantities of
core tablets (120–200 kg), the relatively short processing times required
(1.5–2.5 h for the entire coating process), and the potential for automating the coating process. Microprocessor-controlled systems have been
developed which offer a "turnkey" approach to coating. One major limitation of this technique, however, is the difficulty in obtaining uniform
coatings on very small tablet cores and/or nonpareil-type seeds. This
type of specialized coating is more readily accomplished in a fluidized bed
equipped with a Wurster partition.

Wurster Column Coating

Figure 7 depicts the typical configuration utilized for Wurster coating.
The heat source and agitation for this type of coating is the fluidization
air provided at the bottom of the container. The coating solution is
atomized by the spray nozzle and applied to an ever-changing substrate
by virtue of product passage around the partition in the center of the
processing vessel. This system provides the ideal environment for coating very small tablets, spheres, or other substrates which are relatively
easily fluidized yet possess adequate physical integrity to withstand impact with the partition and walls of the equipment until coated. The
major limitations of this type equipment include smaller (with respect to
the perforated pan) potential batch sizes, constraints on the physical

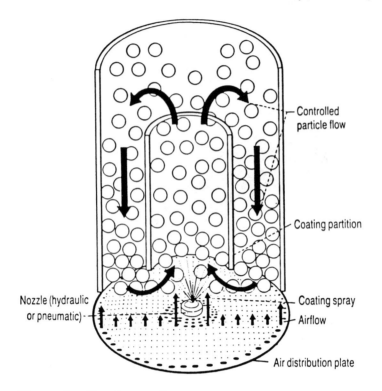

Figure 7   Wurster coating pan.

size and mass of the core tablets, and the capital expense of the equipment
if it is not already available.

I. Validation

A validated process will consistently deliver a dosage form that has a direct relationship to a dosage form on which clinical efficiency and safety
were determined. Thus, comparisons between the manufacturing process,
the raw material used, in-process and finished process test results are in
order. Careful consideration of these factors at the development stage is
a must in the successful scale up to production batches. Again, matching
equipment from laboratory to production helps to eliminate possible validation problems later on. The physical characteristics of the active drug
substance should be controlled. Particle size and crystalline structures
should be evaluated before any substitution of suppliers of drug substance are considered. Direct-compression products must be evaluated
thoroughly for particle size matching of the active drug substance and the
excipients. Special attention should be paid to products in which the
drug substance comprises a very small percentage of the dosage forms.
Wet granulations are susceptible to changes in types of equipment used to
mix and also the methods of drying as well as the amounts of solvent
used to granulate. Bioavailability of the drug over time must be thoroughly investigated before any significant changes are made [4,9].

When reviewing validation of tablet production, the following key elements should be considered.

Raw Materials

The physical characteristics of raw materials play an important role in content uniformity and bioavailability.

The literature has shown that the physical quality (e.g., particle size of raw materials) can sometimes relate to the availability and clinical effect of a product. It would, therefore, seem appropriate that the critical physical characteristics of raw materials be considered in a validation program. It is expected that the physical characteristics of a drug substance be characterized if necessary.

Physical characteristics of raw materials can vary among manufacturers of drug substances and, on occasion, have varied from lot to lot from the same manufacturer. Therefore, it is important whenever changes are being contemplated, or when it is discovered there are changes in particle size or bulk density, that the dissolution rates of granulated products and the content uniformity of direct-compression products be examined very closely.

Particulate solids, once mixed, have a tendency to segregate by virtue of differences in the shape, size, and density of the particles of which they are composed. This process of separation occurs during mixing as well as during subsequent handling of the completed mix. Generally, large differences in particle size, density, or shape within the mixture result in instability. The segregation process normally requires energy input and can be reduced by careful handling following the mixing process.

Control of the physical characteristics of excipients if the oral solid-dosage form is made by direct compression can also be important. One of the most important ingredients in both granulated and direct compression products affecting dissolution is the lubricant. Dissolution rates decrease with increasing lubricant concentration and increasing blending time. For this reason it is normal practice to blend the lubricant briefly prior to compression. Longer blending times of the alkaline stearates increase their distribution and ability to coat particles, resulting in slower dissolution.

Reproducibility of Manufacturing Process

When creating a master formula, particular attention must be paid to certain instructions that may affect the reproducibility of the process (e.g., the amount of granulating liquid and a measurable endpoint such as the measurement of the amperage draw of a particular mixer). The screening procedures are also important. Excipients must be free of lumps and proper screening will aid raw material dispersion. Never leave the option to use improper equipment: It is always safer to specify the size and design of containers and sizing equipment along with the major equipment to be used.

Equipment

The pitfalls to avoid when specifying equipment to be used in the manufacturing process can be briefly addressed by identifying the various types of mixers in general use.

Dry blending is normally accomplished in either tumble blenders or ribbon blenders. When using the tumble blenders, such as the twin-shell or the double-cone blender, care should be taken to avoid lumps of powder by prescreening and by controlling the ambient temperature and humidity. Also, do not exceed recommended volumes to assure adequate tumble action.

Ribbon blenders have two problems which must be addressed. The first is the dead spot at the discharge port. Adequate directions must be given to clear this area once or twice during the mixing cycle and to recycle the powder. The second problem, especially with low-dose actives, may be poor mixing at the shell wall because of blade clearance and also in the bottom portion of the mixer at either end.

Wet granulations are usually done in either low-energy mixers, such as Pony pan mixers, planetary mixers, Sigma or two-blade mixers, or high-energy mixers, such as Diosna, Gral, Lodige, or any number of the high-shear mixers on the market today. Pony mixers and other types of planetary mixers should be avoided when designing a dry blending process.

The low-energy mixers for wet granulations have longer granulating times and usually require larger amounts of granulating solution. When using high-energy mixers, steps must be taken to measure the endpoint so over-granulation is avoided. Also, the very high speed of the various intensifier attachments can generate considerable heat and may damage sensitive materials.

Process Control Testing

With the advent of new manufacturing equipment and changes in process, decisions regarding suitability obviously cannot be made based on historical data. This should be recognized by management, and particularly production personnel, when new equipment is employed. Equipment changes for some products might warrant additional dissolution and/or content uniformity studies.

The validation of a blending operation and blending equipment, particularly in the absence of historical data, occasionally presents problems. As with other elements, the degree and depth of a study is largely dependent upon the specific product.

The Theory and Practice of Industrial Pharmacy states:

> In the evaluation of a mixture, care must be taken that the *scale of scrutiny* is appropriate. That is, the samples chosen must be large enough to contain sufficient particles to accurately represent the region from which they were taken, yet not so large as to obscure important small scale variations in composition. The selection of a scale of scrutiny is also dependent on the ultimate use of the mixture. For example, samples of the same weight as the final tablet are proper for evaluating a tablet granulation. Analysis of multiple samples of this size would allow prediction of tablet to tablet variations due to imperfect mixing [11].

As a general comment, for some products with very good historical content uniformity data coming from a reproducible and controlled process, end product content uniformity test results without in-process sampling of the mix for uniformity could be acceptable.

However, for many of the potent dosage forms, particularly those made by direct compression, sampling of the mix is generally performed. Because of the additional analytical manipulation associated with testing (weighing), there is the tendency to rely more on dose uniformity testing of the tablets than of the blend for assurance of uniformity. However, a validated process would require that the mix be uniform prior to compression.

Finished Product Testing

The next critical element includes finished product testing. For those products with little historical data, as previously pointed out, additional finished product testing might be warranted. This would pertain to dissolution testing as well as content uniformity testing.

It is implied that the finished product test should be meaningful. Individual dose-to-dose content uniformity, dissolution and, where required, release variability must be addressed when modeling validation testing.

J. Tooling Control

Upon receipt of new production tooling ordered from a supplier, punches and dies will be transferred to the appropriate inspection area. Here the individual punches or dies will be inspected to assure that they meet all specifications set forth by the particular drawings for that set of punches or dies.

The following punch specifications should be checked to assure uniform product:

1. Length of punch from tip to head
2. Length of punch from depth of concavity to head
3. Diameter of punch body
4. Diameter of punch tip
5. Overall concentricity
6. Head angles
7. Depth of concavities
8. Embossing dimensions (i.e., depth of monogram, angle, and height of letters)
9. Accuracy of emboss

Die specifications will include:

1. Inside diameters
2. Outside diameters
3. Inside concentricity
4. Outside concentricity

Once a set has been inspected and approved, the individual tools of that set will be assigned a control number and a punch and die record card will be completed for that set (Fig. 8). This card will accompany the set of tools into production and be kept with the set. All production runs will be recorded. The set will be recalibrated at predetermined intervals; usually after approximately 25−50 million tablets.

Any tools that do not meet the required specifications, are damaged, or show abnormal wear will be removed from service. Punch tips will be defaced and the tools will be disposed of in the proper manner. For more detailed information, see the tableting specification manual issued by the Industrial Pharmaceutical Technology Section (IPT) of the Academy of Pharmaceutical Sciences [10].

Superpharm

SUPERPHARM CORPORATION
COMPRESSION DEPARTMENT
PUNCH AND DIE RECORD

SET NUMBER	PRODUCT NAME AND POTENCY			CODE NO.

DATE RECEIVED	PURCHASE ORDER NO.	SUPPLIER		

PUNCH SIZE	SHAPE	TYPE OF METAL	NUMBER OF UPPER	NUMBER OF LOWER

DESCRIPTION

UPPER PUNCHES	LOWER PUNCHES

INSPECTED AND VERIFIED BY: _____ DATE: _____

NOTES AND COMMENTS: _____

_____

_____

DISPOSITION: _____

APPROVED BY: _____ DATE: _____

COMMENTS: _____

DIE SET NO.	SIZE	SHAPE	TYPE OF METAL	NUMBER OF DIES

DATE RECEIVED	PURCHASE ORDER NO.	SUPPLIER		

INSPECTED AND VERIFIED BY: _____

NOTES AND COMMENTS: _____ _____

_____

DISPOSITION: _____

APPROVED BY: _____ DATE: _____

NOTES AND COMMENTS: _____

_____

_____

PIP — FORM NO. MF-401A

Figure 8   Punch and die record card.

K. Packaging

The packaging area calls for great emphasis on type of construction because it is particularly sensitive to mix-ups in either product or labeling. Individual packaging lines should have a minimum separation between each line of 15 ft. Depending on the equipment used, more space may need to be utilized. Consideration should be given to the separation of lines by partitions. The partitions need not be floor to ceiling, but should prevent migration of product by being closed at the floor, and high enough to prevent any crossover of product.

Some companies have started their packaging operations with a prestaging area large enough to contain all required components for that packaging operation. This area is separate but adjacent to or in front of the filling area. The filling area should be equipped, if possible, with air filtered through absolute filters. Dust-collector outlets from the central dust-collector system should be located in the filling area to remove dust from the filling operation. After cleaning by vacuum, bottles move into the filling area, are filled, then moved to the area where cottoning, capping, labeling, etc., takes place. Thus, maximum product protection is exercised in the filling area while the product is exposed, with lesser degrees of control being required in the other areas because the product is now containerized.

Standard operating procedures should be developed for all packaging operations. These include specific procedures for line setup, approval of line before start of operations, periodic line check during operation, close out of line, line clearance at end of operation, and reconciliation of product and components.

Cleaning and Start-Up

Cleaning should be carried out with relative ease and with the use of standard cleaning materials. Vacuum facilities should be available for cleaning and contact parts should be wiped down and sanitized utilizing a sanitizing agent. The equipment should be washed, dried, covered, and stored in an equipment storage area.

As in the case of manufacturing, the packaging operation starts with the generation of the packaging order. This consists of the approved packaging components listed by name and code number, the lot or control number of each component, the batch number of the product to be packaged, and quantities of each. A supervisor verifies the accuraacy and completeness of the packaging order, including expiration date, line being used, and any other special equipment being used for that operation. These steps are accomplished prior to bringing components to the line. The complete line area, including all equipment, is verified as being properly disassembled and cleaned of all product and components from the previous packaging operation. After the Quality Assurance Department verifies that the area has been cleared and cleaned, the components are brought to the line for mechanical setup. After the setup mechanic completes all the adjustments required, a supervisor oversees the prestart procedure, which consists of clearing all product used during the setup, counting labels used in the labler setup, rechecking all components and

lot numbers, verifying the bottle count, verifying all stamps and lot numbers, and signing of the packaging order that all is in readiness to start
packaging operations.

Labeling Operations

Labeling operations must receive very special attention. The use of cut
labels in the pharmaceutical industry is rapidly disappearing. Roll labels,
whether they are glue, thermoplastic, or pressure-sensitive are now the
labels of choice. Electronic label counting and verification is the norm with
bar codes, Universal Product Code (UPC), or Health Industry Bar Code
(HIBC) being used more frequently as label identifiers. The storage of
labels for both security and preservation reasons is very important. The
verification of labeling at the final label application point is also becoming
more popular, as the U.S. Food and Drug Administration (FDA) has
identified labeling errors as the single largest issue in product recalls.

   Standard operating procedures must be developed for label accountability with specific tolerances for accountability spelled out. Provision
must be made for label security, such as locked cabinets on the operating
lines. Accountability sheets for other components must be developed so
that reconciliation between used and finished packages can be developed.
If possible, a cleaning area and shop should be set up for the cleaning of
filters and parts, and the disassembly and assembly of filling machines.

Controls During Run

A packaging department check sheet is prepared each day by the supervisor for each packaging line (Fig. 9). This check sheet indicates the
components being used, the product name and description, packaging production order number, the manufacturing production order number, expiration date, etc. The checklist also includes weight, or tablet count
being filled, line number, appearance of containers, and the effectiveness
of any mechanical controls for detecting empty cartons, missing inserts,
etc. The line and components are checked by the supervisor on all start
ups. In addition, the line and components are checked and initialed approximately every hour during the run by a supervisor.

End of a Packaging Production Order

When a packaging production order (PPO) is completed, the packaging line
will be cleared of all components which are not transferable to the next
order. Those components which can be transferred to the next PPO (i.e.,
components with identical code numbers) will be marked with a sticker
indicating the new PPO number. The supervisor will fill out a clean card
and indicate in the appropriate space if the changeover is to be a product
changeover or a packaging order changeover (no cross-outs will appear in
this section). Clean cards for equipment that is mobile will be attached
directly to the equipment. A complete reconciliation of all labels and
inserts will be performed and any discrepancies outside predetermined
limits will be investigated immediately. Also, for inventory purposes, all
quantities of all components will be recorded. Also, at this time a final
check of product container labels will be performed and recorded.

SUPERPHARM CORPORATION

PACKAGING INSPECTION REPORT
PACKAGED TABLETS

Superpharm

LOT NUMBER

PRODUCT/STRENGTH		CUSTOMER NAME	PACKAGE SIZE	EXPIRATION DATE

SCHEDULED RUN	BULK AMT. REQUIRED	BULK AMT. REQUIRED FOR INSPECTION	TOTAL UNITS REQUIRED	EXAMINATION RATE _____ EVERY _____

RUN COUNT	BULK AMT. FILLED	Q.A. TECHNICIAN(S)	LINE NO.	SUPERVISOR

	LABEL								INSERT			DOSAGE FORM											BOTTLE				SHIPPER			
	INCORRECT ATTACH. EXPLANATION	LOOSE - TORN	SOILED, DEFACED	PRINTING MISSING, SKIPS	LOT. NO./EXP DATE WRONG, MISSING	LOT NO./EXP DATE ILLEGIBLE/SKIPS	LOT NO./EXP DATE MISLOCATED	SMEARED BUT LEGIBLE PRINTING	MISSING	INCORRECT. ATTACH EXPLANATION	TORN, DIRTY	BROKEN	CRACKED	CHIPPED	EDGING	CAPPED	MOTTLED	DYE SPOTS	GREASE SPOTS	PICKING BUT LEGIBLE	FOREIGN OR MIXED PRODUCT	IMPROPER SEAL(S)	MISSING COTTON/CAP/BAND	TORQUE TEST	Count	LOT NO./EXP DATE WRONG, MISSING	LOT NO./EXP DATE LIGHT BUT LEGIBLE	INCORRECT COUNT PER SHIPPER	LINE STARTED / TIME SAMPLE TAKEN
Action Level / Sple No.	1	3	4	2	1	2	5	5	2	1	4	7	7	4	5	3	4	4	4	4	1	2	2	3	6	1	5	1	
Total																														
%																														

REMARKS: _____

_____

_____

PIP FORM NO. QA-PI-2

Figure 9   Packaging check sheet.

IV. DESIGN OF THE PRODUCT

Other considerations relating to tablet production must now be addressed.
As was the case with formulation development activities, good communication
between research, production personnel, quality assurance, and marketing
are essential to the efficient introduction of a product to the manufacturing
environment. The decisions which must be made and the ideal information
which must be supplied are briefly discussed below.

A. Batch Sizes

Aside from the obvious limitations of batch size imposed by the capacities
of the processing equipment, logical choices concerning optimum batch
sizes will depend primarily on marketing projections of sales for the product. Early establishment of accurate batch size translates to more efficient
introduction to production. In today's regulatory environment, process
validation information is required on standard batch sizes for the subject
product. Without firm batch size definition at the outset, not only will any
validation data which is generated have to be repeated if the batch size
changes, but also subsequent decisions relating to equipment utilized for
batch processing, manpower required, raw material procurement/storage
requirements, production scheduling, and a myriad of similar issues will
require redefinition in the case of a change. Therefore, the establishment by the marketing group of a solid sales estimate by unit for any new
product cannot be overemphasized.

An EOQ (economic order quantity) model can be developed to calculate
the theoretical batch size that will generate the least total costs. It is
created by taking the partial derivative with respect to Q of a total cost
equation. The result is usually in the following form:

$$EOQ = \sqrt{\frac{2AD}{vr}}$$

where   EOQ = economic order quantity — that quantity which will generate
               the least total cost of carrying costs plus manufacturing
               costs

        A = set-up costs ($)

        D = demand (number of tablets/unit time)

        v = total manufacturing costs (raw material + value added)
            ($/tablet)

        r = carrying costs ($/$/unit time)

It is clear from the equation that the forecast (D) will directly impact
the EOQ. The development of an EOQ, however, should be used as only
one of the tools for batch sizing. A sensitivity analysis can also be
derived to determine the additional costs incurred by deviating from the
EOQ [3,8].

Within the batch size requirements established by marketing, production, and research personnel is the need to assess operating characteristics of granulation and tableting equipment to determine the most

efficient production cycle. An analysis which addresses marketing's product requirements linked to a temporal projection provides the basis for the manufacturing plan. With this assessment and knowledge of the typical operating cycle time for processing equipment, the impact on existing facilities can be assessed, and the demand for new equipment may be addressed. Careful consideration should be given at this point in the planning stage that delivery times for processing equipment purchase, installation, validation (if required), and similar issues be calculated accurately to assure smooth introduction of the product.

B. Equipment Considerations

In spite of restrictions applied to production based on development decisions with regard to processing equipment and technology, new equipment purchases for the production environment should be evaluated and address the following items.

Construction

Aside from functionality and durability, have the exigencies and growing concerns around "cleanability" and cleaning validation been addressed in the design? This consideration is especially important if the equipment is to be used for multiple products.

Scalability

Does the proposed production equipment operate on the same or similar principle to the pilot-scale equipment? How linear is the scalability from size to size? This factor can be pivotal in successful scale up to production-size batches.

Capacity/Output Requirements

If this equipment will augment or supercede existing equipment, will its output meet the required demand? It is wise to remember that in the case of tablet presses, a factor of 0.6−0.7 times the maximum rated output would logically provide a value for the optimum output of the equipment. Analysis based on using the manufacturer's stated maximum output will overstate the machine's practical capabilities in some cases by 30−40%.

Installation/Operating Requirements

Assess the equipment's space, utility, and any other special requirements and determine the feasibility of the proposed installation. In addition, if special features (i.e., explosion-proof electrics, etc.) are required, verify that the equipment vendor's interpretation will address local requirements.

Processing Test

Even though production equipment is technically similar to the R&D equipment used, verify, if possible, that the equipment will perform up to expectations at production scale. Very careful evaluation should precede any equipment purchase. An integral step in the prepurchase process should include actual equipment testing with tests products representative of typical production batches.

Availability of Quantitative In-Process Data

The regulatory climate regarding process validation continues to require ever-increasing amounts of quantitative manufacturing process data. Whether it is amperage measurements on a high-shear mixer taken during the granulating process or compression force monitoring from a tablet press, equipment should be evaluated with the anticipation that this information will be utilized and likely required at some point during its useful lifetime.

V. DESIGN OF THE FACILITY

A. Layout of Facilities

The overall facility as well as the individual process areas should always take into consideration the most simplistic route of material flow and the control of cross contamination. As previously noted, the prime objective at all stages of inventory is to separate released materials from quarantined or rejected materials. Several typical layouts for pharmaceutical manufacturing follow.

Figure 10 depicts one of the more popular solid-dosage form layouts. Basically, the center, or core, of the facility is a storage of warehouse area for raw materials, packaging components, and bulk stocks, with the manufacturing and packaging operations located at the outer perimeter. As can be observed, the flow of raw materials and components is from the receiving and quarantine areas into approved storage. Materials are weighed into batch quantities in dispensing, and then moved into the manufacturing area. After completion of manufacturing, the finished tablets are placed in quarantine, and moved to bulk stock upon release. When the packaging run is scheduled, tablets and packaging components are delivered from the bulk stock and approved storage areas.

This layout has the advantage of space conservation by virtue of having the supply areas close to the areas being supplied. However, a significant disadvantage is the crossover traffic pattern of materials, with the ensuing potential for contamination or mixup.

A second layout consisting of receiving, approved raw materials and components storage, and dispensing on one side, with manufacturing, quarantine, bulk stock, and packaging across a central corridor is depicted in Figure 11. The movement of materials from one area to another is the same as in Figure 10. However, owing to the modified layout, the flow is basically circular, eliminating much of the crossover traffic previously shown.

The third layout in Figure 12 consists of a basic straight-line flow to minimize contamination or mixup, moving the materials along a critical path. The principal advantage over the other layouts is minimal crossover of materials, thus minimizing the potential for contamination or mixup. One disadvantage is the additional space required to accommodate this configuration.

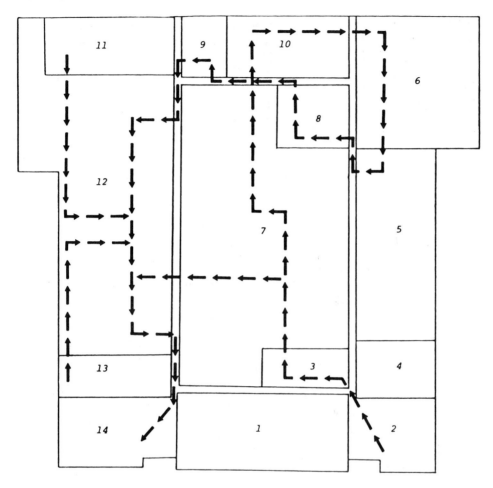

Figure 10   Perimeter manufacturing, center warehouse. (1) Administrative offices, (2) receiving area, (3) receiving quarantine, (4) tablet coating, (5) tablet compression, (6) tablet granulation, (7) approved materials warehousing, (8) in-process quarantine, (9) approved bulk materials, (10) pharmaceutical dispensing, (11) liquids, creams, ointment manufacturing, (12) packaging area, (13) label room operations, (14) shipping area.

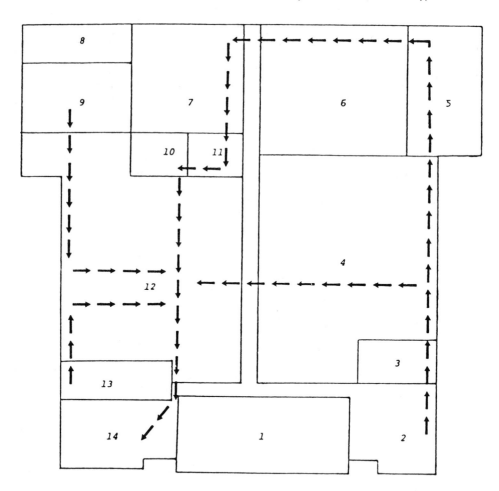

Figure 11   Circular flow: (1) administrative offices, (2) receiving area,
(3) receiving quarantine, (4) approved materials warehousing, (5) pharmaceutical dispensing, (6) tablet granulation, (7) tablet compression,
(8) tablet coating, (9) liquids, creams, ointment manufacturing, (10) approved bulk materials, (11) in-process quarantine, (12) packaging
area, (13 label room operations, (14) shipping area.

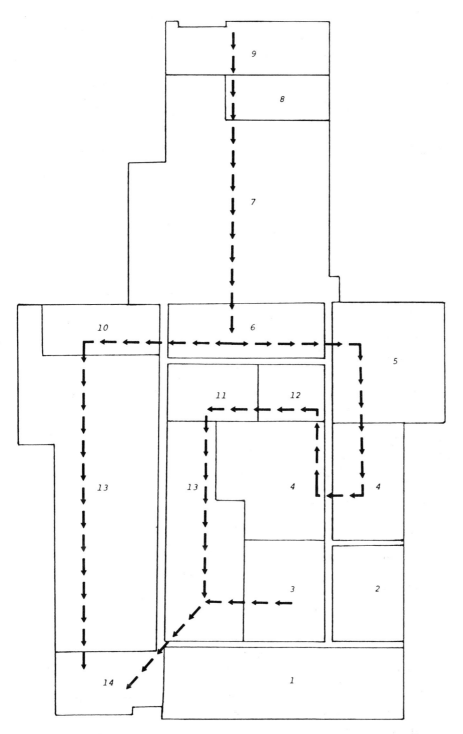

Figure 12 Straight line flow: (1) administrative offices, (2) tablet coating, (3) label room operations, (4) tablet compression, (5) tablet granulation, (6) pharmaceutical dispensing, (7) approved materials warehousing, (8) receiving quarantine, (9) receiving area, (10) liquids, creams, ointment manufacturing, (11) approved bulk materials, (12) in-process quarantine, (13) packaging area, (14) shipping area.

B. Control of Cross Contamination

Air-Handling Systems

One of the most important considerations in the design of a solid dosage
facility is the air-handling system. In considering air systems from the
standpoint of CGMPs, one begins with the supply of outside air, and then
moves on to the filtration systems that will be utilized, determining where
positive and negative air pressures are necessary, whether to recirculate
or exhaust spent air 100%, and finally dust collection and exhaust systems.
The CGMP regulation 211.46 section c specifically mandates that

> Air filtration systems, including prefilters and particulate matter
> air filters, shall be used when appropriate on air supplies to pro-
> duction areas. If air is recirculated to production areas, measures
> shall be taken to control recirculation of dust from production. In
> areas where air contamination occurs during production, there shall
> be adequate exhaust systems or other systems adequate to control
> contaminants [6].

A typical design involves one or more bag or cartridge filters located
close to the area of dust generation. Either of these coarse filtration
units will remove at least 95% of the dust generated from normal pharmaceutical manufacturing operations. The prefiltered air is then mixed with
10–15% outside make-up air and passed through a HEPA filter and re-
enters the rooms through the supply plenum diffuser.

Dust Collection

SAMPLING AND WEIGHING. The first area that must be addressed is
the raw material sampling rooms and the pharmacy or dispensing area.
Both these functions can be handled with the same illustration. Figure 13
shows a typical layout for sampling or weighing. The area should be an
enclosed facility with separate booths or hoods where the individual
weighing or sampling can take place. These areas may be designed using
horizontal laminar flow or appropriate hoods and other dust pickup devices. The supply air to these stations will, therefore, either be HEPA
filtered at the pickup stations, or HEPA filtered after the dust collector
prior to returning to the general area or supply air.

GRANULATING. The next area to be addressed is granulating. In
designing a granulating area the material flow should again be carefully
considered. Easy movement of materials into separate processing rooms
will minimize the potential of cross-contamination. A typical design is
shown in Figure 14. Here again there are two basic methods of air-
system design. In this illustration, the mixing rooms are negative to the
main corridor. This prevents airborne particles from escaping into the
main area and migrating to the other rooms.

COMPRESSION. Figures 15 and 16 illustrate a tablet-compression room
design using slightly negative pressure in the corridors to preclude contamination of other booths through open doorways. Both methods, designed and maintained properly, will work equally as well. The important
point being the supply air is prefiltered through a dust collector and
final filtered through a HEPA filter.

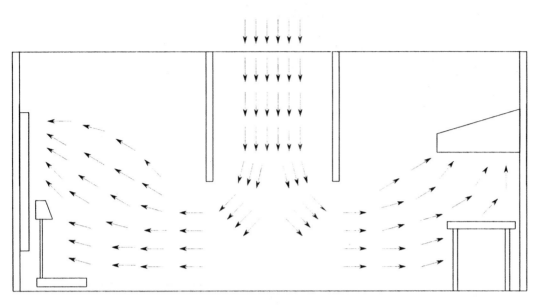

Figure 13   Dust collection for sampling and weighing stations.

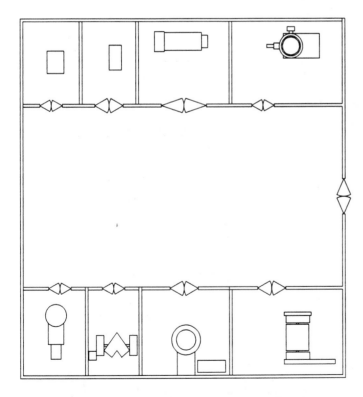

Figure 14   Layout of mixing and granulating areas.

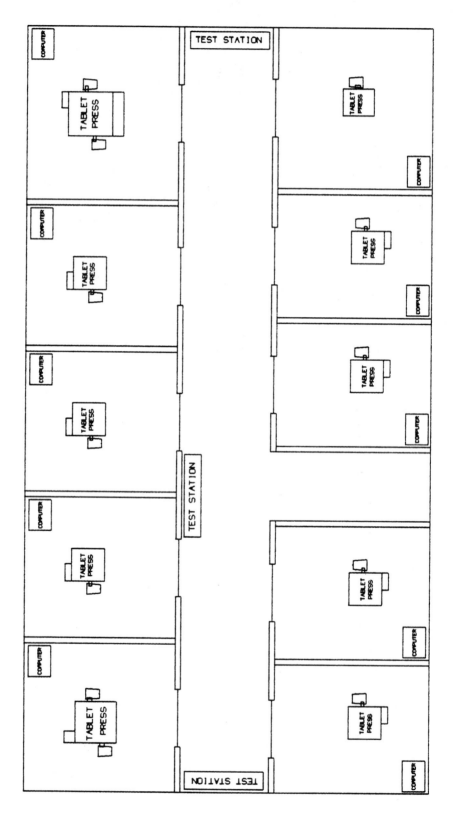

Figure 15   Layout of compression area.

398

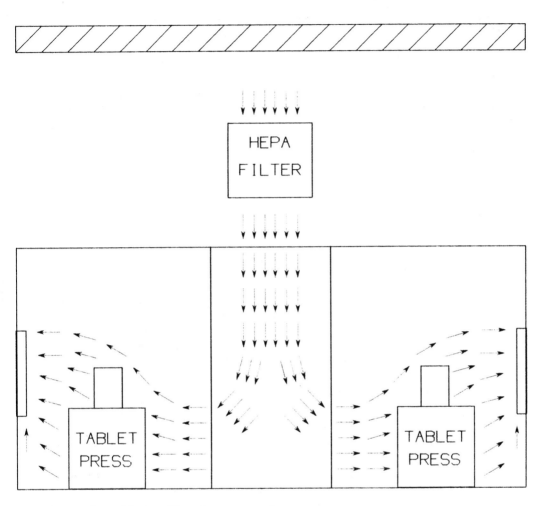

Figure 16   Air handling in compression area.

PACKAGING.   Some tablet-filling machines are designed with a self-
contained vacuum system that returns the air, filtered through an absolute
filter, back to the packaging area.   There should also be some provisions
made at the cottoning stations.   If the filling machine being used does not
have an air-filtering system, dust pcikups of approximately 300 cfm
should be provided at the hopper station and 50 CFM at the bottle chute.

C. Humidity/Temperature Controls

From the standpoint of both product protection and employee comfort,
careful consideration must be given to humidity and/or temperature controls.   Unless otherwise indicated, conditions of 45% RH and 70°F are
generally adequate for critical manufacturing areas such as compression
and coating.   Comfort conditioning should be provided for weighing,

granulation, compression, and packaging operations. However, temperature controls should be such that little or no variation will be caused by external ambient temperatures. Thus, comfortable working conditions are achieved and there should be no impact on characteristics of in-process materials, such as granulation, raw materials, etc. Warehousing operations should have some adequate type of ventilation, particularly in areas of high storage, either pallet racks or pallet-to-pallet-type storage. The ventilation could be provided by large roof fans to circulate air. In addition, some form of supplemental air heating, such as hot-air blowers, should be provided for cold areas, such as shipping or receiving docks.

D. Water Systems

Although water systems are not covered to any great extent in the CGMPs, CGMP regulation 211.48 states that the supply of potable water in a plumbing system must be free of defects that could contribute contamination to any drug product [6]. Thus, an effective water system is a necessity. In recent years, various techniques have been developed for producing the high-quality water required in ever-increasing quantities in pharmaceutical manufacturing operations. These include ion-exchange treatment, reverse osmosis, distillation, electrodialysis, and ultrafiltration. In fact, the *United States Pharmacopeia* (USP) XXI defines purified water, USP, as water obtained by these processes or other suitable processes. Unfortunately, there is no single optimum system for producing high-purity water, and selection of the final system(s) is dependent on such factors as raw-water quality, intent of use, flow rate, cost, etc. [1].

In the pharmaceutical industry, the classes of water normally encountered are well water, potable water, USP (which complies with Public Health Service Drinking Water Standards), purified water, USP, and specially purified grades of water, such as water for injection, USP, or FDA water for cleaning and initial rinse in parenteral areas (as defined in the CGMPs for large-volume parenterals). For purposes of this chapter, only the first three classes will be addressed because these are the classifications encountered in processing for solid- and semisolid-dosage forms.

Well Water

Well water, as the title indicates, is water drawn directly from a well. The water may not be either chemically or microbiologically pure because it is untreated. Therefore, the use of well water should be restricted to nonmanufacturing operations, such as lawn sprinklers, fire protection systems, utilities, and the like.

Potable Water

Potable water, USP, is city water or private well water that has usually been subjected to some form of microbiological treatment, such as chlorination, to meet the United States Public Health Service Standard with respect to microbiological purity. Potable water is fit for drinking, and is generally used in processing operations for cleaning and sanitation purposes. Periodic monitoring of use points should be conducted to ensure adequate residual chlorine levels and the absence of microbial contamina-

tion. If necessary, additional chlorine should be added to the water
supply as it enters the plant, or a suitable flushing program should be
implemented to ensure adequate chlorine levels at point of use.

Purified Water

Purified water, USP, is usually prepared from water that meets the potable
water standard. Purified water is treated to attain specified levels of
chemical purity and it is the type of water used in most pharmaceutical
processing operations. However, this class of water is not without problems in that the requirements of no chlorides presents special concerns
from a microbial contamination standpoint.

Purified water, USP, generally is produced by deionization or distillation, although reverse osmosis or ultrafiltration systems might be utilized
if the required chemical purity could be achieved. As a starting point in
these processes, water softening or activated carbon filtration frequently
is employed as a pretreatment process to remove calcium and magnesium
ions or chlorine and organic materials. Ion exchange and demineralization
through deionization is a very common method of obtaining the purified
water, USP, used in the pharmaceutical industry.

Water-Treatment Equipment

Deionization equipment should be sized to ensure frequent regeneration and
a recirculating system should be installed on the unit that approaches the
rated flow of the deionization unit. Procedures should be written to ensure that all water-treatment equipment is properly operated, monitored,
maintained, and sanitized on a regular basis.

WATER FILTRATION. Water filtration generally is approached on the
basis of two major considerations: prefiltering to prevent large particulates
from entering the system and microfiltering to remove bacteria. Prefilters
are generally the replaceable cartridge type with porosities ranging as
high as 25 μ. Microfiltering is usually accomplished with a 0.2-μ absolute
filters, which will remove most bacteria.

A proliferation of filters within the system should be avoided, since
what might be implemented as a protective measure could readily develop
into a problem wherein retained bacteria are given the opportunity to
multiply. In any system employing filters for the control of bacteria, the
filters and all of the downstream piping must be effectively sanitized on a
regular basis. There should be procedures written for filter inspection,
replacement, integrity testing, and monitoring on a scheduled basis.

SANITIZATION PROCEDURES. Sanitization is best accomplished
through several methods. After periods of low usage of water, the system should be flushed with a supply of water that has residual chlorine.
Periodic hyperchlorination also is recommended. Effective microbial control can be maintained by storing water at 80°C. However, this approach
is expensive and presents some hazards to personnel and material. Ultraviolet radiation may be used, but it has limited application because of the
many factors which can reduce its effectiveness. Written instructions
should be developed for sanitization procedures for water-treatment equipment on a regular, prescribed basis.

E. Plant Pest Control

The CGMP regulation 211.56a states that

> Any building used in the manufacture, processing, packing, or
> holding of a drug product shall be maintained in a clean and san-
> itary condition. Any such building shall be free of infestation by
> rodents, birds, insects, and other vermin (other than laboratory
> animals). Trash and organic waste matter shall be held and dis-
> posed of in a timely and sanitary manner [6].

A pest-control program should be developed that will ensure the integrity and quality of products produced and comply with existing legislation. The program should be written to include a general statement of
purpose and the company position. Effectiveness of the program should be
assured by defining the plant individual with overall responsibility for the
program and how the responsibility will be carried out. The training and
experience requirements of the extermination staff should be delineated,
whether they be in-house or subcontracted personnel. Assistance in supporting the program may be gained from other plant personnel by their
pointing out problem areas.

The program should be issued to line management personnel and
periodically updated in order to keep the program current. The program
should contain a list of approved pesticides to be used in the plant. Individual sheets should be prepared for each specific item of use [5].
Basic information should be spelled out as follows:

1. Trade name of the pesticide
2. Classification
3. Type of action
4. Chemical name and concentration of active ingredient
5. Effective for:
6. To be used for:
7. Area of usage
8. Mode and frequency of application
9. Toxicities and any specific toxic symptoms, if known
10. Status of government approval
11. Specific restrictions and cautions

The development of sheets as indicated above will serve a twofold purpose. First, the sheets can be subjected to approval by the plant safety
organization to determine if the materials comply with the Occupational
Safety and Health Administration (OSHA) requirements and the requirements of other state or local agencies. Second, the sheets would also
facilitate compliance with CGMP regulation 211.56c, which states the
following:

> There shall be written procedures for use of suitable rodenticides,
> insecticides, fungicides, fumigating agents, and cleaning and
> sanitizing agents. Such written procedures shall be designed to
> prevent the contamination of equipment, components, drug prod-
> ucts containers, closures, packaging, labeling materials, or drug
> products and shall be followed. Rodenticides, insecticides, and

fungicides shall not be used unless registered and used in accordance with the Federal Insecticide, Fungicide, and Rodenticide Act (7 U.S.C. 135) [6].

Written records of regularly scheduled inspections and preventive treatments should be maintained. Emergency or special services should be documented specifying the type of problem encountered, the service rendered, effectiveness of the treatment, and any follow-up that might be required.

The program should also specify when production interruptions might be necessary, either due to the presence of a specific pest or to avoid possible contamination during the treatment to exterminate a pest.

All manufacturing areas should be constructed using nonporous materials on the walls and floors. Any protrusions such as pipes and electrical boxes should be minimized. Space should be allocated carefully to provide sufficient rooms for all operations. There should be adequate lighting and the areas should be remote from any openings to the outside. Care should be taken that adequate training in understanding CGMPs be given to all personnel. Outside contractors must also be trained and understand CGMPs before embarking on any construction or remodeling efforts having to do with pharmaceutical manufacturing.

VI. EQUIPMENT SELECTION

A. Granulation

There are a multitude of equipment manufacturers, each with a specific advantage. But, more importantly, the initial formulations coming from the scale-up laboratory should be done in equipment that most closely mimics the final processing equipment that will be used in production. The success or failure of a manufacturing process depends on the time and effort put into the formulation design and equipment selection.

Selection of equipment for dry blending, dry granulation, or wet granulation is a process that must start at the time the formulation is first conceptualized. There are numerous types and designs for each processing technique.

Dry Blending

The first choice for dry mixing is in tumble-type blenders, and here, as elsewhere in this section, an effort will be made to identify the more commonly used designs and some of the manufacturers of that equipment. This information is intended as a guide and is not proported to be a complete listing. Figure 17 shows some configurations of a double-cone blender, both straight and offset.

Figure 18 illustrates both the conventional twin-shell or Vee blender, and the newer cross-flow or short-leg Vee blender. Double-cone and twin-cone blenders are supplied by Gemco, J. H. Day Corp., and Patterson Kelly Co., among others.

The important considerations to take into account when developing a formulation for these type mixers are deagglomeration of the raw materials prior to charging the blender, not exceeding the rated capacities which is approximately 60% of the total capacity, particle size uniformity, dry and humid conditions, reducing vibration, and avoiding over mixing.

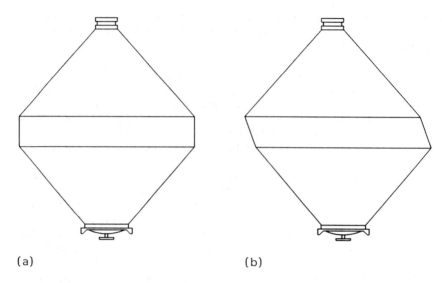

(a)   (b)

Figure 17   (a) Double-cone blender, (b) slant-cone blender.

Ribbon blenders of the type shown in Figure 19 may also be used for dry blending. However, care must be exercised here when formulating low-dosage products. Dead spots such as discharge ports must be cleared and the materials recycled. Samples must be taken from multiple locations when validating this process. Some ribbon blender suppliers are Marion Mixers, Inc., J. H. Day Corp., Charles Ross & Son Co., and S. Howes Co., among others.

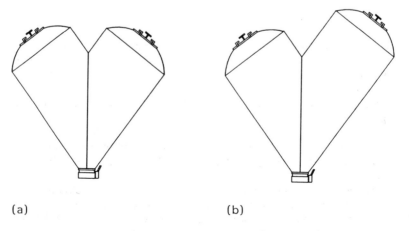

(a)   (b)

Figure 18   (a) Vee blender, (b) short-leg vee blender.

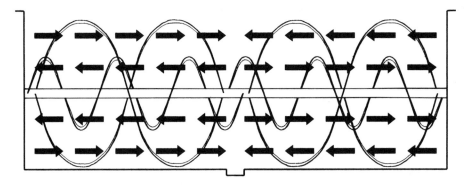

Figure 19   Ribbon blender.

Dry Granulation

Dry granulation is becoming more popular as equipment improvements continue to accelerate. Moisture-sensitive actives and some heat-sensitive
actives can now be prepared as efficiently as less sensitive products. A
combination of roll compaction and sizing coupled with improved cleanability
of the equipment have encouraged formulators to look at this method more
closely than in the past.

Figure 20 shows a typical design for roll compaction. Again, equipment manufacturers have realized the importance of being able to precisely control feed rates, compaction force, and particle size, and have
carefully addressed these parameters when scaling from lab equipment to
production equipment. Some roll compaction equipment suppliers are
Vector Corp., Fitzpatrick Corp., Alexanderwerke, and Bepex, among
others.

Wet Granulation

The wet-granulation technique is benefiting from improved processing
equipment. High-shear granulating equipment is being developed and improved upon. Equipment manufacturers are studying changeover times,
clean up, end point measurement, ease of discharge, and many more points
to improve quality and productivity. Granulator/dryer combinations are
also becoming more available. Fluid-bed drying, microwave drying, and
vacuum-drying equipment are rapidly replacing the traditional tray
dryers.

B. Compression

Introduction of the high-speed, computer-controlled tablet press has had a
profound impact on the industry. With capacities of over 800,000 doses/hr,
presses no longer need to be dedicated to a single product. Many products may be manufactured on one machine to utilize excess capacity and to
justify the high costs. Depending on the manufacturing strategies of a
particular company, different criteria would be used to select their equipment. Large production rate capacities become important as the batch size

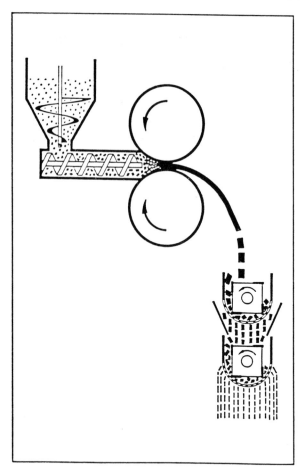

Figure 20   Roll compactor.   (Courtesy of Alexanderwerke.)

increases and the number of different products decreases.   Cleanability
and change-over time become important as the batch size decreases and
the number of products increases.   Some manufacturers claim as little as
4 h for a complete changeover to a different product.

Theory of Computer-Controlled Presses

If every particle and granule were the same size and shape, and if every
die cavity were filled with exactly the same amount, and if every punch
were exactly the same, etc., the compression force for each tablet produced would be identical from die cavity-to-die cavity, from revolution-to-
revolution, and from the beginning to the end of a batch.   Unfortunately,
the particle size distribution may vary slightly from die cavity-to-die
cavity, from revolution-to-revolution, and from the beginning to the end
of a batch.   Therein lies one of the sources of variation of weight and
hardness from tablet-to-tablet.

Consider two identical die cavities, A and B. A is filled with small particles, whereas B is filled with larger particles. While both die cavities are filled, the weight of the powder in A is heavier than the weight of the powder in B. The compression force will be larger for A than for B as they pass under the same compression rollers. Obviously, the tablet resulting from A will be heavier than the tablet resulting from B. The compression forces can therefore be directly correlated to tablet weights.

The basic assumption used by all computer controlling systems is that all significant variations in compression forces are resultant from the actial weight of the material being compressed, hence tablet weight. The target tablet weight can be correlated to a target compression force that is determined during the setup operation. This target compression force can then be used to control the compression operation.

During the prestart operation, a target compression force will be determined. As the press begins production, it will warm up and its operating condition will change. As the punches warm, they will elongate slightly. As the electronic components warm, their signals may vary slightly. The sum of the press's varying operating conditions is a drift in the compression force/target weight correlation.

Until recently, it was up to the operator to verify that the target compression force correlated to the target tablet. If this was found not to be the case, an adjustment needed to be made before compression could continue. With the introduction of tablet measurement/feedback systems, control is taken a step further and the loop is closed. Compression forces are periodically referenced to actual produced tablet measurements. All necessary adjustments, including weight and hardness adjustments, are then performed automatically and the compression force/tablet weight correlation is adjusted automatically as necessary.

Instrumentation Strategies

There are currently two basic strategies used by the many tablet manufacturers to computer-control their presses. The first is to set up the press to produce tablets with the desired weight, hardness, thickness, friability, etc. The next step is to convert the compression force signal to a reference value. This reference value corresponds to the target tablet, and is usually displayed as an average per revolution of each station's actual compression force. This reference value must be established at the start up for each batch and is then used to control the tablet weights. When the average force value drifts from the reference value and reaches an adjustment value, a signal is sent to the weight-control motor to adjust the filling depth appropriately. Some manufacturers provide for the duration of the weight-control signal to be set so that the adjustment brings the force value back to the reference value. Compression forces of individual stations are measured, and if their force values are within a set reject range, the tablet is accepted as a good tablet. If the force value is outside the reject range, the tablet is rejected as an out-of-spec tablet.

The second strategy, which most tablet manufacturers are using or moving toward, is the use of internal calibrations so that actual compression forces are measured and displayed. The benefits include a simplfied computer setup and a standard/common base by which batches of the same product can be compared for compression characteristics and statistical analysis. The adjustment range settings and the reject range settings initiate the same responses as they do in the first strategy. The difference is that they are set and displayed as actual compression forces.

Rejection Strategies

The rejection mechanisms are also of two basic strategies, pneumatic reject and mechanical reject. The pneumatic reject relies on a timed burst of air to direct a bad tablet to a reject chute. The disadvantages with a dusty product are clogging of the jets and inducing airborne dust particles. Also, depending on the speed of the press, up to six or more tablets may be rejected for each bad tablet. The advantages are no moving parts and the timing is fixed and not varied owing to table speed changes.

The mechanical reject is usually a gate or arm that swings out to divert the bad tablet to the reject chute. The timing is critical and must be set correctly. As the table speed changes, the timing may need to be changed. Also, tablets of different sizes and shapes will require different timings and gate settings. Abrasive dusts can interfere with proper rejection by causing sluggishness. On the other hand, mechanical mechanisms can be set to reject only one tablet, regardless of speed.

Induced Die Feeder (IDF) Strategies

Another distinguishing feature of high-speed machines is the induced die feeder (IDF). The IDF is basically a mechanism to ensure adequate and uniform filling of the die cavities as they pass the feeder at high speeds. It uses a combination of paddles which pushes or plows the powder over the dies. Virtually every combination of paddle placement and blade configuration is represented by some manufacturer. Different IDF configurations and speeds may induce different compression characteristics of the same material. Because the IDF agitates the powder, and its speed can be varied, some additional mixing may be considered to occur in the feeder for some formulations. This can sometimes become a source of problems rather than a solution.

Power Delivery Systems

Some manufacturers offer a powder feed controller which maintains a constant level of powder that feeds the IDF. The effects of the sudden increase of weight by adding a scoop full of powder to a hopper can be seen very clearly on computer monitoring/controlling devices that have graphical displays. These effects are eliminated by the powder feed controller, and help to create more uniform products by eliminating the powder level variable.

Future Trends

Most press manufacturers currently have on the market presses and controlling systems which provide a complete loop for controlling all of the tablet parameters. Tablet sampling and checking systems take a sample of tablets at specified intervals, automatically perform weight, hardness, and thickness measurements, perform statistical calculations, and feedback the appropriate signals to the press to adjust the weight and/or hardness. These signals include readjusting the target compression force and the

Manufacturer	Elizabeth Hata	Kilian	Kikusui	Korsch	Manesty	Stokes
Model	AP-38-SU	T300	Libra	Pharmapress 336	Novapress 45	Stokes 454
Station No.	38	32	36	36	45	45
Output/Hr: Max(M)	160	240	216	216	222	270
Min(M)	34.6	9.6	21.6	71.3	54	96
Main Comp	9	80 kN	8	8	6.5	6
Pre Comp	3.5	28 kN	8	2	–	2
Computerized: Monitoring	Y	Y	Y	Y	Y	Y
Control by Force	Y	Y	Y	Y	Y	Y
Control by Weight	Y	Y	Y	Y	Y	N

Figure 21   General comparison of currently available tablet presses.

window of limits. The target compression force is therefore being constantly verified against actual tablet parameters.

Some manufacturers currently offer systems where all of a product's parameters are stored on a disk and the operator loads the information in a computer. The computer will tell the press where the initial settings are, produce some tablets for automatic testing, make any necessary adjustments until the tablets are at target, and then begin production. Figure 21 is a general comparison of some of the tablet presses currently available and is not all inclusive.

VII. PERSONNEL

A. Training

Operators

This group includes the mixing and granulating operators and the compression operators. The training of the mixing and granulation operators should include the following:

1. Cleaning procedures
2. Familiarization with and ability to identify the codes and names of the raw materials being used in the product being mixed
3. Proper label control and reconciliation
4. Handling, usage, and operation of equipment in area
5. Proper handling of raw materials in each operation
6. Importance of precise mixing times and geometric dilutions
7. Proper labeling and handling of mixed materials
8. Quality assurance and validation procedures
9. Training to observe and look for foreign matter in the raw materials
10. Product reconciliation
11. Ability to check mathematics required by the formula

The training of the compression operators should include the following:

1. Cleaning procedures
2. Ability to identify and distinguish from quarantine and released materials
3. Proper label control and reconciliation
4. Handling, usage, and operation of equipment in the area
5. Proper handling and hopper loading of mixed material
6. Proper handling of bulk tablets produced
7. Quality assurance and validation procedures
8. Training to observe and look for foreign matter in the mixed material and bulk tablets
9. Product reconciliation
10. Ability to check mathematics required by the formula

Mechanics

Mechanics have specialized training in addition to the same training as the operators. During their setup operation, mechanics operate the machine and, also during periods where there are no setups to be performed, they may be asked to operate a machine. The training of mechanics, in addition to operator training, should therefore include the following:

1. Cleaning procedures for tooling and machinery
2. Breakdown and setup of machinery
3. Complete operation of the machines
4. Proper handling of the tooling
5. Theory behind computer-controlled tablet presses
6. Setup and control of computerized units
7. Maintenance and repair of machinery
8. Troubleshooting of machinery

Supervisors

Supervisors need to have the necessary training and background to lead and direct their operators and mechanics. They must have an intimate knowledge and preferably some hands-on experience of the operators' and mechanics' jobs. In addition, supervisors must also possess the supervisory skills necessary to maintain the high standards demanded by the pharmaceutical industry.

In addition to the job-specific responsibilities outlined above, all manufacturing employees must be versed and trained in CGMPs and in the appropriate standard operating procedures (SOPs) governing their area.

VIII. ROLE OF MANUFACTURING

A. Marketing Support

Marketing is usually the only organizational link to the customer, and any feedback on the sales impact of quality and delivery comes through as marketing requests. Also, the direction that applied R&D takes should be driven by the marketing function. Marketing should encourage the development of products that would generate the highest potential revenues with the greatest margin. Each product developed or produced should fit into an overall marketing plan. Without insight to the marketing plan, the R&D and Production Departments might question the wisdom of their directions, creating unnecessary, undesirable boundaries between departments.

The importance of marking to an organization is obvious. However, the importance of accurate, timely information from marketing to various other departments cannot be stressed enough. The role of manufacturing, therefore, is to support the marketing function. Successful support might be defined by improving quality, reducing manufacturing lead times, lowering costs, and hastening manufacturing response to changing demands. The role of all other departments in the organization is to support, in one way or another, manufacturing [7].

B. The Production Plan

A finished goods requirements plan should drive the master production schedule, which provides a detailed action plan from placing purchase orders to final packaging schedules.

The master schedule is the operations statement for production and related activities. It is a positive commitment to perform certain activities within the required time span. In the packaging area, the master schedule states that the Packaging Department will package X amount of a put-up during week N on day Y. In order to fulfill this commitment, the Quality Control Department must release the bulk during week N-1. For quality control to meet its commitment, the Manufacturing Department must have the bulk produced in time for the former to perform its functions. In order for the Manufacturing Department to produce the product, approved materials must be available X number of weeks before the manufacturing is to be completed, the number of weeks being dependent on the manufacturing cycle time (including dispensing time). Having approved material available to manufacturing requires that quality control perform their analysis in the stated time span for quality control lead time. For this to happen the material must be received as scheduled. The Purchasing Department must, therefore, place the order X weeks before the material is to be received, where X is the vendor lead time. Purchasing must also follow up with the blendor to assure the material will be received on time. If the material is rejected, purchasing must issue a replacement order. In order for purchasing to issue the order on time, production planning must requisition the material at least 1 week before the order is to be placed.

Given the large number of components and materials involved in pharmaceutical production operations, the task of manually performing the above "time-phasing" routine would be virtually impossible. This time phasing of the production, quality control, and purchasing processes is one of the functions performed by materials requirement planning (MRP).

C. Materials Requirement Plan

Materials requirement planning starts with the master schedule. Using the bill of materials, lead time, capacities, and other product-related database information, together with information on inventory, open production orders, and open purchase orders, the materials requirement planning system will determine the quantity of materials and the date they are needed for each phase of the production process. The logic used in making the determination is basically the same as that described under the master schedule. The master schedule states which put-ups are scheduled to be packaged during the weekly time periods. By applying the bills of material for the put-ups to the quantities to be packaged, the system can determine the quantities of packaging components and bulk that are needed. Working within the established lead times, the system will show a demand for the items in the correct time segment. In turn, the system will plan replacement orders to maintain specified levels of inventory. The planned order will be shown as being available in the time frame needed and will be placed "on order" by considering the purchasing, production, and quality control lead times. The procedure is carried out for each phase of production and the release of a planned order at one level generates requirements at the next level. For example, if finished products were assigned to 0 level code, items used to produce finished stock would be assigned a 1, products used to produce bulk would be assigned a 2, and so on until the purchased materials are reached.

The MRP lends itself well to computerization and can perform other functions, such as alerting management to items with excessive inventory. It can suggest corrective actions (such as delaying or canceling open orders) and can predict inventory levels and investments for each time period in the planning horizon [2].

D. Production Scheduling

All of the elements previously described could be categorized as planning elements. From the planning phase one must move into the execution phase, with the transition being supplied by the master schedule.

The development of a production schedule is of prime importance because this is the basic means for monitoring production activities. Progress can be checked and results reported based on the production or planning period. The production planning schedule forms a basis for decision making during the production cycle. Production scheduling is one of the most detailed and demanding tasks in the organization.

Scheduling may be performed in an adequate manner either manually or mechanically, depending on the size and scope of the organization. Any scheduling system requires basic input data from the production plan consisting of *What?*, *When?*, and *How many?* Regardless of the circumstances, monitoring production activities with the production schedule becomes the key to successful fulfillment of the production plan. This is the method by which control is exercised over the production operation. A proper schedule can optimize production and inventory costs by proper sequencing of order quantities and time phasing. No matter how small the organization, the development of a sound production schedule is a tool which cannot be neglected. The production schedule is the cement which creates the foundation for an effective production organization that can meet sales demands.

IX. INDUSTRY OUTLOOK

The advances over the next decade in equipment, design, instrumentation, and process control techniques will certainly be significant. The nature of these advancements are difficult to predict. Certainly, computer-integrated manufacturing will come into its own in the pharmaceutical manufacturing industry as a whole and most assuredly in tablet production. Statistical process-control techniques will become widespread throughout the industry. Numerous data-collection devices and computer systems are currently available and in use as a means of implementing statistical process control. Computer-controlled tablet presses and automated material handling devices are available that virtually remove the operator from the need to control the operation.

The general state of the industry is that there exists many islands of automation. The challenge for the future is to first integrate these islands with a computer network so that process data can be easily collected, and so that the inventory position and scheduling can be optimized on a real-time basis. The second challenge is that of validation of these systems to the complete satisfaction of the individual manufacturers and of the U.S. Food and Drug Administration.

The authors stated in the introduction to this chapter that "ours is an evolving technology-based science that requires canstant attention." With this in mind, the professionals of our industry must stay abreast of current practices and recognize the emerging trends. Only in this way, will the industry continue to be profitable and provide an important service in an increasingly competitive world market.

APPENDIX: LIST OF SUPPLIERS

A C Compacting Presses
North Brunswick, New Jersey

Aeromatic, Inc.
Towaco, New Jersey

Alexanderwerke
Remscheid, West Germany

Bepex Corp.
3 Crossroads of Commerce
Rolling Meadows, Illinois

Charles Ross & Son Co.
Hauppauge, New York

Diosna
Osnabruck, West Germany

Elizabeth Hata Int., Inc.
North Huntingdon, Pennsylvania

Fitzpatrick Corp.
Elmhurst, Illinois

Fluid Air, Inc.
Napersville, Illinois

Gemco (The General Machine Co.
  of N.J.)
Middlesex, New Jersey

Glatt Air Techniques, Inc.
Ramsey, New Jersey

Glen Mills, Inc.
Maywood, New Jersey

Gral-Collette
Northbrook, Illinois

H. C. Davis Sons Mfg. Co., Inc.
Bonner Springs, Kansas

Holland-McKinley
Malvern, Pennsylvania

Indupol Filtration Assoc., Inc.
Cresskill, New Jersey (Torit)

Inppec, Inc.
Milford, Connecticut (Kilian)

J. H. Day Corp.
Cincinnati, Ohio

Jaygo, Inc.
Mahwah, New Jersey

Kemutec, Inc.
Bristol, Pennsylvania

Korsch Tableting, Inc.
Somerset, New Jersey

Lightnin Mixing Equipment Co.
Rochester, New York

Littleford Bros., Inc.
Florence, Kentucky

Manesty, Thomas Engineering, Inc.
Hoffman Estates, Illinois

Marion Mixers, Inc.
Marion, Iowa

Micropul
Summit, New Jersey

Millipore Corp.
Bedford, Massachusetts

Mocon (Modern Controls, Inc.)
Minneapolis, Minnesota

Natoli Engineering
Chesterfield, Missouri

Patterson-Kelly Co.
East Stroudsburg, Pennsylvania

Raymond Automation Co., Inc.
Norwalk, Connecticut

S. Howes Co., Inc.
Silver Creek, New York

Scientific Instruments &
Technology Corp.
Piscataway, New Jersey

Stokes-Merrill
Warminster, Pennsylvania

Thomas Engineering, Inc.
Hoffman Estates, Illinois

United Chemical Machinery
Supply, Inc.
Toms River, New Jersey

(Kikusui)

Urschel Laboratories, Inc.
Valparaiso, Indiana

Vector Corp.
Marion, Iowa

SUGGESTED READINGS

Alessi, P. Operational MRP vs. Integrated MRP, P&IM with APICS
News, June 1986.
Anton, C. J. and Malmborg, C. J. *The Integration of Inventory
Modeling and MRP Processing: A Case Study*, Production and
Inventory Management, 2nd Quarter, 1985.
Ballou, Ronald H. Estimating and auditing aggregate inventory
levels at multiple stocking points. *J. Operations Management*
1(3):143−154 (Feb. 1981).
Bryson, W. L. *Profit-Oriented Inventory Management.* APICS
22nd Annual Conference Proceedings, 1979, pp. 88−91.
The Competitive Status of the U.S. Pharmaceutical Industry.
National Academy Press, Washington, D.C., 1983.
Hadley, G. and Whitin, T. M. *Analysis of Inventory Systems.*
Prentice-Hall, New York, 1963.
Lotenschtein, S. Just-in-Time in the MRP II Environment, P&IM
Review with APICS News, Feb. 1986.
Mehta, N. *How to Handle Safety Stock in an MRP System.* Produc-
tion and Inventory Management, 3rd Quarter, 1980.
Ott, E. T. *Process Quality Control.* McGraw-Hill, New York,
1975.

REFERENCES

1. Artiss, D. H. and Klink, A. E. *Good Manufacturing Practices
for Water: Methods of Manufacturing, Testing Requirements
and Intended Use.* AIChE 70th Annual Meeting, New York,
Nov. 1977.
2. Berry, W. L., Whybark, D. C., and Vollmann, T. E. *Manufacturing Planning and Control Systems.* Irwin, Homewood,
Illinois, 1984.

3. Boucher, T. O. and Elsayed, E. A. *Analysis and Control of Production Systems*, Prentice-Hall, New York, 1985.
4. *Guideline on General Principles of Process Validation.* U.S. Food and Drug Administration, Washington, D.C., May 1984.
5. *Guidelines for Plant Pest Control Program.* PMA, Washington, D.C., Jan. 1975.
6. Hitchings, W. S., IV, Tuckerman, M. M., and Willig, S. H. *Good Manufacturing Practices for Pharmaceuticals.* Marcel Dekker, Inc., New York, 1982.
7. Hutt, M. D. and Speh, T. W. *Industrial Marketing Management.* Dryden Press, Chicago, 1981.
8. Peterson, R. and Silver, E. A. *Decision Systems for Inventory Management and Production Planning.* Wiley, New York, 1985.
9. *Pharmaceutical Process Validation.* Marcel Dekker, New York, 1984.
10. *Tableting Specification Manual, IPT Standard Specifications for Tableting Tools.* Academy of Pharmaceutical Sciences and American Pharmaceutical Association, 1981.
11. *The Theory and Practice of Industrial Pharmacy.* Lea & Febiger, Philadelphia, 1976.

7
The Essentials of Process Validation

Robert A. Nash

St. John's University, Jamaica, New York

I. INTRODUCTION

The U.S. Food and Drug Administration (FDA) in its most recently proposed guidelines has offered the following definition for process validation [1]:

> Process validation is a documented program which provides a high degree of assurance that a specific process (such as the manufacture of pharmaceutical solid dosage forms) will consistently produce a product meeting its predetermined specifications and quality attributes.

According to the FDA, assurance of product quality is derived from careful (and systemic) attention to a number of (important) factors, including: selection of quality (components) and materials, adequate product and process design, and (statistical) control of the process through in-process and end-product testing.

Thus it is through careful design and validation of both the process and its control systems that a high degree of confidence can be established that all individual manufactured units of a given batch or succession of batches that meet specification will be acceptable.

According to FDA's Current Good Manufacturing Practices (21CFR 211.110)

> Control procedures shall be established to *monitor* output and to *validate* performance of the manufacturing processes that may be responsible for causing variability in the characteristics of in-process material and the drug product. Such control procedures

shall include, but are not limited to the following, where appropriate [2]:

1. Tablet or capsule weight variation
2. Disintegration time
3. Adequacy of mixing to assure uniformity and homogeneity
4. Dissolution time and rate
5. Clarity, completeness, or pH of solutions

The first four items listed above are directly related to the manufacture
and validation of solid dosage forms. Items 1 and 3 are normally associated
with variability in the manufacturing process, while items 2 and 4 are
usually influenced by the selection of the ingredients in the product formulation. With respect to content uniformity and unit potency control (item 3)
adequacy of mixing to assure uniformity and homogeneity is considered to
be a high-priority concern.

Conventional quality control procedures for finished product testing
encompass three basic steps:

1. Establishment of specifications and performance characteristics
2. Selection of appropriate methodology, equipment, and instrumentation to ensure that testing of the product meets specification
3. Testing of the final drug product, using validated analytical and
   test methods in order to insure that finished product meets
   specifications.

With the emergence of the pharmaceutical process validation concept, the
following four additional steps have been added

4. Qualification and validation of the processing facility and its
   equipment
5. Qualification and validation of the manufacturing process through
   appropriate means
6. Auditing, monitoring, sampling, or challenging the key steps in
   the process for conformance to specifications
7. Requalification and revalidation when there is a significant change
   in either the product or its manufacturing process [3]

II. TOTAL APPROACH TO PHARMACEUTICAL
PROCESS VALIDATION

It has been said that there is no specific basis for requiring a separate
set of process validation guidelines since the essentials of process validation are embodied within the purpose and scope of the present Current
Good Manufacturing Practices (CGMPs) regulations [2]. With this in mind,
the entire CGMP document, from subpart B through subpart M, may be
viewed as being a set of principles applicable to the *overall process* of
manufacturing, i.e., solid dosage forms or other drug products and thus
may be subjected, subpart by subpart, to the application of the principles
of qualification, validation, control, as well as requalification and revalidation, where appropriate. Although not a specific requirement of current

regulations, such as comprehensive validation approach with respect to each subpart of the CGMP document has been adopted by many drug firms.

A checklist of validation and control documentation with respect to CGMPs is provided in Table 1. With the exception of subpart M (sterilization), the rest of the CGMPs are directly applicable to the manufacture of solid dosage forms.

Table 1   Checklist of Validation and Control Documentation

Subpart	Section of CGMP	Validation and control documentation
A	Introduction	Establishment of QA & PV functions
B	Organization and personnel	Establishment and facility installation and qualification [4,5]
C	Buildings and facilities	Plant and facility installation and qualification [4,5] Maintenance and sanitation [6] Microbial and pest control [7]
D	Equipment	Installation and qualification cleaning methods [8]
E	Control of raw materials, in-process material, product	Incoming components [9] Manufacturing non-sterile products [10]
F	Production and process controls	Process control systems [11] (instrumentation and computers)
G	Packaging and labeling controls	Depyrogenation, sterile packaging, filling, and closing [12,13]
H	Holding and distribution	Facilities [14]
I	Laboratory controls	Analytical methods [15]
J	Records and reports	Computer systems [16]
K	Returned and salvaged drug product	Batch reprocessing [17]
L	Air and water quality	Water treatment and steam systems air, heat, and vacuum handling [18-20]

Table 1 (Continued)

Subpart	Section of CGMP	Validation and control documentation
M	Sterilization	LVPs [21,22]
		Autoclaves and process
		Parametrics [23−25]
		Aseptic facilities [26]
		Devices [27]
		Sterilizing filters [28,29]

Table 2 Process Validation Matrix or Checklist of Activities to be Considered

	Qualification: Installation Calibration Certification	Validation: Proving	Control: Monitor Sample Audit Testing	Requalification and revalidation
Personnel (manpower) (people systems)				
Parts (components, in-process, finished product)				
Process (machines) (buildings, facilities, equipment, support systems)				
Procedures (methods) (manufacturing and control, documentation, records)				

The CGMPs may also be viewed as consisting of the following four essential elements:

1. *Personnel.* The people system and manpower required to carry out the various tasks within the manufacturing and control functions.
2. *Parts.* The raw materials and components used in connection with the manufacture and packaging of the drug product as well as the materials used in association with its control.
3. *Process.* The buildings, facilities, equipment, instrumentation, and support systems (heat, air, vacuum, water, and lighting) used in connection with the manufacturing process and its control.
4. *Procedure.* The paperwork, documentation, and records used in connection with the manufacturing process and its control.

Thus the four elements of CGMPs listed above may be combined with the four elements of pharmaceutical process validation (i.e., qualification, validation, control, and revalidation) to form a 4 × 4 matrix with respect to all the activities that may be considered in connection with the manufacture and control of each drug product. An example of such a process validation matrix provides a simple checklist of activities to be considered in connection with the general principles of process validation (Table 2).

III. ORGANIZING FOR VALIDATION

The mission of quality assurance in most pharmaceutical companies today has grown in importance with the advent of process validation. The process validation concept, which started as a subject noun (validation) in

Table 3   Specific Responsibilities of Each Organizational Structure within the Scope of Process Validation

Engineering	Install, qualify, and certify plant, facilities, equipment, and support systems.
Development	Design, optimize, and qualify manufacturing process within design limits, specifications, and/or requirements. In other words, the establishment of process capability information.
Manufacturing	Operate and maintain plant, facilities, equipment, support systems, and the specific manufacturing process within its design limits, specifications, and/or requirements.
Quality assurance	Establish approvable validation protocols and conduct process validation by monitoring, sampling, testing, challenging, and/or auditing the specific manufacturing process for compliance with design limits, specifications, and/or requirements.

Source: Ref. 31.

Table 4   Validation Progress Gantt Chart

Key elements	Design stage	Qualification stage		Validation stage	
		Installation	Operational	Prospective	Concurrent
Facilities and equipment		Engineering phase → Manufacturing start-up			
		(Validation protocols)		(Batch records and validation documentation)	
Process and product		Developmental phase (formula definition and stability testing) →	Scale-up phase (process optimization and pilot production) →		QA and manufacturing phase (full production)

Time line for new product introduction →

the late 1970s, has been turned into an action verb (to validate) by the quality assuance function of many drug companies. Quality Assurance was initially organized as a logical response to the need to assure that CGMPs were being complied with. Therefore, it is not surprising that process validation became the vehicle through which quality assurance now carries out its commitment to CGMPs [30].

The specifics of how a dedicated group, team, or committee is organized in order to conduct process validation assignments is beyond the scope of this chapter. It is clear, however, that the following responsibilities must be carried out and that the organizational structures best equipped to handle each assignment is presented in Table 3.

The concept of divided validation responsibilities can be used for the purpose of constructing a validation progress time chart (Table 4). Such a chart is capable of examining the logical sequence of key events or milestones (both parallel and series) that take place during the time course of new product introduction and is similar to a Gantt chart constructed by Chapman [32].

In Table 4, facilities and equipment are the responsibility of Engineering and Manufacturing, while process and product are the responsibility of the product and process development function(s). The engineering and development functions in conjunction with quality assurance come together to prepare the validation protocols during the qualification stage of product and process development.

IV. PROCESS VALIDATION — ORDER
OF PRIORITY

Because of resource limitation, it is not always possible to validate an entire company's product line at once. With the obvious exception that a company's most profitable products should be given a higher priority, it is advisable to draw up a list of product categories that are to be validated.

The following order of importance or priority with respect to validation is suggested to the reader:

Sterile Products and Their Processes

    1. Large-volume parenterals (LVPs)
    2. Small-volume parenterals (SVPs)
    3. Ophthalmics and other sterile products

Nonsterile Products and Their Processes

    4. Low-dose/high-potency tablets and capsules
    5. Drugs with stability problems
    6. Other tablets and capsules
    7. Oral liquids and topicals

V. PILOT — SCALE-UP AND PROCESS VALIDATION

The following operations are normally carried out by the development function prior to the preparation of the first pilot-production batch. The development activities are listed as follows:

1. Formulation design, selection, and optimization
2. Preparation of the first pilot-laboratory batch
3. Conduct initial accelerated stability testing
4. If the formulation is deemed stable, preparation of additional pilot-laboratory batches of the drug product for expanded non-clinical and/or clinical use

The pilot program is defined as the scale-up operations conducted subsequent to the product and its process leaving the development laboratory and prior to its acceptance by the full-production manufacturing unit. For the pilot program to be successful, elements of process validation (i.e., product and process qualification studies) must be included and completed during the developmental or pilot-laboratory phase of the work.

Thus product and process scale-up should proceed in graduated steps with elements of process validation (such as qualification) incorporated at each stage of the piloting program [33].

1. *Laboratory Batch.* The first step in the scale-up process is the selection of a suitable preliminary formula for more critical study and testing based upon certain agreed-upon initial design criteria, requirements and/or specifications. The work is performed in the development laboratory. The formula selected is designated as the (1X) laboratory batch. The size of the (1X) laboratory batch is usually 3−5 kg of a solid or semi-solid, 3−5 liters of a liquid or 3000 to 5000 units of a tablet or capsule.

2. *Laboratory−Pilot Batch.* After the (1X) laboratory batch is determined to be both physically and chemically stable based upon accelerated, elevated temperature testing (i.e., 1 month at 45°C or 3 months at 38°C or 38°C/80% RH), the next step in the scale-up process is the preparation of the (10X) laboratory−pilot batch. The (10X) laboratory−pilot batch represents the first replicated scale-up of the designated formula. The size of the laboratory−pilot batch is usually 30−50 kg, 30−50 liters or 30,000 to 50,000 units.

It is usually prepared in small-size, pilot equipment within a designated CGMP approved area of the development laboratory. The number and actual size of the laboratory−pilot batches may vary in response to one or more of the following factors:

a. Equipment availability
b. Active drug substance availability
c. Cost of raw materials
d. Inventory requirements for clinical and nonclinical studies

Process qualification or process capability studies are usually started in this important second stage of the pilot program. Such qualification or capability studies consist of process ranging, process characterization, and process optimization as a prerequisite to the more formal validation program that follows later in the piloting sequence.

3. *Pilot Production.* The pilot-production phase may be carried out either as a shared responsibility between the development laboratories and its appropriate manufacturing counterpart —or as a process demonstration by a separate, designated pilot-plant or process-development function. The two organizational piloting options are presented separately in Figure 1. The creation of a separate pilot-plant or process-development unit

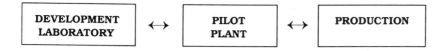

JOINT PILOT OPERATION

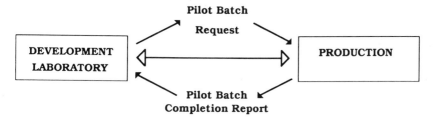

Figure 1   Main piloting options. (top) Separate pilot plant functions—engineering concept. (bottom) Joint pilot operation.

has been favored in recent years for it is ideally suited to carry out process qualification and/or validation assignments in a timely manner. On the other hand, the joint pilot-operation option provides direct communication between the development laboratory and pharmaceutical production.

The objective of the pilot-production batch is to scale the product and process by another order of magnitude (100×) to, for example, 300–500 kg, 300–500 liters, or 300,000–500,000 dosage-form units (tablets or capsules) in size. For most drug products this represents a full production batch in standard production equipment. If required, pharmaceutical production is capable of scaling the product and process to even larger batch sizes should the product require expanded production output. If the batch size changes significantly (say to 500× or 1000×) additional validation studies would be required.

Usually large production batch scale-up is undertaken only after product introduction. Again, the actual size of the pilot-production (100×) batch may vary due to equipment and raw material availability. The need for additional pilot-production batches ultimately depends upon the successful completion of a first pilot batch and its process validation program. Usually three successfully completed pilot-production batches are required for validation purposes.

In summary, process capability studies start in the development laboratories and/or during product and process development continue in well-defined stages until the process is validated in the pilot plant and/or pharmaceutical production.

An approximate timetable for new product development and its pilot scale-up program is suggested in Table 5.

Table 5   Approximate Timetable for New Product Development and Pilot
Scale-Up Trials

Event	Calendar months
Formula selection and development	2 − 4
Assay methods development and formula optimization	2 − 4
Stability in standard packaging 3-month read-out (1× size)	3 − 4
Pilot-laboratory batches (10× size)	1 − 3
Preparation and release of clinical supplies (10× size) and establishment of process qualification	1 − 4

Additional stability testing in approved packaging
   6 − 8-month read-out (1× size)
   3-month read-out (10× size)
	3 − 4

Validation protocols and pilot batch request	1 − 3
Pilot-production batches (100× size)	1 − 3

Additional stability testing in approved packaging
   9 − 12-month read-out (1× size)
   6 − 8-month read-out (10× size)
   3-month read-out (100× size)
	3 − 4

Interim approved technical product manual with approximately 12-months stability (1× size)	1 − 3
Totals	18 − 36

VI. PROCESS CAPABILITY DESIGN AND TESTING

Process validation trials are never designed to fail. Process validation
failures, however, are often attributable to an incomplete picture of the
manufacturing process being evaluated. Upon closer examination of the
problem, often failures appear to be directly related to an incomplete
understanding of the process's capability or that the process qualification
trials were not properly defined for the job to be done.

Process capability is defined as studies that are carried out to determine the *critical* process parameters or operating variables that influence
process output and the range of numerical data for each of the critical
process parameters that result in acceptable process output.

Thus, the objectives of process capability design and testing may be
listed as follows:

1. To determine the number and relative importance of the critical
    parameters in a process that affect the quality of process output
2. To show that the numerical data generated for each critical
    parameter are within at least statistical quality control limits (i.e.,

±3 standard deviations and that there is no drift or assignable
cause of variation in the process data

If the capability of a process is properly delineated, the process should
consistently stay within the defined limits of its critical process parameters
and product characteristics [34].

Process qualification, on the other hand, represents the actual studies
or trials conducted to show that all systems, subsystems, or unit operations of a manufacturing process perform as intended. Furthermore, that
all critical process parameters operate within their assigned control limits
and that such studies and trials, which form the basis of process capability design and testing, are verifiable and certifiable through appropriate documentation. Process qualification is often referred to as Operational or Performance Qualification.

The manufacturing process is briefly defined as the ways and means
used to convert raw materials into a finished product. The ways and
means also include: people, equipment, facilities, and support systems
that are required in order to operate the process in a planned and an
effectively managed way. Therefore, let us assume that all people, equipment, facilities, and support systems that are required to run the process
qualification trials have been themselves qualified and validated beforehand.

The steps and the sequence of events required in order to perform
process capability design and testing are outlined in Table 6.

Using the basic process for the manufacture of a simple tablet dosage
form, we will attempt here to highlight some of the important elements of
the process capability and qualification sequence.

1. Basic information is obtained from the (1×) size laboratory
batch.

    a. Quantitative formula is scaled to (10×) size batch and rationale for
       inert ingredient selection provided.
    b. Critical specifications, test methods, and acceptance criteria for
       each raw material used in the formula are provided.
    c. List of proposed specifications, test methods, and acceptance cri-
       teria for the finished dosage form are provided.
    d. Interim stability report on (1×) size laboratory batch is provided.
    e. Detailed operating instructions for preparing the (10×) size batch
       are provided.

2. Preparation of a simple flow diagram of the process should be provided. A good flow diagram should show all the unit operations in a
logical sequence, the major pieces of equipment to be used, and the
stages or operations at which the various ingredients are added. The
flow diagram, shown in Figure 2, outlines the sequence of unit operations used to prepare a typical tablet dosage form by the wet granulation
method. In Figure 3, the enclosed large rectangular *modules* represent
the various unit operations in the manufacturing process. The arrows
represent transfers of material into and out of each unit operation. Each
large rectangular module or box indicates the particular unit operation,
the major piece of processing equipment employed, and the facility in
which the operation takes place. The sequential arrangement of unit

Table 6   Protocol for Process Capability Design and Testing

Objective of piloting program	Process capability design and testing
Types of process	Batch, intermittent, continuous
Typical processes	Chemical, pharmaceutical, filling, and packaging
Definition of process	Flow diagram, equipment/materials in-process, finished product
Definition of process output	Potency, yield, physical parameters
Definition of test methods	Methods, equipment, calibration traceability, precision, accuracy
Analysis of process	Definition of process variables, influence matrix, fractional factorial analysis
Review and analysis of data	Data plot (x−y plots, histogram, control chart) time sequence, sources of variation
Pilot batch trials	Define stable/extended runs, define sample and testing, remove sources of variation
Pilot batch replication	Different shifts and days, different materials, different facilities and equipment
Need for process capability redefinition	Data analysis, modification of influence matrix, reclassification of variables
Process capability of evaluated process	Stability and variability of process output, conformance to defined specifications, economic limits of process
Final report and recommendations	Recommended SOP, limits on process adjustments, recommended specifications

operations should be analogous to the major sequential steps in the operating instructions of the manufacturing process.

3. Using the flow chart (Fig. 2) as a guide, a list of process or control variables are next drawn up for each unit operation or step in the process. A test parameter or response to be objectively measured is then assigned to each process variable. The control parameters (i.e., process variables plus their test parameters) for the manufacture of compressed tablets by the wet granulation method are shown in Table 7. According to the data presented in Table 7, there are six unit operations or processing steps, with from two to five process variables for each unit operation and, with the exception of tablet compression (finished tablet analysis), one key test parameter for each of the processing steps. Please note that the first unit operation, i.e., the weighing of active and inert ingredients, was eliminated from Table 7. Weighing operations are a general consideration in all manufacturing processes. Balances and measuring devices are normally qualified and validated separately on a routine basis as required by CGMP's guidelines.

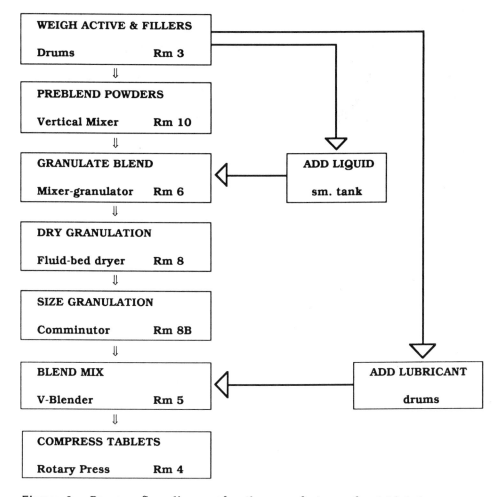

Figure 2   Process flow diagram for the manufacture of a tablet dosage form by the wet granulation method.

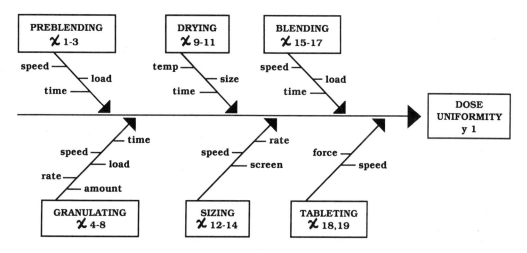

Figure 3   A simple "fishbone" diagram of the processing steps and in-process variables during tablet manufacture that may influence the quality and consistency of final product-dose uniformity.

Table 7 Control Parameters for the Manufacture of a Tablet Dosage Form by the Wet Granulation Method

Unit operations	Process variables	Test parameters
Preblend powders	Blending time Blender speed Load size	Assay for blend uniformity
Granulate blend	Granulating time Granulator speed Load Size Liquid addition rate Amount of liquid	End-point by wattmeter
Dry granulation	Drying time Inlet temperature Load size	Moisture content
Size granulation	Feed rate Mill speed Screen size	Granule size distribution
Blend mix	Blending time Blender speed Load size	Assay for blend uniformity
Compress tablets	Compression force Press speed Dissolution time	Dose uniformity Weight uniformity Dissolution time Disintegration time Hardness

4. The question arises, how do we determine which process variables and/or unit operations are *critical* with respect to the product outcomes or attributes (i.e., dose uniformity, weight variations, dissolution time, disintegration time, and tablet hardness)? Even among these finished tablet attributes, dose uniformity (potency), dissolution time, and/or tablet hardness are usually considered to be more important than weight uniformity or disintegration time.

In order to determine the critical process parameters, *process characterization* and *process ranging* studies should be carried out in connection with the performance qualification trials. Process characterization represents the methods used to determine the critical processing steps and process control variables that affect the quality and consistency of the product outcomes or attributes. While process ranging represents the studies that are used to identify the critical process or test parameters and their respective control limits which also will affect the quality and consistency of the product outcomes or attributes.

There are several ways to determine the critical processing steps and processing variables that influence product outcomes. One of these, is to construct a *cause and effect* or "*fishbone*" diagram [35].

VII. CAUSE-AND-EFFECT OR "FISHBONE" DIAGRAM

The "fishbone" diagram represents all possible relationships and inter-relationships that may exist among the various process variables (possible causes) and the single response or product attribute (effect) affected during the manufacture of a tablet dosage form by the wet granulation method. The central line of the cause and effect diagram shown in Figure 3 is a composite of all the possible factors (19 in all) that may influence the quality and consistency of dose uniformity of the tablet (y_1 response). Branches off the central line represent the influence of the six unit operations or process steps. The principle process variables for each process step that can cause or influence the final outcome are depicted as sub-branches off each of the six main branches. The diagram shows six possible critical process steps and 19 possible critical process variables. If required and using the same 19 factors, similar "fishbone" diagrams could also be constructed for dissolution time (y_2 response) or tablet hardness (y_3 response).

The unit operations are next broken down into six subsystems for cause and effect analysis. Where the process variables have been described previously and the test parameters listed in Table 7 now serve as the measured output response (effect) to the various input control variables (causes). In the case of tablet compression, where there are only two key input variables (compression force and press speed) and five possible output responses to select from (dose uniformity, weight variation, dissolution time, disintegration time, or tablet hardness) from experience, tablet hardness is often chosen as the most representative test parameter for tablet compression analysis.

VIII. CONSTRAINT ANALYSIS

The factor that makes the subsystem evaluations and performance qualification trials manageable is the application of constraint analysis. Boundary limits of the technology and restrictions as to what constitutes a well-blended powder, a well-formed granule, or a well-made tablet will often constrain the number of process variables and product attributes that require analysis. Constraint analysis will also limit and restrict the operational range of each process variable or the specification limits of each product attribute.

Take, for example, the fluid-bed drying of the wet granulation. The inlet temperature for producing rapid drying of granules without exposing

Table 8 Constraint Analysis of the Key Process Variables Required in the Manufacture of a Tablet Dosage Form by the Wet Granulation Method

Unit operations	Process variables	Control limits	
		Lower	Upper
Preblending	Blending time (at 8 RPM and 50% load)	10 min	20 min
Granulating	Impeller speed	200 RPM	400 RPM
	Chopper speed	2000 RPM	4000 RPM
	Granulating time (rapid addition of 5 liter of water)		
Drying	Inlet temperature	50°C	60°C
	Air velocity ratio	7 CFM/lb	10 CFM/lb
	Drying time	20 min	40 min
Sizing	Mill speed	1200 RPM	5400 RPM
	Feed rate (knives forward, no screen)	500 g/min	1000 g/min
Blending	Blending time (at 8 RPM and 50% load)	10 min	20 min
Tableting[a]	Compression force	1500 lb	2500 lb
	Press speed (7/32 – 13/32-in. oval punches)	32 RPM	68 RPM

[a]Data from the work of Williams and Stiel [36].

the material to undue thermal stress may range between 50 and 60°C. The air velocity per load ratio may range between 7 and 10 CFM/lb. Therefore, setting inlet air temperature at 55 ± 2°C and incoming air velocity per load at 8.5 ± 0.5 CFM/lb should, in most cases, produce acceptable product (i.e., moisture content below 2%) in a usual drying time of 30 min ± 10 min. Conducting qualification trials, with different lots of raw material on different days while exercising control of the inlet air temperature and air velocity, may be all that is required in order to qualify the drying step in the manufacturing process.

Using the constraint analysis concept, the practical upper and lower control limits for each of the key process variables associated with each of the unit operations required to make simple uncoated tablets by the wet granulation method are presented in Table 8.

Table 9 A simplified Analysis of the Input – Output Values Expected During the Manufacture of a Tablet Dosage Form by the Wet Granulation Method

Unit operations	Key process variables	Selected inputs	Measured responses	Expected outputs
Preblending	Blend time	15 min	Blend uni-formity	95 – 105% L.P.
Granulating	Impeller speed	300 RPM	Moisture content	25 – 35%
	Chopper speed	3000 RPM		
	Granulating time	4 min		
Drying	Inlet tempera-ture	55°C	Moisture content	Less than 2%
	Air velocity	8.5 CFM		
	Drying time	30 min		
Sizing	Mill speed	2700 RPM	Granule size distribution	Majority 40 – 60 mesh
	Feed rate	750 g/min		
Blending	Blend time	15 min	Blend uni-formity	95 – 105% L.P.
Tableting	Compression force	2000 lb	Dose uni-formity	95 – 105% L.P.
	Press speed	48 RPM	Dissolution time	t90% NMT 15 min
			Tablet hard-ness	14 – 18 SCU

A comparison of the process variables listed in Table 7 and in Table 8 indicates that application of constraint analysis reduced the number of key process variables by seven from 19 to 12. Next, using the mean or central value in the range that lies between the control limits for each key process variable or control parameter, Table 9 was constructed containing average input values for each control parameter and the expected output response for each unit operation and the final finished tablet.

IX. QUALIFICATION TRIAL OPTIONS

There are several ways to carry out the process capability qualification trials. The options are discussed as follows:

A. Replication of Optimum or Midrange Values

Using the selected midrange input values presented in Table 9, the
process may be run as a pilot-laboratory batch (10×-size) in accordance
with an agreed upon standard operating procedure and the protocol for
in-process testing. Expected outputs are then measured after each unit
operation and if the results are within in-process specifications, the
process is permitted to continue to the next processing step. After tablet
compression has been successfully completed (i.e., tablet hardness, tablet
weight, and tablet dimensions are within specifications), representative
sample of final finished tablets are next subjected to end product testing
for dose uniformity and compliance with established dissolution time specifications. Having completed an acceptable run, the process may be repeated several times more in order to establish process reproducibility.

In the course of this work, if one or more of the processing steps
fail to comply with the expected in-process outcomes, additional development time will be spent to get these particular unit operations up to
standard operating conditions. The first option is, therefore, a simple
go — no go approach, where the process qualification proceeds upon the
completion of each unit operation and each pilot batch. In this simple,
straight-forward qualification procedure, control limits are never tested
and critical steps in the overall process are never fully established.

B. Fractional Factorial Design

An experimental design is a series of statistically sufficient qualification
trials that are planned in a specific arrangement and include all processing
variables that can possibly affect the expected outcome of the process
under investigation. In the case of a factorial design, n, equals the
number of factors or process variables, each at two levels (i.e., the
upper- and lower-control limits). Such a simple design is known as a 2^{11}
factorial. Using the process variables found in Table 8 we could, for example, run 2^{12} or 4096 qualification trials.

The fractional factorial is designed to reduce the number of qualification trials to a reasonable number, say eight, while holding the number
of processing variables to be evaluated to a reasonable number as well,
again eight. The technique was developed as a nonparametric test for
process evaluation by Box and Hunter [37] and reviewed by Hendrix
[38].

Each processing variable, however, is studied at both its control
limits. The positive (+) symbol is used for the upper control limit and
the negative (−) symbol is used for the lower control limit. In this way
a full factorial of 2^8 may be reduced from 256 experiments to only eight
(see the design in Table 10).

Following the design, eight pilot-laboratory batches (10×-size) are
next prepared for testing and evaluation. Trial No. 1 is run where each
process variable X_1 through X_8 is at its lower control limit (LCL), while
in trial No. 8 each process variable is at its upper control limit (UCL).

The design is so constructed that the total number of +'s and −'s are
the same for each process variable (4&4). With the exception of trail
No. 1 and No. 8, the total number of +'s and −'s is also the same for
each trial run (4&4).

Table 10   Fractional Factorial Design (8 Variables in 8 Experiments)

Trial No.	X_1	X_2	X_3	X_4	X_5	X_6	X_7	X_8
1	−	−	−	−	−	−	−	−
2	+	−	−	−	−	+	+	+
3	−	+	−	−	+	−	+	+
4	−	+	−	+	−	+	−	+
5	+	−	+	−	+	−	+	−
6	−	+	+	+	+	−	−	−
7	+	−	+	+	−	+	−	−
8	+	+	+	+	+	+	+	+

Next eight pilot-laboratory batches (10× size each) of tablets are prepared following the design given in Table 10 and the conditions established for each trial run in Table 11. For example, according to the conditions established for trial No. 4, powder preblend time is 10 min, granulating time is 5 min, inlet temperature in the dryer is set at 50°C, mill speed is set at 5400 RPM, feed rate to Fitzmill is 500 g/min, blend time is 20 min, compression force during tableting is 1500 lb, and press speed is set at 68 RPM.

Table 11   Process Variables and Control Limits Selected for Fractional Factorial Design of Eight Qualification Trials

	Process variable	LCL (−)	UCL (+)
X_1	Preblend time	10 min	20 min
X_2	Granulating time	3 min	5 min
X_3	Inlet temperature	50°C	60°C
X_4	Mill speed	1200 RPM	5400 RPM
X_5	Feed rate	500 g/min	1000 g/min
X_6	Blend time	10 min	20 min
X_7	Compression force	1500 lb	2500 lb
X_8	Press Speed	32 RPM	68 RPM

Focusing our attention on the key processing variables listed in Tables 8 and 9, the number selected for analysis have been reduced to eight in the following manner:

X_1 = preblend time

X_2 = granulating time (at 300 RPM and 3000 RPM)

X_3 = inlet temperature (at 8.5 CFM)

X_4 = mill speed

X_5 = feed rate

X_6 = blend time

X_7 = compression force

X_8 = press speed

The processing conditions to be evaluated using a fractional factorial experimental design are presented in Table 11.

When all trial runs have been completed, the finished tablets are then subjected to end-product testing for compliance to content uniformity, weight uniformity, tablet hardness, disintegration time, and dissolution time specifications. Tablet hardness data were chosen for analysis of fractional factorial experimental design for the following reasons:

1. A direct correlation between tablet hardness and dissolution time had been previously established for the product
2. Variability for tablet hardness among trial runs was greater than for the other output parameters
3. Four batches (trial Nos. 3, 4, 5, and 7) were out of specification with respect to the proposed limits for tablet hardness (i.e., not less than 12 SCU and not more than 16 SCU)

The results of the analysis of the tablet hardness data are presented in Table 12.

Simple analysis of the data presented in Table 12 reveals the following useful information:

1. The mean tablet hardness for all trial runs is 14 SCU. Three batches (Nos. 1, 4, and 7) fall below this mean, while three batches (Nos. 3, 5, and 8) are above the mean. Two batches (Nos. 2 and 6) have a mean value of 14 SCU. The batches appear to be normally distributed about the value 14 SCU.

2. If the process variables (Xs) have no effect on the process outcome and if the experimental design is reasonably balanced, one would expect that the contrasting sum of + and − tablet hardness values in each process variable column would approach a minimum numerical value and that the resultant average contrasting sum would approach a value of zero. Therefore on this basis, the following process variables appear to have little or no effect upon tablet hardness. These variables are preblending, granulating, drying, and press speed. On the other hand, the following process variables appear to influence the outcome, i.e., tablet hardness. These latter variables are mill speed and feed rate during comminution, blending time during lubricant addition, and compression force during tableting.

Table 12 Nonparametric Analysis of Fractional Factorial Experimental Design Using Tablet Hardness as the Measured Response

Trial No.	X_1	X_2	X_3	X_4	X_5	X_6	X_7	X_8	Tablet hardness[a]
1	−13	−13	−13	−13	−13	−13	−13	−13	13
2	+14	−14	−14	−14	−14	+14	+14	+14	14
3	−18	+18	−18	−18	+18	−18	+18	+18	18
4	−10	+10	−10	+10	−10	+10	−10	+10	10
5	+17	−17	+17	−17	+17	−17	+17	−17	17
6	−14	+14	+14	+14	+14	−14	−14	−14	14
7	+11	−11	+11	+11	−11	+11	−11	−11	11
8	+15	+15	+15	+15	+15	+15	+15	+15	15
Sum of column	+2	+2	+2	−12	+16	−12	+16	+2	
Sum/4[b]	+0.5	+0.5	+0.5	−3.0	+4.0	−3.0	+4.0	+0.5	

[a] Using a calibrated electronic hardness tester, mean of 20 representative tablets (rounded to 2 significant numbers) is reported in Strong Cobb Units (SCU).

[b] The sum of each column is divided by 4, since there are 4 values at each control limit (i.e., 4 +'s and 4 −'s).

3. The overall design does not balance to zero because there is a constant +2 for each process variable. Since there are, this is due to the fact that in our design eight −13s in trial No. 1 and eight +15s in trial No. 8 were created.

The advantage of the fractional factorial experimental design is that, using No. 8 qualification trial, eight important process variables were tested at both their lower and upper control limits. In addition, three processing steps [dry milling, lubricant addition (blending), and tablet compression] were all shown to be *critical* with respect to a measured response, namely tablet hardness. Since tablet hardness also influences tablet dissolution, this second outcome was also indirectly evaluated by the experimental design chosen.

Using a larger fractional factorial experimental design, 12 or even 16 process variables could be tested by expanding the qualification trials to say 12 or 16 pilot runs. But in practice, eight pilot-laboratory batches is most likely the maximum number that is reasonable to produce for this purpose. Those unit operations that were found, by fractional factorial experimental design, to be critical with respect to process capability design and testing (size reduction, blending, and tablet compression) could then be subjected to more extensive investigation during the laboratory stage of product and/or process development.

C. Optimization Techniques

Optimization techniques are used to find either the best possible quantitative formula for a product or the best possible set of experimental conditions (input values) that are needed to run the process. Optimization techniques may be employed in the laboratory state to develop the most stable, least sensitive formula, or in the qualification and validation stages of scale-up in order to develop the most stable, least variable process within its proven acceptable range(s) of operation, Chapman's so-called PAR principle [39]

Optimization techniques may be classified as Parametric Statistical Methods and Nonparametric Search Methods.

Parametric Statistical Methods

Parametric Statistical Methods, usually employed for optimization, are full-factorial designs [40], half-factorial designs [41], simplex design [42], and Lagrangian multiple-regression analysis [43]. Parametric methods are best suited for formula optimization in the early stages of product development. The application of constraint analysis, which was described previously, is used to simplify the testing protocol and the analysis of experimental results.

The steps involved in the parametric optimization procedure for pharmaceutical systems have been fully described by Schwartz [44]. The optimization technique consists of the following essential operations:

1. Selection of a suitable experimental design
2. Selection of variables (independent Xs and dependent Ys) to be tested

Table 13   Results of a Three-Components Simplex Design for Tablet Hardness

Run no.	Excipient components			Transformed proportions			Average tablet hardness (SCU)
	X_1	X_2	X_3	X_1	X_2	X_3	
1	55	10	10	1	0	0	6.1
2	10	55	10	0	1	0	7.5
3	10	10	55	0	0	1	5.3
4	32.5	32.5	10	0.5	0.5	0	6.6
5	32.5	10	32.5	0.5	0	0.5	6.4
6	10	32.5	32.5	0	0.5	0.5	6.9
7	25	25	25	0.33	0.33	0.25	7.3
8	32.5	21.25	21.25	0.5	0.25	0.25	7.2

3. Performance of a set of statistically designed experiments (i.e., 2^3 or 3^2 factorials)
4. Measurement of responses (dependent variables)
5. Development of a predictor, polynomial equation based upon statistical and regression analysis of the generated experimental data
6. Development of a set of optimized requirements for the formula based upon mathematical and graphical analysis of the data generated

According to Bolton, one of the most useful methods of defining optimal regions of formulation characteristics is based upon the application of *simplex matrix design* [45]. For example, formulations may be constructed, using constraint analysis, so that the total amount of excipients (Xs) to be added to the powder mix is never more than 75 mg of a total tablet weight of 300 mg. A brief outline of the simplex technique, used in connection with this example is shown in Table 13.

In the transformations shown in Table 13, the highest excipient concentration, 55 mg, is assigned a value of one and the lowest excipient concentration, 10 mg, equals 0 is assigned a value of zero. Coefficients for X_1, X_2, and X_3 in the following polynomial equation are the hardness values from run Nos. 1, 2, and 3. Simple equations for calculating coefficients for the following terms: $X_1 X_2$, $X_1 X_3$, $X_2 X_3$, and $X_1 X_2 X_3$ are given in the reference [45].

where

$$Y = 6.1 X_1 + 7.5 X_2 + 5.3 X_3 - 0.8 X_1 X_2 + 2.8 X_1 X_3 + 2.0 X_2 X_3$$

$$+ 15 X_1 X_2 X_3$$

Example (run no. 8):

$$Y = 6.1\ (0.5) + 7.5\ (0.25) + 5.3\ (0.25) - 0.8\ (0.125) + 2.8\ (0.125)$$
$$+ 2\ (0.0625) + 15\ (0.03125)$$

$$Y = 3.05 + 1.875 + 1.325 - 0.1 + 0.35 + 0.125 + 0.47 = 7.1$$

The best tablet hardness (7.4 value SCU) containing all three excipients is obtained at $X_1 = 0.25$, $X_2 = 0.5$, and $X_3 = 0.25$, where $X_1 = 18.75$ mg, $X_2 = 37.5$ mg, and $X_3 = 18.75$ mg.

Nonparametric Search Methods

Nonparametric Search Methods are relatively simple techniques used to fine-tune or optimize a process by varying the critical process parameters that were found during the qualification and validation stages of process development. The procedure is so constrained that no process variable is ever permitted to exceed its lower or upper control limit. In searching a given process, it is assumed that there is optimum peak (set of experimental conditions or inputs) where the process operates most efficiently. There are two basic search methods that are used for this purpose. The first method is called *evolutionary operation* (EVOP) and a second method is called *random evolutionary operation* (REVOP). The difference between the two methods, EVOP and REVOP, is not objectivity but simplicity of the experimental design chosen.

Process Improvement Through EVOP

The process variables whose perturbation or slight change might lead to improvement in process performance are usually identified during the qualification trials where the operational and control limits for the process have been developed. Next, initial perturbation steps away from the present operational inputs are selected for each of the critical process variables. These steps must be sufficiently small so that no input goes beyond the control limits of the process and no output goes out of product and process specification. In the traditional box EVOP design [46] a simple two-factor, two-level design is created about the present condition or input values (see Fig. 4).

Analysis of the data presented in Figure 4 shows that the *path of steepest ascent* to improve tablet hardness is in the direction of run No. 1 to run No. 4, which is a change of +3 SCU in tablet hardness. A second two-factor, two-level box is constructed about run No. 4 where one corner of the box is the original condition, run No. 1. Following the same procedure, a series of from 8 to 24 runs, using the path of steepest ascent, is usually required to ascertain the optimum input values for tablet hardness and rapid tablet dissolution.

By using a *simplex EVOP design* [47] where connecting triangles are created from 2 additional experimental conditions, it is possible to complete the optimization search in fewer trial runs than Box EVOP (see Fig. 5).

Process Improvement Through REVOP

Random evolutionary operation (REVOP) is a comparatively little-used method for process and product optimization [48]. The technique,

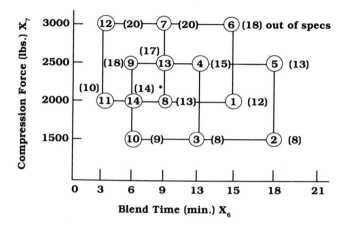

Figure 4   Optimization by box Evolutionary Operation. Tablet hardness (SCU shown in parenthesis). Optimum conditions (2000 lbs and 6 min).

developed by F. E. Satterthwaite, employs a random direction of movement under constraint analysis to discover a probable pathway of ascent to peak process performance. If the linear direction chosen is not promising, the direction is reversed and the opposite pathway is chosen in an effort to improve performance. Movement continues along the new path in direction previously established, as long as the results are positive. Movement will then proceed at right angles when progress ceases on the previously chosen pathway. Peak performance is almost always achieved in less than 20 trials runs (see Fig. 6).

In summary, process capability studies and qualification trials should be underaken during the first stage of pilot scale-up, i.e., with the preparation of the pilot-laboratory batch (10×) size). The objective of such

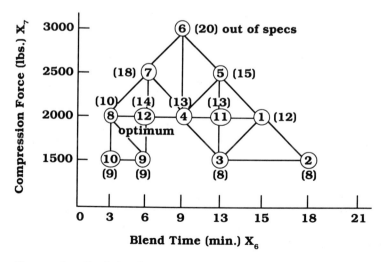

Figure 5   Optimization by simplex evolutionary operation. Tablet hardness (SCU) shown in parenthesis.

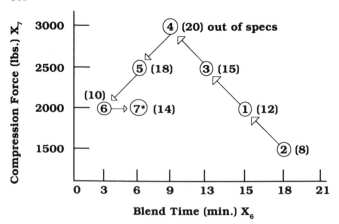

Figure 6   Optimization by random evolutionary operation. Tablet hardness (SCU) shown in parenthesis.

studies is to test the proposed upper and lower control limits and to determine those critical processing steps and process variables that affect end-product performance. In this connection, nonparametric methods, such as fractional factorial experimental designs and search methods like EVOP and REVOP should prove useful in connection with process optimization and process capability testing which should be carried out prior to the start of the more formal process-validation program.

X. PROCESS VALIDATION

The topic, process validation of tablets and other solid dosage forms has been covered in separate articles by Nash [49,50], Simmons [51], von Doehren et al. [52], Rudolph [53], and Avallone [10]. Chapman writes about the possibility of conducting three different types of validation programs [39]. They may be defined briefly as:

  1. *Prospective Process Validation*. Where an experimental plan called the *validation protocol* is executed (following completion of the qualification trials) before the process is put to commercial use. Most validation efforts require some degree of prospective experimentation in order to generate validation support data.
  2. *Concurrent Process Validation*. Establishing documented evidence that the process is in a *state of control* during the actual implementation of the process. This is normally performed by conducting in-process testing and/or monitoring of critical operations during the manufacture of each production batch.
  3. *Retrospective Process Validation*. Where historic data taken from the records of the completed production batches are used to provide documented evidence that the process has been in a state of control prior to the request for such evidence.

XI. PROSPECTIVE PROCESS VALIDATION

This particular type of process validation is normally carried out in connection with the introduction of new drug products and their manufacturing processes. *The formalized process validation program should never be undertaken unless and until the following operations and procedures have been completed satisfactorily.*

1. The facilities and equipment, in which the process validation is to be conducted, meets CGMP requirements (completion of *installation qualification*)
2. The operators and supervising personnel, who will be "running" the validation batch(es), have an understanding of the process and its requirements
3. The design, selection, and optimization of the formula have been completed
4. The qualification trials, using (10×-size) pilot-laboratory batches have been completed, in which the critical processing steps and process variables have been identified and the provisional operational control limits for each critical test parameter have been provided.
5. Detailed technical information on the product and the manufacturing process have been provided, including documented evidence of product stability
6. Finally, at least one qualification trial of a pilot-production (100×-size) batch has been made and shows, upon scale-up, that there were no significant deviations from the expected performance of the process

The steps and sequence of events required in order to carry out a process-validation assignment are outlined in Table 14. The first half of

Table 14   Outline for Program Process Validation

Objective of program	A proving or demonstration that the process works
Types of validation	Prospective, concurrent, retrospective
Typical processes	Chemical, pharmaceutical, fabrication packaging, sterilization
Definition of process	Flow diagram, equipment/materials inprocess, finished product
Definition of process output	Potency, yield, physical parameters
Definition of test methods	Methods, equipment, calibration traceability, precision and accuracy
Analysis of process	Critical modules and variables defined by process capability design and testing program

Table 14   (Continued)

Control limits of critical variables	Defined by process capability design and testing program
Preparation of validation protocol	Facility, equipment, process, product number of validation trials and type sampling frequency, type, size tests to be performed, method, criteria definition of successful validation
Organizing for validation trials	Responsibility, authority
Planning validation trials	Timetable and PERT chart, availability, material acquisition and disposal
Validation trials	Supervision/administration, process documentation
Validation findings	Data summary, data analysis, conclusions
Final report and recommendations	Process validated, further trials, requires more process capability design and testing

the procedure is similar to that developed for process capability design and testing which was shown previously in Table 6. The objective of prospective validation is to prove or demonstrate that the process will work in accordance with validation protocol prepared for the pilot-production (100×-size) trials.

In practice, usually two or three pilot-production (100×-size) batches are prepared for validation purposes. The first batch to be included in the sequence may be the already successfully concluded first qualification trial at 100× size, which should be prepared under the direction of the organizational function directly responsible for pilot scale-up activities. Later, replicate batch manufacture may be performed by the Pharmaceutical Production function.

XII. STRATEGY FOR PROCESS VALIDATION

The strategy selected for process validation should be simple and straightforward. The following five points are presented here for the reader's consideration:

1. The use of different lots of raw materials should be included, i.e., active drug substance and major excipients.
2. Batches should be run in succession and on different days and shifts (the latter condition, if appropriate).
3. Batches should be manufactured in the equipment and facilities designated for eventual commercial production.

4. Critical process variables should be set within their *operating ranges* and should not exceed their upper and lower control limits during process operation. Output responses should be well within finished product specifications.

5. Failure to meet the requirements of the validation protocol with respect to process input and output control should be subjected to process *requalification* and subsequent *revalidation* following a thorough analysis of process data and formal discussion by the validation team.

XIII. CONCURRENT VALIDATION

In-process monitoring of critical processing steps and end-product testing of current production can provide documented evidence to show that the manufacturing process is in a *state of control*. Such validation documentation can be provided from the following test parameters and data sources:

Test parameter	Data source
Average unit potency	End-product testing
Content uniformity	End-product testing
Dissolution time	End-product testing
Powder-blend uniformity	In-process testing
Moisture content	In-process testing
Particle or granule size distribution	In-process testing
Unit weight variation	In-process testing
Tablet hardness	In-process testing
Disintegration time	In-process testing

Not all of the in-process tests enumerated above are required to demonstrate that the process is in a state of control. Selections should be made on the basis of the *critical* processing variables to be evaluated. On the basis of the example presented in this chapter (Table 12), the critical in-process test parameters would be particle or granule size distribution, blend time, and tablet hardness. Subsequent data analysis of these three parameters coupled with end-product testing should provide sufficient documented evidence of concurrent validation.

The following example is taken from my work in solids blending and is used to illustrate a method for obtaining concurrent validation data [54].

FDA investigators, during their plant inspections, will often ask to see validation information with respect to solids blending and mixing operations in connection with solid dosage form manufacture. A simple validation protocol has been designed here to supply validation documentation for the mixing of 40% penicillin G powder and 60% lactose diluent in a 50 ft^3 V-shaped production blender. The validation protocol for solids blending is given in Table 15. If the blending of penicillin G and lactose

Table 15   Protocol for the Concurrent Validation of a Solids Blending
Operation in a 50 ft^3 V-Shaped Blender

		Action
Parts	Active/diluent ratio	40% active (assayed as 100% label potency)
	Powder properties	Evaluate different lots of active and diluent
	Preblending option	Not required for "high actives"
Process	Blender type	V-shaped
	Blender size	50 ft^3 equivalent to 1400-liters working capacity
	Load size	65% capacity equivalent to 450 kg of powder mix (bulk density equals 0.6 g/cm^3)
	Blend speed	8 RPM
	Loading pattern	Layered (through exit port inverted)
	Intensifier	Additional agitation is not required
	Blend time	Qualification trials showed that the best mix was achieved in 15 min
Procedure	Assay method	HPLC for penicillin content
	Sample weight for assay	350 mg, same as for finished capsule
	Sample number for assay	30
	When sampled	After powder is dumped into 5 × 90 kg drums
	How sampled	6 samples are taken from each drum for assay (top, middle, and bottom)
Criterion for batch acceptance	The requirement is met if the potency of all 30 samples falls within the limits of 75.0% and 125.0% of label potency and the assay of not less than 27 samples falls within the limits of 85.0% and 115.0% of label potency	

was determined to be a critical processing step in the manufacture of penicillin hard-shell capsules, then the protocol presented in Table 15 could
be used to monitor blend uniformity on either a regular or intermittent
basis. In either case the in-process test method so devised from the following protocol could be considered to be an example of concurrent
validation.

XIV. RETROSPECTIVE VALIDATION

The retrospective validation option is chosen for established products where
their manufacturing processes are considered to be stable (i.e., long
history state-of-control operation) and where, on the basis of economic
considerations alone and resource limitations, prospective qualification, and
validation experimentation cannot be justified. Prior to undertaking retrospective validation, wherein the numerical in-process and/or end-product
test data of historic production batches are subjected to statistical analysis,
the equipment, facilities, and subsystems used in connection with the manufacturing process must be qualified and validated in conformance with
CGMP requirements.

The concept of using accumulated final product as well as in-process
numerical test data and batch records to provide documented evidence of
product and/or process validation was originally advanced by Meyers [55]
and Simms [56] of Eli Lilly and Company in 1980. Retrospective validation
has gained wide acceptance since that time, and the topic has been covered adequately in separate articles by Agalloco [57] and Trubinski and
Majeed [58]. The concept is also recognized in FDA's Guideline on General Principle of Process Validation [1].

Using either data-based computer systems [59,60] or manual methods,
retrospective validation may be conducted in the following manner:

1. Gather the numerical values from the completed batch record and
   include assay values, end-product test results, and in-process
   data.
2. Organize these data in a chronological sequence, according to
   batch manufacturing data using a spread-sheet format.
3. Include data from at least the last 20 – 30 manufactured batches for
   analysis. If the number of manufactured batches is less than 20,
   then include all manufactured batches in your analysis.
4. Trim the data by eliminating test results from noncritical processing steps and delete all gratuitous numerical information.
5. Subject the resultant data to statistical analysis and evaluation.
6. Draw conclusions as to the state of control of the manufacturing
   process based upon the analysis of retrospective validation data.
7. Issue a report of your findings (documented evidence).

The following output data (measured responses) from the manufacturing process are usually selected for statistical analysis:

1. Individual assay results from content uniformity testing
2. Individual tablet hardness values
3. Dissolution time at $t_{50\%}$

The statistical methods that may be employed to analyze numerical output data from the manufacturing process are listed as follows:

1. Basic statistics (mean, standard deviation, and tolerance limits) [45]
2. Analysis of variance (ANOVA and related techniques) [45]
3. Regression analysis [45]
4. Cumulative sum analysis (Cusum) [61]
5. Cumulative difference analysis [56]
6. Control charting (averages and range) [62,63]

Control charting, with the exception of basic statistical analysis, is probably the most useful statistical technique one might use to analyze retrospective and concurrent process data. Control charting forms the basis of modern statistical process control.

XV. CONTROL CHARTING

A detailed discussion of control charting and its use for the analysis of retrospective production-batch data are given in the following references [56,63–65]. The control chart is used to decide periodically whether a process is in *statistical control*. The use of such a technique facilitates the detection and possible elimination of assignable causes of process variation. The use of control charts (for averages) is considered to be the best statistical tool available for establishing, monitoring, and verifying a validated product and/or manufacturing process. The control chart, as devised by Shewhart (Bell Telephone Labs) in 1930, is a graphic presentation on which the numerical values of the test parameters (process outputs) of for example a tablet (potency, hardness, disintegration time, dissolution time, or weight variation) under investigation are plotted sequentially.

The control chart consists of a central line or grand average ($\bar{\bar{X}}$) and a control limit line above (UCL) and below (LCL) the central line. These two control or action limits represent ±3 sigma (standard deviations) about $\bar{\bar{X}}$. Occasionally ±2 sigma warning or inner control limits are used to alert the user of possible trends or systematic deviations in the process data. In either case, the distribution of the plotted numerical values (one value for each lot or batch) with respect to the control limits provides valuable statistical information about the quality of the process outputs and the process itself.

In theory, using ±3 sigma control limits, if the individual lot of batch averages were plotted over time on the graph or chart, one would expect, according to this statistic, that 99% of the individual lot averages would lie within the control limits. If appreciably more than 1% fell outside these limits, one could then conclude that the process was not in (statistical) control on a lot-to-lot or batch-to-batch basis. If, on the other hand, all of the 99% of the batch averages were within the limits, it then would provide supportive documented evidence of state-of-control process validation.

In addition, the following rules have been developed to detect shifts or trends in the process batch-to-batch averages in order to avoid the possibility of a process tending to go out of control:

1. Whenever, in seven successive points on the control chart, all are on the same side of the central line, this is not considered to be a random occurrence.
2. Whenever, in 18 successive points on the control charts, at least 12 are on the same side of the central line, this too is not considered to be random occurrence.
3. Whenever, in 20 successive points on the control chart, at least 16 are on the same side of the central line, this too is not considered to be a random occurrence.

Nevertheless, the above rules for trend analysis may be less instructive than the occurrence of 2, 3, or 4 data points outside the ±3 sigma control limits.

The mechanics of developing control charts for process data is beyond the objectives and scope of this chapter. The statistical techniques employed for control charting, however, are fairly simple and straightforward. Control charting and its analysis can be done manually or with the aid of a computer program [66].

The following illustration of control charting is taken from the powder blending example presented in Table 15. A control chart of blend uniformity was prepared from the results of penicillin G assay data. Each data point represents the average of six individual assayed samples, expressed in percent label potency per drum following the 15-minute blend time in the V-shaped mixer. Five drums containing 90 kg of powder each represents penicillin G mixed with lactose diluent prior to encapsulation. The averages for each drum were plotted in accordance with the method of constructing control charts. The results of five consecutive batches (25 drums) are presented in Figure 7. None of the data points were found to lie outside the 3-sigma control limits. Control charts can be used to monitor and

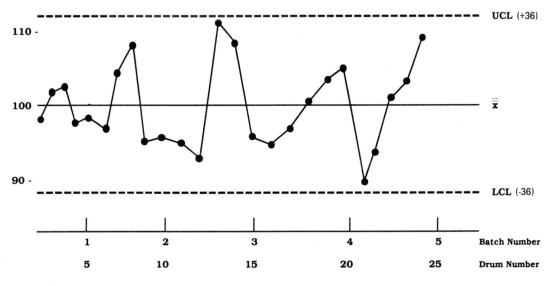

Figure 7   Quality control chart of mixing data.

analyze output data obtained in connection with either concurrent or retrospective validation studies. Validated products and processes can be
shown by appropriate statistical means —such as control charting—to be
uniform within a lot or batch, consistent among lots or batches, and able
to meet design criteria within defined control limits.

XVI. CONCLUSIONS

Process validation represents an important, final stage of a broader, more
fundamental engineering concept called *process quality control* or *statistical
quality control*. *Pharmaceutical process validation* for either sterile or
nonsterile drug products (whether liquid, semisolid, or solid) can never be
completely successful unless prior stages in the product and process development sequence have been successful as well. In this connection, engineering as well as statistical principles and practices are used effectively
in order to obtain a desired outcome.

The essential or key steps or stages of a successful product and
process development program are presented in Table 16. According to the
key steps or stages in product and process development shown in Table 16,
pharmaceutical process validation comes only at the end of this sequence as
a simple proving and documenting procedure to show that the process for
the manufacture of the drug product works, i.e., process consistently produces a product that has characteristics that fall within defined limits of
acceptability [34,39].

Since process validation is a requirement of CGMP regulations for finished pharmaceuticals (21 CFR parts 210 and 211) and for medical devices

Table 16 Key Stages in Product and Process
Development

Development stage	Pilot scale-up phase
Product design	1× size
Product characterization	
Product selection	
Process design	
Product optimization	10× size
Process characterization	
Process optimization	
Process qualification	
Process qualification	100× size
Process validation	
Product certification	

(21 CFR part 820), compliance with CGMPs also can be used to establish compliance with process validation requirements as well [1].

The reader of this chapter should realize that there is *no one way* to establish proof or evidence of process validation (i.e., a product and process in control). If a manufacturer is certain that its products and processes are under statistical control and in compliance with CGMP regulations it should be a relatively simple matter to establish documented evidence of process validation through the use of either prospective, concurrent, or retrospective pilot and/or production quality information and data. The choice of procedures and methods to be used to establish validation documentation is left with the manufacturer.

The Essentials of Process Validation were written simply to aid the manufacturer of pharmaceutical solid dosage forms with respect to the selection of procedures and approaches that may be employed in order to achieve a successful outcome with respect to product performance and process validation.

GLOSSARY OF TERMS

The terminology of validation used in this chapter was developed initially by Chapman [67].

Acceptable mean range	All values of a given control parameter that fall between proven high and low worst case conditions.
Batchwise control	The use of validated in-process samples and testing methods in such a way that results prove the process has done what it purports to do for the specific batch concerned, assuming control parameters have been appropriately respected.
Calibration	Demonstrating that a measured device produces results within specified limits of those produced by a reference standard device over an appropriate range of measurements.
Certification	Documentation by qualified authorities that a system's qualification, validation, or revalidation has been performed appropriately and the results are acceptable.
Concurrent process validation	Establishing documented evidence that a process does what it purports to do based on information generated during actual implementation of the process.
Control parameters	Those operating variables which can be assigned values that are used as control levels.
Control parameter range	Range of values for a given control parameter that lies between its two limits, or control levels.

Critical process parameter	Those process parameters which are deemed important to product fitness-for-use.
Edge-of-failure	Control parameter value which, if exceeded, means adverse effect on state-of-control and/or fitness-for-use.
GMP	Good manufacturing practices.
Installation qualification	Documented verification that all key aspects of the installation adhere to approved design intentions and that manufacturer's recommendations are suitably considered.
Module	Subdivision of system or process into unit operations or tasks.
Operating variables	All factors, including control parameters, which may potentially affect process state-of-control and/or fitness-for-use of the end product.
Operation qualification	Documented verification that the system or subsystem performs as intended throughout all anticipated operating ranges; sometimes called *performance qualifications*.
Policy	A directive usually specifying *what* is to be accomplished.
Procedure	A directive usually specifying *how* certain activities are to be accomplished.
Process life cycle	Time span from early stages of development until commercial use of the process is discontinued.
Process parameters	Those process operating variables which can be assigned values that are used as control levels or operating limits.
Process validation	Establishing documented evidence that a process does what it purports to do.
Process validation program	Collection of activities which include and are specifically related to process validation itself.
Prospective process validation	Establishing documented evidence that a process does what it purports to do based on a preplanned validation protocol.
Protocol	A prospective experimental plan which, when executed, is intended to produce documented evidence that the system has been validated.
Quality assurance	The activity of providing, to all concerned, the evidence needed to establish confidence that the quality function is being performed adequately.

Quality function	The entire collection of activities from which industry achieves fitness-for-use, no matter where these activities are performed.
Retrospective process validation	Establishing documented evidence that a process does what it purports to do based on review and analysis of historic information. It is important that the terms retroactive and retrospective are not confused. *Retroactive validation* would imply that a process is validated after its product has entered the marketplace.
Revalidation	Repetition of the validation process or a specific portion of it.
State-of-control	A condition in which all process parameters that can affect performance remain within such ranges that the process performs consistently and as intended.
Sterilization process	Treatment process from which probability of a microorganism's survival is less than one in a million (10^{-6}).
Validation	Establishing documented evidence that a system does what it purports to do.
Validation change control	Formal monitoring system by which qualified representatives of appropriate disciplines review proposed or actual changes that might affect validated status and cause corrective action to be taken that will ensure that the system retains its validated state-of-control.
Worst case	Highest or lowest value of a given control parameter actually evaluated in a validation exercise.

REFERENCES

1. *Guidelines on General Principles of Process Validation*, Division of Manufacturing and Product Quality (HFN-320) Center for Drugs and Biologics (FDA), Rockville, Maryland, May 1986.
2. Current Good Manufacturing Practices in Manufacture, Processing, Packaging and Holding of Human and Veterinary Drugs, *Federal Register* 43(190), 45085 and 45086, September 1978.
3. *Pharmaceutical Process Validation*, B. T. Loftus and R. A. Nash, eds., Marcel Dekker, New York, 1984.
4. Ralston, A. H. and Ricigliano, J. V., Planning for commissioning and validation of pharmaceutical building systems, *Pharm. Eng.*, July/Aug. (1988).
5. Estes, G. K. and Luthell, G. H., An approach to process validation in a multiproduct pharmaceutical plan, *Pharm. Tech.*, April (1983).
6. Hess, A., An integrated approach to validation, *BioPharm.*, March (1988).

7. Cipriano, P. A., Designing clean rooms for FDA process validation, *BioPharm.*, June (1983).
8. Harder, S. W., The validation of cleaning procedures, *BioPharm.*, May (1984).
9. Berry, I. R., Process validation of raw materials, *Pharmaceutical Process Validation, Op. Cit.*
10. Avallone, H. L., The primary elements of validation of solid oral and topical dosage forms, *Pharm. Eng.*, January (1985).
11. Motise, P. J., What to expect when FDA audits computer-controlled processes, *Pharm. Mfg.*, July (1984).
12. Wolber, P. and Dosmar, M., Depyrogenation of pharmaceutical solutions by ultrafiltration: Aspects of validation, *Pharm. Tech.*, September (1987).
13. Stellon, R. C., Sterile packaging: Process validation and GMP requirements, *MD&DI*, October (1986).
14. Cipriano, P. A., Process validation begins with initial plant design, *Pharm. Eng.*, May/June (1982).
15. Williams, D. R., An overview of test method validation, *BioPharm.*, November (1987).
16. Kahan, J. S., Validating computer systems, *MD&DI*, March (1987).
17. Concepts for reprocessing drug products, PMA Committee Report, *Pharm. Tech.*, September (1985).
18. Protection of water treatment systems: Validation and control, PMA Committee Report, *Pharm. Tech.*, September (1984).
19. Validation and control concepts for water treatment systems, PMA Committee Report, *Pharm. Tech.*, November (1985).
20. Cattaneo, D. J., HVAC and the clean room, *Pharm. Eng.*, November/December (1984).
21. Proceedings of Third PMA Seminar on Validation of Sterile Manufacturing Processes, Lincolnshire, Illinois, February 1980.
22. *Validation of Aseptic Pharmaceutical Processes*, F. J. Carleton and J. P. Agalloco, eds., Marcel Dekker, New York, 1986.
23. Simmons, P. L., Sterilizer validation, *Pharm. Tech.*, April (1979).
24. Vogel, D. G., Schmidt, W. C., and Sanford, B. G., A computer interface for sterilization validation, *Pharm. Tech.*, June (1984).
25. Nash, R. A., A method for calculating thermal sterilization conditions based upon process parametrics, *J. Parent. Sci. Tech.*, 39: 251–255 (1985).
26. Wasynczuk, J., Validation of aseptic filling processes, *Pharm. Tech.*, May (1986).
27. Cabernoch, J. L., Materials qualification and design for medical device packaging, *MD&DI*, August (1982).
28. Olson, W. P., Validation and qualification of filtration systems for bacterial removal, *Pharm. Tech.*, November (1979).
29. Goldsmith, S. H. and Grundelman, G. P., Validation of pharmaceutical filtration products, *Pharm. Mfg.*, November (1985).
30. Bader, M. E., Quality assurance and quality control (in four parts), *Chem. Eng.* (1980).
31. *Organizing for Validation*, Proceedings of PMA Seminar on Validation of Solid Dosage Form Processes, Atlanta, Georgia, May 1980.
32. Chapman, K. G., a private communication.

33. Nash, R. A., Product formulation, *CHEMTECH*, April (1976).
34. Concept Development in Process Validation Seminars by R. F. Johnson, P.E., Quality Systems & Tech., P.O. Box 29, Naperville, Illinois 60566.
35. Chao, A. Y., St. John Forbes, F., Johnson, R. F., and von Doehren, P., Prospective process validation, *Pharmaceutical Process Validation, Op. Cit.*
36. Williams, J. J. and Stiel, D. M., An intelligent tablet press monitor for formulation development, *Pharm. Tech.*, March (1984).
37. Box, G. E., Hunter, W. G., and Hunter, J. S., *Statistics for Experimenters*, Wiley, New York, 1978.
38. Hendrix, C. D., What every technologist should know about experimental design, *CHEMTECH*, March (1979).
39. Schwartz, J. B., Klamholz, J. R., and Press, R. H., Computer optimization of pharmaceutical formulations, *J. Pharm. Sci.*, *62*: 1165−1170 (1973).
41. Cooper, L. and Steinberg, D., *Introduction to Methods of Optimization*, Saunders, Philadelphia, 1970.
42. O. L. Davies (ed.), *The Design and Analysis of Industrial Experiments*, Macmillan (Hafner), New York, 1967.
43. Fonner, D. E., Buck, J. R., and Banker, G. S., Mathematical optimization techniques in drug product design and process analysis, *J. Pharm. Sci.*, *59*:1587−1596 (1970).
44. Schwartz, J. B., Optimization techniques in product formulation, *J. Soc. Cosmet. Chem.*, *32*:287−301 (1981).
45. Bolton, S., *Pharmaceutical Statistics, Practical and Clinical Applications*, 2nd Ed., Marcel Dekker, New York, 1990.
46. Hill, R. A., Process improvement by evolutionary operation, *Amer. Perf. Cosm.*, September (1965).
47. Hahn, G. J., Process improvement through simplex EVOP, *CHEMTECH*, May (1976).
48. F. E. Satterthwaite, Seminars on REVOP, Statistical Engineering Institute, Wellsley Hills, Massachusetts (1970).
49. Nash, R. A., Process validation for solid dosage forms, *Pharm. Tech.*, June (1979).
50. Nash, R. A., Process validation: Solid dosage forms, *Drug Cosm. Ind.*, September (1981).
51. Simmons, P., Solid process validation, *Pharm. Eng.*, August/October (1981).
52. von Doehren, P. J., St. John Forbes, F., and Shively, C. D., An approach to the characterization and technology transfer of solid dosage form processes, *Pharm. Tech.*, June (1984).
53. Rudolph, J. S., Validation of solid dosage forms, *Pharmaceutical Process Validation, Op. Cit.*
54. Nash, R. A., A validation experiment in solids blending, *Pharm. Eng.*, July/August (1985).
55. Meyer, R. J., Validation of products and processes from a production, quality control viewpoint, PMA Seminar on Validation of Solid Dosage Form Process, Atlanta, Georgia, May 1980.
56. Simms, L., Validation of existing products by statistical evaluation, *Op. Cit.*

Nash

57. Agalloco, J. P., Practical considerations in retrospective validation, *Pharm. Tech.*, June (1983).
58. Trubinski, C. J. and Majeed, M., Retrospective process validation, *Pharmaceutical Process Validation, Op. Cit.*
59. Kuzel, N. R., Fundamentals of computer system validation and documentation in the pharmaceutical industry, *Pharm. Tech.*, September (1985).
60. Fraade, D. J., The application of digital control systems in the pharmaceutical industry, *Pharm. Mfg.*, May (1984).
61. Butler, J. J., Statistical quality control with CUSUM charts, *Chem. Eng.*, August (1983).
62. Deming, S. N., Quality by design, *Chemtech*, September (1988).
63. Contino, A. V., Improved plant performance with statistical process control, *Chem. Eng.*, July (1987).
64. Ott, E. R., *Process Quality Control*, McGraw-Hill, New York, 1975.
65. Cheng, P. H. and Dutt, J. E., Analysis of retrospective production data using quality control charts, *Pharmaceutical Process Validation, Op. Cit.*
66. Ouchi, G., Control charting with Lotus 1-2-3, *Amer. Lab., 19*(2): 82-95 (1987).
67. Chapman, K. G., A suggested validation lexicon, *Pharm. Tech.*, September (1985).

8
Stability Kinetics

Samir A. Hanna

Bristol-Myers Squibb Company, Syracuse, New York

I. INTRODUCTION

Moral, legal, and economic reasons have been advanced for the need to verify the stability of drug products. Tablets of a particular formulation in a specific container are defined as stable if they remain within their physical, chemical, therapeutic, and toxicological specifications during their designated shelf life.

II. CURRENT GOOD MANUFACTURING PRACTICES REQUIREMENTS

The legal requirements stem from the Federal Food, Drug, and Cosmetic Act and the Current Good Manufacturing Practices Regulations (CGMPs) as published in the *Federal Register* on March 28, 1979, and Title 21, Code of Federal Regulations. The CGMPs state that there shall be assurances of stability of the finished product and suitable expiration date, based on appropriate stability studies and related to specific storage conditions placed on the label. Stability tests are to be performed on tablets in their finished marketed container using reliable and specific test methods. Effective September 28, 1979, all drug labels for tablets, prescription and nonprescriptions, are required to state the product's expiration date; i.e., the time after which the drug can no longer be considered within the legal potency requirement.

III. COMPENDIAL REQUIREMENTS

The *United States Pharmacopeia/National Formulary* (USP/NF) has required expiration dates on all monograph drugs since January 1, 1976. The

USP/NF states that for pharmacopeia tablets, the label shall bear an expiration date limiting the period during which the tablet may be expected
to retain the full label potency of the active ingredient provided the tablet
is stored as directed. A set of label storage temperatures is provided by
the USP/NF to cover the various types of storage conditions. These include: store in a freezer not exceeding $-10°C$, store in a refrigerator
held between 2 and 8°C, store in a cool place between 8 and 15°C, store
at controlled room temperature between 15 and 30°C, store at room temperature which is the temperature prevailing in a working area, protect
from excessive heat as any temperature above 40°C, protect from light,
protect from freezing, and protect from moisture or keep tightly closed.

IV. U.S. FOOD AND DRUG ADMINISTRATION
REQUIREMENTS

In 1971, the Food and Drug Administration (FDA) published a set of *Guidelines: Manufacturing and Controls for IND's and NDA's* which defines in
greater detail the stability information required for a new drug application.
The guidelines were subsequently republished as part of the book, *FDA
Introduction to Total Drug Quality* in November 1973. In July 1976, the
Bureau of Veterinary Medicine published a set of proposed stability study
guidelines in greater detail. As an example of such detailed requirements,
the stability data generated from a tablet formulation under accelerated
conditions must be statistically related to shelf-life storage conditions. It
would be desirable to have the degradation products quantitatively identified, the precurosors and degradation kinetics presented. Tablet physical
parameters recommended for testing at IND phase III are surface appearance, friability, fragility, hardness, disintegration, color, weight variation,
odor, moisture, and dissolution rate.

In February 1987, the FDA published *Guideline for Submitting Documentation for the Stability of Human Drugs and Biologics*. These guidelines recommended that tablets stability studies should include tests for appearance, friability, hardness, color, odor, moisture, strength, and
dissolution.

Stability and expiration dating for antibiotics has been required since
their advent in the 1940s. The stability requirements are covered in a general way in the federal regulations for each antibiotic. Section 4 (Forms
5 and 6) requests a complete description and data derived from stability
studies of the potency and physical characteristics of the drug. Data were
to be accumulated on at least three batches of the exact formulation. Separate data on different types of containers, if any, were also requested.
The marketing container is to be used for all the stability studies and
under the same conditions of storage and reconstitution time as specified
on the label. A sufficient number of assays must be run at each time interval to establish an accurate result, especially at the initial assay. Accelerated data could be submitted only as supporting evidence.

V. REACTION KINETICS IN SOLID-DOSAGE FORMS

When evaluating the stability of a tablet formulation, both physical and
chemical properties must be thoroughly considered. The chemical causes

of tablet deterioration are incompatibility, oxidation, reduction, hydrolysis, racemization, epimerization, and dehydration. The chemical reactions involved occur at definite rates. These rates are influenced by such factors as temperature, light, pH, humidity, radiation, and pressure. The study of the rates of change and the factors that influence them is called reaction kinetics. By studying the manner in which the rate of a reaction varies with the concentration of the reactants, the order of the reaction can be defined. This process is helpful in evaluating the stability of tablet formulation, predicting shelf life, and creating optimum storage conditions.

Zero-order, first-order, and pseudo–first-order reaction kinetics are the most frequently encountered in tablet degradation, although more complex reactions have been also observed. Moreover, for shelf-life calculations in which the concentration change is generally no more than $10-20\%$, the differentiation between orders is relatively unimportant, leading to data treatment simplification. Therefore, only the zero-, first-, and pseudo-first-order reactions will be discussed here.

A. Zero-Order Reaction

When the reaction rate is affected not by the concentration of the reacting substance(s), but by some other limiting property, such as photolysis and solubility, then the rate is dependent on the zero power of the reactant. The rate at which a drug decomposes can be written mathematically:

$$\frac{-dC_a}{dt} = K_0$$

where C_a = concentration of reactant a

K_0 = reaction rate

t = time

Integrating from $t = 0$ to $t = t$ with $C_a = C_0$ at $t = 0$:

$$C_a = C_0 - K_0 t \tag{1}$$

Therefore, for data that follow a zero-order reaction, a plot of concentration against time produces a straight line whose slope is equal to K_0, which represents the quantity of drug that degrades in a given unit of time. The half-life equation is

$$t_{1/2} = \frac{0.5 C_0}{K_0} \tag{2}$$

and the shelf-life equation is

$$t_{90} = \frac{0.1C_0}{K_0} \tag{3}$$

Example: A zero-order rate of degradation of a vitamin in a mixture of 25 mg per tablet and solubility of 2.5 mg ml^{-1} (C_0) is shown in Figure 1. Using equation 1:

$$K_0 = \frac{C_0 - C_a}{t}$$

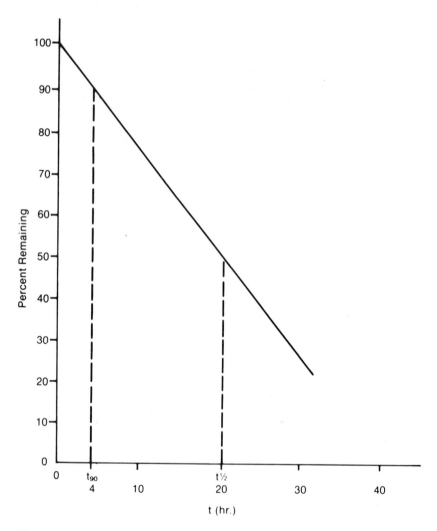

Figure 1   Percent of vitamin remaining as a function of time for a zero-order reaction.

where $C_0 = 2.5$ and $C_a = 0$ at time (t) = 40 h. Then

$$K_0 = \frac{2.5 - 0}{40} = 0.0625$$

And using equation 2:

$$t_{1/2} = \frac{0.5C_0}{K_0}$$

$$= \frac{0.5 \times 2.5}{0.0625} = 20 \text{ h}$$

And using equation 3:

$$t_{90} = \frac{0.1C_0}{K_0}$$

$$= \frac{0.1 \times 2.5}{0.0625} = 4 \text{ h}$$

B. First-Order Reaction

When the reaction rate depends on the first power of concentration of a single reactant and the drug decomposes directly into one or more products, then the reaction rate is directly proportional to the concentration of the reactant and can be written mathematically as

$$\frac{-dC_a}{dt} = KC_a \tag{4}$$

by integrating the rate from t = 0 to t = t, where C_a at t = 0 is C_0:

$$\ln C_a = \ln C_0 - Kt \tag{5}$$

Converting from the natural logarithm (ln) yields

$$\log C_a = \log C_0 - \frac{Kt}{2.303} \tag{6}$$

or

$$K = \frac{2.303}{t} \left(\log \frac{C_0}{C_a} \right) \tag{7}$$

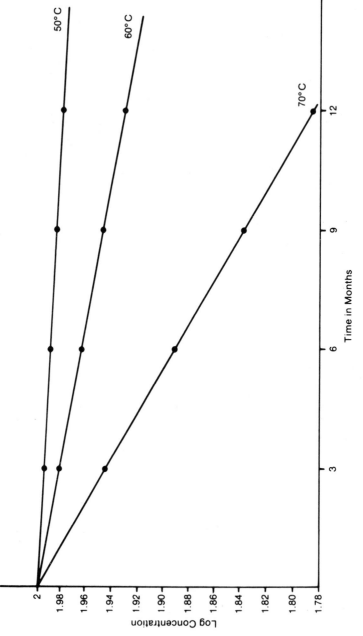

Figure 2   Percent of alkaloid remaining as a function of time for a first-order reaction.

Table 1 Percent of Alkaloid[a] in Tablet Formulation

Temperature (°C)	Time (months)			
	3	6	9	12
50	98.92	97.83	96.70	95.72
60	96.16	92.47	88.92	85.51
70	88.41	98.16	69.10	61.09

[a]Initial 100%.

As log C_0 is a constant, then a plot of log (drug concentration) against time will produce a straight line whose slope is equal to $-K/2.303$.

The constant, K. is the reaction velocity constant or specific reaction rate, which expresses the fraction of material that reacts in a given unit of time expressed in reciprocal seconds, minutes, or hours. For example, let $K = 0.01$ h^{-1}; then the rate at which the drug is degrading is 1% h^{-1}.

The half-life equation is

$$t_{1/2} = \frac{0.693}{K} \tag{8}$$

and the shelf-life equation is

$$t_{90} = \frac{0.105}{K} \tag{9}$$

Example: A first-order rate of hydrolysis degradation of an alkaloid at 1 mg per tablet manufactured by aqueous wet granulation technique is shown in Table 1, which, if graphically plotted, should give a straight line as shown in Figure 2.

C. Pseudo-First-Order Reaction

When the reaction rate depends on the concentration of two reactants or a bimolecular reaction that is made to act like a first-order reaction, then it is called pseudo-first-order reaction, for example, when one reactant is present in greater quantity than the other or when the first is kept at a constant concentration in relation to the second. Under these circumstances, one reactant appears to control the rate of reaction even though two reactants are present because the concentration of the second reactant does not change significantly during the degradation. An example of such a reaction is the degradation of sodium hypochlorite tablets in aqueous solution, which is highly pH dependent and follows a pseudo-first-order reaction because the hydroxyl ion concentration is high compared to the concentration of the carboxylic ion.

VI. KINETIC STUDIES

Solid-dosage forms that are tablets and capsules constitute a large majority of pharmaceutical products. However, few kinetic studies and studies on rates of drug degradation in solid state have been published. Drug solid degradation in absence of excipients and moisture generally follows a nucleation chemical reaction rate which may approximate a first-order reaction rate. In the presence of moisture and excipients, the reaction rate could be either zero-, first-, or pseudo-first-order. It should be noted that there is little difference in degradation rates estimated by the zero- or first-order reactions when less than 15% degradation has occurred. When the amount of degradation found is in excess of 15% the order of the reaction which accounts for the degradation should be established.

Stability study at room temperature is the surest method of determining the actual shelf life of a product. Unfortunately, it is difficult to make an accurate expiration date prediction until 2 or 3 years of data are generated, a situation which can be further complicated by the frequent need for tablet formulation changes that would require additional long shelf-life study at actual shelf-life conditions.

The principles of chemical kinetics for the evaluation of drug stability are based on the fact that reaction rates are expected to be proportional to the number of collisions per unit time. Since this number increases with the increase of temperature, it is necessary to evaluate the temperature dependency of the reaction. Experimentally, the reaction rate constant is observed to have an exponential dependence on temperature as expressed by the Arrhenius equation:

$$K = A^{(-Ha/RT)} \tag{10}$$

or

$$\log K = \log A - \frac{\Delta H}{2.303RT} \tag{11}$$

or

$$\log \frac{K_1}{K_2} = \frac{Ha}{2.303R} \left(\frac{1}{T_2} - \frac{1}{T_1} \right) \tag{12}$$

where K = specific rate of degradation

R = gas constant (1.987 cal deg^{-1} mol^{-1})

A = frequency factor (constant)

T = absolute temperature (t°C + 273.16°C)

Ha = activation energy of the chemical reaction

A plot of log K against $1/T$ will produce a straight line whose slope is equal to $-\Delta Ha/R$ (2.303), and is known as an Arrhenius plot (Fig. 3). The resulting line obtained at higher temperatures is extrapolated to obtain

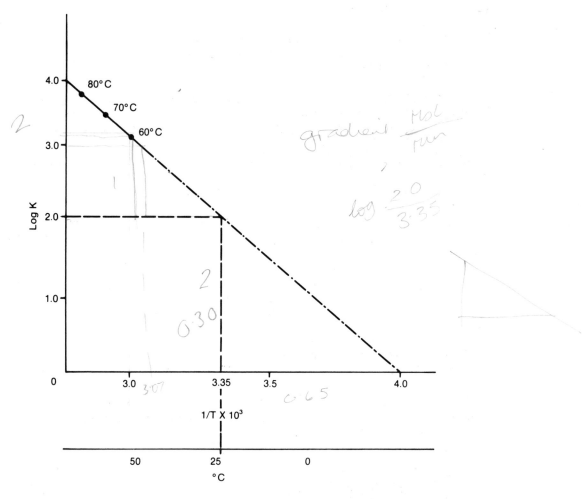

Figure 3 Arrhenius plot of log K against reciprocal of absolute temperature.

room temperatures and K_{25} is generally used to obtain a measure of the stability of the drug under ordinary shelf conditions at room temperature; however, any other desired temperature can be equally obtained.

From Figure 3, log K_{25} is 2 and K_{25} will be 100 months or 8.3 years under shelf conditions at room temperature (25°C) if the original points at 60, 70, and 80°C in the Arrhenius plot were calculated from monthly stability points. Activation energy can also be calculated from an Arrhenius plot by using the slope of the line which is equivalent to $-Ha/2.303R$. From Figure 3, the slope of the line is -3.5×10^3. Then

$$-3.5 \times 10^3 = \frac{Ha}{2.303 \times 1.987}$$

and

$$Ha = (-3.5 \times 10^3)(2.303)(1.987)$$

$$= 16.0 \text{ kcal/mol}^{-1}$$

Arrhenius projection enables predictions to be made that are based on accelerated data in such a way that any change in the relationship between the degradation at different temperatures will be detected and estimated. For example, using equation 10 for the prediction of a tablet product expiration date at shelf storage (25°C) from accelerated stability study at 40°C and activation energy of 10 kcal/mol:

$$K_{40} = A^{(-Ha/RT_1)}$$

and

$$K_{25} = A^{(-Ha/RT_2)}$$

then

$$\frac{K_{40}}{K_{25}} = \frac{A^{(-Ha/RT_1)}}{A^{(-Ha/RT_2)}}$$

Assuming that $Ha = 10 \text{ kcal/mol}^{-1}$, then $T_1 = 273.15 + 40 = 313.15$ and $T_2 = 273.15 + 25 = 298.15$.

$$\frac{K_{40}}{K_{25}} = \frac{A^{-10,000/1,987(313.15)}}{A^{-10,000/1.987(298.15)}}$$

$$= 2.24465$$

Shelf stability at 25°C = 12 × 2.245 = 26.94 months. Tablet product with 10 kcal/mol^{-1} activation energy of the chemical reaction and stable at 40°C for 12 months will have an expiration date at shelf life (25°C) of 27 months.

When reactant molecules, e.g., A + B, in a tablet formulation proceeds to products, e.g., C + D, the energy of the system must change higher than that of the initial reactant and is defined as the activation energy (Ha) (Fig. 4).

The usual range for activation energies for tablet formulation decomposition is about 10-20 kcal/mol^{-1}, except if diffusion or photolysis is rate determining. Then the rate is about 2 to 3 kcal/mol^{-1}, which rarely occurs in tablet degradation. For reactions in which the heat activation energies range is more than 50 kcal/mol^{-1}, the rate of degradation is not of any practical significance at the temperature of shelf-life storage of tablet formulations. For tablets with activation energy values higher than

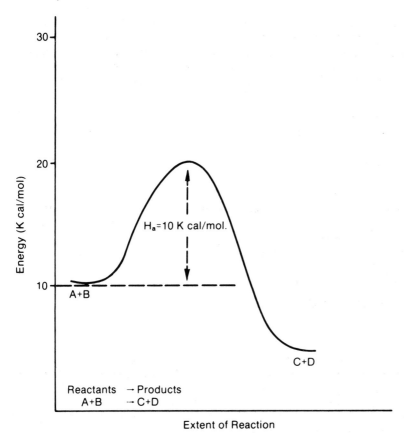

Figure 4   Activation energy.

20 kcal/mol^{-1}, the error in shelf-life prediction will be on the conservative side. For example, using equation 10, for a tablet product with 20 kcal/mol^{-1} activation energy and stable at 40°C for 3 months:

$$\frac{K_{40}}{K_{25}} = \frac{A^{(-Ha/RT_1)}}{A^{(-Ha/RT_2)}}$$

$$= \frac{A^{-20,000/1.987(313.15)}}{A^{-20,000/1.987(298.15)}}$$

$$= \frac{A^{-32.14250}}{A^{-33.75960}}$$

$$= 5.03847$$

Shelf stability at 25°C = 3 × 5.03847 = 15 months. For this tablet product we will predict an expiration date of 15 months at shelf-life storage. If in reality the activation energy of the chemical reaction of these tablet product was on the higher side, that is, 25 kcal/mol^{-1} instead of the previously assumed 20 kcal/mol^{-1}, then using equation 10

$$\frac{K_{40}}{K_{25}} = \frac{A^{-25,000/1.987(313.15)}}{A^{-25,000/1.097(298.15)}}$$

$$= 7.54867$$

and the predicted shelf stability at 25°C will be 3 × 7.54867 = 22.5 months, which indicates that our original prediction of 15 months expiration date was on the conservative side. On the other hand, if the real activation energy of the chemical reaction was on the lower side, that is, 15 kcal/mol^{-1} rather than the originally assumed 20 kcal/mol^{-1}, then by using equation 10

$$\frac{K_{40}}{K_{25}} = \frac{A^{-15,000/1.987(313.15)}}{A^{-15,000/1.987(298.15)}}$$

$$= 3.36296$$

and the predicted shelf stability at 25°C will be 3 × 3.36296 = 10 months, which indicates that our original prediction of 15 months expiration date was a risky prediction.

To use the Arrhenius equation, three stability storage temperatures are obviously the minimum as the more additional temperatures are used the more the accuracy of extrapolation is enhanced.

Table 2 gives an example of the application of the Arrhenius equation to predict the stability of tablet product Z, Lot No. X, containing active ingredient A.

1. Determine the potency of active A in the tablet product at appropriate intervals of time when held at three temperatures, 50, 60, and 70°C, as shown in Table 2, make two plots to determine if the degradation reaction is zero- or first-order.

2. First, plot potency (y) against time (t) in weeks for the three temperatures on normal graph paper, as shown in Figure 5. Then plot log potency (log y) against time (t) in weeks for the three temperatures on semilogarithmic graph paper as shown in Figure 6.

Table 2 Percent of Active A in Tablet Z Lot No. X

Temperature (°C)	Time (weeks)									
	0	5	10	15	20	30	40	60	90	120
50	107	—	—	—	—	85	—	58	35	10
60	107	—	86	—	60	38	13	—	—	—
70	107	85	70	40	20	—	—	—	—	—

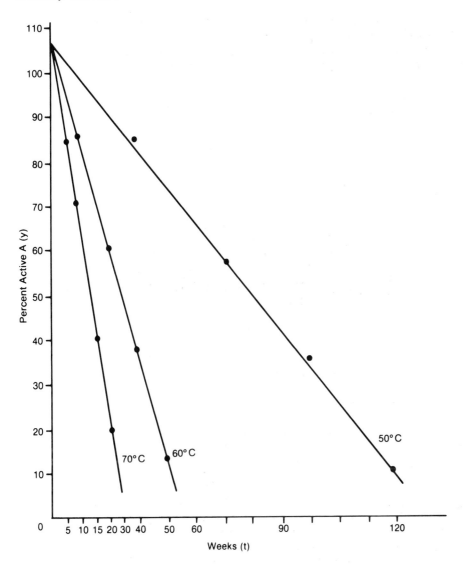

Figure 5   Zero-order plot for Active A Tablet Z Lot No. X.

3. Draw a straight line of best fit through the five points in both graphs. Select the plot in which the line most closely fits the determined points, including the original potency determined at zero time, which should agree with the potency estimated by extending the degradation lines back to zero time. In this example, these two conditions are met by the first plot figure (y versus t or a zero-order reaction).

4. Determine for each of the three temperatures the slope of the degradation rates (K_0) in units of y (in case of first-order reaction K_1 in units of log y) by selecting two points lying on the line to determine the slopes for each of the three temperatures, as shown in Table 3. The slope of a line is defined as change in y divided by the change in x.

5. Plot the log values of K_0 on semilogarithmic graph paper against the reciprocal of absolute temperature as shown in Figure 7.

Table 3 K_0 Values for Active
A in Tablets Z Lot No. X

Temperature (°C)	K_0
50	−0.53
60	−2.5
70	−4.28

6. Draw a straight line of best fit through the three points and ex-
trapolate it to the lower temperatures.
7. Estimate the rate of degradation at the desired temperature. If
this is 25°C, then the K_0 from the graph is 0.33.
8. Calculate the expiration data (t_x) from equation 13.

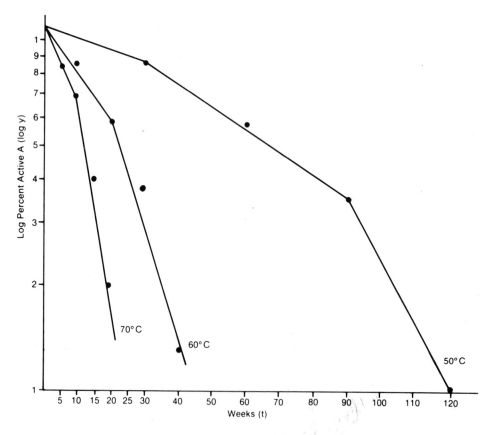

Figure 6   First-order plot for active A Tablet Z Lot No. X.

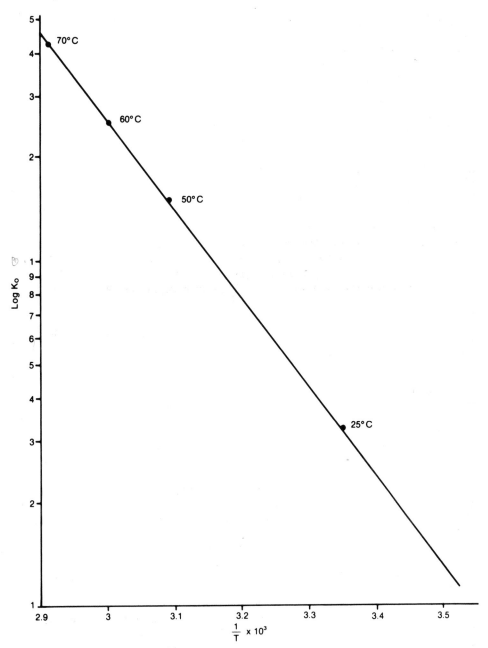

Figure 7   Arrhenius plot for Active A Tablet Z Lot No. X.

$$t_x = y_0 - y_x/K_0 \quad \text{for zero-order} \tag{13}$$

$$= \frac{\text{initial potency} - \text{minimum potency}}{\text{reaction rate}}$$

or

$$t_x = \log y_0 - \log y_x/K_1 \quad \text{for first-order} \tag{14}$$

Expiration date at $25°C = (107 - 90)/0.33 = 51.5$ weeks.

An understanding of the limitations of the collected stability data and heat of activation values is important in stability prediction, as the obtained data may not fit the Arrhenius relationship. By using the Arrhenius plot, few assumptions are made regarding linearity extending to room temperature; that is, A and Ha independent of T, and the same chemical reaction is being considered at different stability-elevated temperatures. This means that it is necessary to obtain the heats of activation for all bimolecular rate constants involved in a two or more mechanism of degradation at a pH value as the apparent heat of activation is not necessarily constant with temperature. For example, the rate of degradation after 24 h of 1% sodium ampicillin in 5% dextrose solution at $-20°C$ is 46%, which is equivalent to the same degradation at $27°C$, whereas the degradation at 0 to $5°C$ is only 28%. In photolysis degradation, no advantage is gained by higher temperature studies as the activation energy of the reaction is small and consequently the effect of temperature is small. Many tablet actives contain functional groups that are derivatives of carboxylic acids, e.g., esters as in aspirin or lactones as in penicillin occasionally exhibit complex degradation reaction.

In lieu of these limitations of the application of the Arrhenius method, a number of statistical methods for stability prediction, which is easily adapted to a computer, have been developed. One method is to use simple linear regression to calculate the regression line for each of a number of batches. The resulting slopes are pooled if homogeneous and the standard error of the grand slope is used to establish a confidence slope for stability prediction.

A second method is to obtain the stability results at various stability points at room temperature and then calculate the standard error of the results at each discrete point to estimate confidence in potency being above a certain value at a given point.

The most commonly used method involves the calculation of the regression for an ingredient from all batches of a tablet formulation available. The standard error of the line is then calculated and the confidence shelf life is determined or the standard error of the predicted value is calculated whereby the time predicted (t_{90}) is the time at which the regression line reaches not less than 90% of potency claimed (Fig. 8).

For example: A vitamin tablet formulation, at a potency of 75 mg per tablet and overage of 33%, was released initially at 100 mg per tablet. The batch was put on stability at $40°C$ and assay results obtained with their upper and lower limits are tabulated in Table 4. From Table 4 using the lower limits, we are 95% confident that the average potency of the vitamin tablet will be not less than 90% of the label claim (67.5 mg per tablet) at

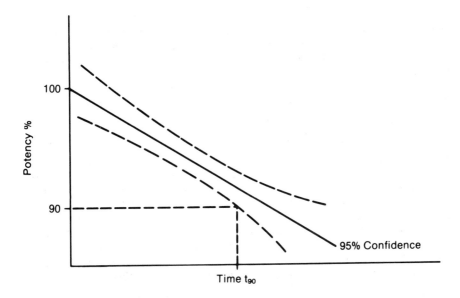

Figure 8   Plot of ln potency against time showing 95% confidence limit line.

Table 4   Vitamin Tablets Stability Confidence
Intervals at 40°C

Time (months)	Results (mg/tablet)	Lower limit	Upper limit
0	100.0	95.2	104.9
1	91.2	88.7	93.8
3	83.1	79.3	87.3
6	75.8	69.8	82.5
9	69.1	61.2	78.2
12	63.0	53.6	74.0

where estimate of the standard error of regression(s)

$$= \sqrt{\frac{\Sigma (y_i - \hat{y}_i)^2}{n - 2}}$$

y_i = predicted value at t_i

n = sample size

Sy = standard error of the line

$\alpha = 0.1$ two-sided
    0.05 one-sided

6.75 months if the tablets were held at 40°C in a stability storage cabinet. Knowing that the log of the potency versus time is a straight line, we interpolate that we are 95% confident that the average potency of the vitamin tablet will be above the 90% of the label claim at 8.75 months if the tablet is stored at 25°C.

The covariance analysis statistical method is sometimes chosen over regression analysis because it gives the average rate of loss for each lot and allows a statistical test for parallelism of rates of loss prior to the pooling of lots within a given product line. In the covariance technique the relationship between potency and time is considered to be a first-order degradation reaction and a minimum of three lots of product is required. The least-squares line is calculated with three assay points or more in addition to the original release zero-time point. Four computation steps are required for mathematical calculation. In step one, for each individual lot calculate the individual rate of loss (ROL) per month, intercept (a), and residual mean square (RMS). In step two, determine validity of combining all data by performing Bartlett's test of homogeneity of variance (χ^2 test) and parallelism test of between versus within mean squares for slopes (F-test). In step three, calculate for combined lots data the statistically valid ROL ($\hat{B}$) per month variance of B $\left(\delta\frac{2}{b}\right)$, intercept of combined lots ($\hat{A}$), and variance of average intercept $\left(\delta\frac{2}{b}\right)$. In step four, perform the best line fit (BLF) with 95% confidence levels.

The above-mentioned four computation steps can be mathematically detailed as follows:

1. Step one (for each lot):

    a. Obtain the sums of

        Σx, y_2, x_2, y, and xy

    b. Calculate sum squares of x (S_{xx}), xy (S_{xy}), y (S_{yy}), and residual sum squares

        $[RSS = S_{yy} - (S_{xy})^2/S_{xx}]$

    c. Calculate rate of loss $[ROL = S_{xy}/S_{xx}]$

        intercept ($a = \bar{y} - b\bar{x}$) and residual mean square for the lot

        $[RMS = RSS/(n - 2)]$

        where x = time of assay (months), y = loss of percent retained, n = number of (x,y) values for a lot.

2. Step two

    a. Using Bartlett's test of homogeneity of residual variances test the validity of combining all lots data

    b. Test for parallelism of loss rates

Table 5A Single Vitamin Tablet Stability Data at 37°C

Lot No.	Months	Potency assay (mg/tablet)	X	Log Y
A	0	130	—	—
	2	130	2	0.0000000
	4	126	4	−0.0312525
	6	129	6	−0.0077220
	9	125	9	−0.0392207
	12	126	12	−0.0312525
	18	130	18	0.0000000
	24	132	24	+0.0152674
	36	117	36	−0.1053605
B	0	132	—	—
	3	123	3	−0.0706175
	6	125	6	−0.0544881
	8	122	8	−0.0787808
	12	128	12	−0.0307716
	18	117	18	−0.1206279
	24	115	24	−0.1378697
C	0	133	—	—
	2	137	2	+0.0296317
	4	130	4	−0.0228146
	6	133	6	0.0000000
	10	122	10	−0.0863280
	12	122	12	−0.0863280
	18	124	18	−0.0700675
D	0	120	—	—
	2	114	2	−0.0512932
	4	131	4	+0.0877055
	8	119	8	+0.1177830
	12	130	12	+0.0800427

3. Step three

   a. Calculate the values of the parallelism and chi-square tests using the values obtained in 2.a. above.

   b. The smallest value for the parallelism test would indicate the lot data to be deleted. If this value is not significant, the pooled slope and intercept will be calculated minus the deleted lot.

4. Step four

   a. Calculate the pooled rate of loss and intercept using $\hat{B}$, δ 2/b, and $\hat{A}$.

   b. Calculate and sum for each lot

5. Step five

   a. Calculate the best line fit with 95% confidence levels

$$x = \frac{\sum\limits_{1}^{k} x}{\sum\limits_{1}^{k} n}$$

where K = the number of lots in analysis.

For example: A single vitamin tablet formulation at a potency of 130 mg per tablet and at 37°C, four different lots were put on stability for 3 years. Stability results are presented in Table 5A. Upper and lower limits are tabulated in Table 5B and presented graphically in Figure 9.

Table 5B   Single Vitamin Tablet Stability at 37°C
Confidence Intervals

Time (months)	Results (mg/tablet)	Lower limit (mg/tablet)	Upper limit (mg/tablet)
0	130.00	123.22	137.17
6	128.11	121.20	135.42
12	126.25	119.63	133.23
18	124.05	117.09	131.42

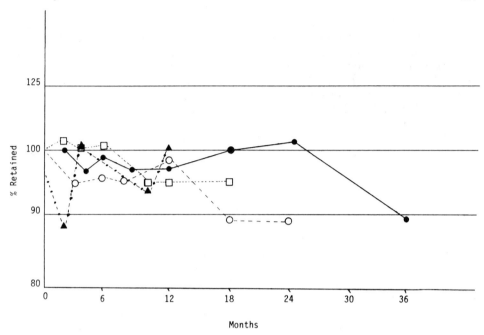

Figure 9   Single vitamin tablet stability at 37°C.

VII. SOLID-DRUG DEGRADATION

The degradation of pure solid drugs can be illustrated by two equations:

(a)   Solid ⟶ solid + gas

(b)   Solid ⟶ liquid + gas

In the first equation, the degradation can be initially steep, then slow, until 100% degradation, which is usually due to geometrical contractive consideration, or can start with an induction period, then accelerates, which is usually due to either nucleation or liquid layer. There are few published examples of this, such as the degradation of aspirin anhydride [1]. In the second equation, the degradation is sometimes related to the melting point of the solid, such as the degradation of p-substituted benzoic acids [2].

VIII. SOLID-SOLID DEGRADATION

Active solid-solid or active excipient degradation reactions in tablet formulations have been reported in many cases. Acylation and subsequent loss of potency has been reported for aspirin-codeine [3] and aspirin-phenylephrine [4] combinations in solid dosage forms. Dextroamphetamine sulfate and spray-dried lactose will react quantitatively in solid-dosage forms [5].

The stability of various vitamins with different tablet excipients was studied [6]. The influence of antacid compounds and other excipients in aspirin, alone or with other actives, has been published [7–10]. The absorption of some antirheumatics on antacids has been shown [11]. The effect of excipients on salicylamide [12] and amphetamine [13] sulfate discoloration has been investigated. The influence of tablet excipients on color fading [14] and other physical tablet parameters, e.g., disintegration [15], has been demonstrated.

The detection of such active solid–solid or possible excipients interactions or incompatibilities is achieved through tablet preformulation studies. A detailed program for such studies is given in Volume 1.

IX. SOLID-DOSAGE FORM DEGRADATION

Solid dosage forms are solid heterogeneous systems whereby the active ingredents tend to decompose at a slower rate than the liquid heterogeneous or homogeneous systems. Since most tablet formulations are complex, the degradation reaction may be complicated by possible interaction of the active and inert ingredients in the formulation. Therefore, it is more difficult to apply chemical kinetics and the Arrhenius relationship to stability data for tablet systems, and it is sometimes impractical to perform through basic kinetics studies on the final tablet formulation to predict the shelf life of the product.

Because of the great structural variety of actives and the complexity of tablet formulations, many kinds of drug degradation reactions are possible. Although the degradation of active ingredients in tablet formulations can occur through several degradative pathways, e.g., oxidation, hydrolysis, racemization, and photolysis, perhaps most of those that occur in tablet degradation are either oxidation or hydrolysis.

X. MECHANISMS THAT AFFECT TABLET STABILITY

A. Oxidation

Oxidative degradation is one of the major causes of tablet instability. One of the main reasons is that oxygen need not present in more than trace quantities to produce significant degradation. Another aspect is that oxidative reactions are influenced by light and metal ions (copper, iron, cobalt, and nickel) and many drugs either form colored products or produce objectionable off-odors. Oxidation cannot happen without reduction. Oxidation/reduction reactions involve the transfer of one or more oxygen or hydrogen atoms or the transfer of electrons.

In inorganic compounds, oxidation is a loss of electrons and reduction is a gain of electrons.

$$Fe^{2+} \rightleftarrows Fe^{3+} + e^{-}$$

Ferrous $\rightleftarrows$ ferric + electron

In organic compounds, oxidation is governed by the number of bonds from carbon to oxygen. The greater the number of carbon –oxygen bonds, the more highly oxidized is the molecule and, since oxygen is added, the aldehyde is more oxidizable than alcohol. Also, in organic compounds a change in molecular structure, e.g., proton transfer, accompanies the electron transfer.

Autooxidation which involves a free-radical chain process is the most common form of oxidative degradation in tablet formulations. The majority of autoxidation reactions involve any material with molecular oxygen. Free radicals are atoms or molecules that have one or more unshared valence electrons. This can be illustrated as in the formation of methyl radicals:

$$CH_3 : CH_3 \longrightarrow 2\ CH_3^{\cdot}$$

These radicals are unsaturated and readily take electrons from other substances causing oxidation.

The first step in the autoxidation of a hydrocarbon (RH) by a free-radical chain process is written as

$$RH \xrightarrow[\text{light and/or heat}]{\text{activation}} R^{\cdot} + H^{\cdot} \qquad \begin{array}{c} \text{initiation} \\ \text{or} \\ \text{induction} \end{array}$$

The second step, a hydrogen peroxide formation:

$$R^{\cdot} + O_2 \longrightarrow RO_2^{\cdot}$$

$$RO_2^{\cdot} + RH \longrightarrow ROOH + R^{\cdot} \qquad \text{propagation}$$

$$ROOH \longrightarrow RO^{\cdot} + HO^{\cdot}$$

The final step, the chain break:

$$RO_2^{\cdot} + X \longrightarrow \text{inactive products}$$

$$\qquad\qquad\qquad\qquad \text{termination}$$

$$RO_2^{\cdot} + RO_2^{\cdot} \xrightarrow{\text{coupling}} \text{inactive products}$$

where X = free radical inhibitor, such as sulfite, aromatic amine. Sometimes the product of recombination of radicals contains sufficient energy to redissociate the molecule.

Autoxidation requires only that a small amount of oxygen initiate the reaction, which is catalyzed by heavy-metal ions possessing a valence of 2 or more. These metals reduce the length of the induction step and increase the maximum rate of oxidation by increasing the rate of formation of free radicals. As little as 0.0002 M copper ion has been shown to increase the rate of vitamin C oxidation by a factor of 10,000 [16]. To reduce the effect of metallic ions on tablet formulations, water used for granulation should be free of heavy metals, and special manufacturing equipment that will reduce the direct contact of the tablets during manufacturing with metals are recommended. Protection from light can also reduce autoxidation.

The speed of autoxidation reactions depends on temperature, radiation, oxygen, and drug concentration in addition to the catalyst.

Autoxidation reactions have been reported for tablet formulations of the following drugs: steroids (e.g., prednisolone [17]), vitamins (e.g., vitamins C [18], B_1 [19], A [20], and E [21]), phenothiazine derivatives (e.g., chlorpromazine [22]), alkaloids (e.g., physostigmine [23]), antibiotics (e.g., tetracyclines [24]). Because oxidation reactions are complex processes and sensitive to many other factors, such as trace metals and impurities, it is difficult to reproduce them and usually it is difficult to carry out kinetics studies on oxidative processes in a general-stability program.

B. Hydrolysis

Although the solid-dosage form stabilizes drug hydrolysis by limiting the access of the drug to water, compounds containing ester or amide linkage are still prone to hydrolysis even in tablet form.

Drug compounds that possess an acyl group also tend to hydrolysis degradation reactions.

Acyl compounds can be illustrated as follows:

$$R-\underset{\substack{\| \\ O}}{C}-X$$

and the chemical behavior of these compounds depends greatly on the nature of this X atom or group. The most important groups of such compounds in tablet formulations that facilitate hydrolysis degradation are as follows:

$R-\overset{O}{\underset{\|}{C}}-OR'$ ester $R-\overset{O}{\underset{\|}{C}}-NHR'$ amide

$R-\overset{O}{\underset{\|}{C}}-OH$ carboxylic acid $R-\overset{O}{\underset{\|}{C}}-Cl$ acid chloride

$R-\overset{O}{\underset{\|}{C}}-O\overset{O}{\underset{\|}{C}}-R$ acid anhydride $R-CH\underset{(CH_2)_n}{\overset{\|}{|}}\,C{=}O\,\underset{NH}{|}$ lactam

The hydrolysis reaction will involve cleavage of the C—X bond and the acyl transfer to water:

$$R-\overset{O}{\underset{\|}{C}}-X + H_2O \qquad R-\overset{O}{\underset{\|}{C}}-OH + HX$$

Although hydrolysis can be effected by pure H_2O, the presence of catalyst, for example, acid or alkalies that are capable of supplying hydrogen or hydroxyl ions to the reaction, will enhance the reaction.

The hydrolysis of an ester for either acid- or alkaline-catalyzed reaction involves the covalent linkage between the carbon atom and the oxygen atom to form an acid and alcohol as follows:

$$R-\overset{\overset{\displaystyle O}{\|}}{C}-OR' + H^+ + OH^- \qquad R-\overset{\overset{\displaystyle O}{\|}}{C}-OH + HOR$$

$$\qquad\qquad\qquad\qquad\qquad\qquad\qquad\text{acid}\qquad\text{alcohol}$$

In case of alkaline-catalyzed reactions:

$$R-\overset{\overset{\displaystyle O}{\|}}{C}-OR' + OH^- \rightleftharpoons R-\overset{\overset{\displaystyle O^-}{\|}}{\underset{\underset{\displaystyle OH}{|}}{C}}-OR' \longrightarrow RCOO^- + R'OH$$

In case of acid-catalyzed reactions:

$$R-\overset{\overset{\displaystyle O}{\|}}{C}-OR' + H^+ \rightleftharpoons R-\overset{\overset{\displaystyle O}{\|}}{\underset{\underset{\displaystyle H}{|}}{C}}-\overset{+}{OR'} \longrightarrow R-\overset{\overset{\displaystyle O}{\|}}{C}-OH + R'OH$$

The hydrolysis of an amide is similar to that of an ester-type compound, except that the hydrolytic cleavage in this case will result in the formation of an acid and an amine:

$$R-\overset{\overset{\displaystyle O}{\|}}{C}-NHR' + H_2O \longrightarrow R-\overset{\overset{\displaystyle O}{\|}}{C}-OH + R-NH_2$$

$$\qquad\qquad\qquad\qquad\qquad\quad\text{acid}\qquad\qquad\text{amine}$$

The general form of the reaction kinetic equation used to express such types of hydrolysis is the first- or pseudo-first-order reaction. This is based on the assumption that the OH^- or H^+ concentration is essentially kept constant or is kept at a considerably higher concentration than the ester concentration during the reaction.

As previously discussed, hydrolysis degradations are catalyzed by both hydrogen and hydroxyl ions, the latter usually has the stronger effect, and pH is an important factor in determining the rate of the reaction. Therefore, the choice of excipients for any particular tablet formulation must be made only after a thorough evaluation of the influence of these excipients on the stability of drug product has been carried out. For example, atropine sulfate is most stable at pH 4 and excipients that will impart alkalinity to the tablet formulation, for example, sodium phosphate dibasic or calcium carbonate, should be avoided.

Hydrolysis reactions have been reported for tablet formulation of the following drugs: atropine [25], aspirin [26], thiamine [27], penicillins [28], cephalosporins [29], and barbituric acid derivatives [30].

C. Photolysis

Photolysis is a surface phenomenon and in most cases the interior of the
tablet will be unaffected. Photolysis of a surface molecule should give rise
to first-order degradation. However, many variables may be involved in
photolysis degradation; for example, intensity and wavelength of light,
size, shape, composition and color of container, so that the kinetics of reactions is complex and zero-, first-, or pseudo-first-order reactions are
possible. An active will exhibit photolysis degradation if it absorbs radiation at a particular wavelength or the energy exceeds a threshold. Thus,
not all absorbed radiation produces photolysis degradation, as part may
change to heat, inducing a thermal reaction that is identical or opposite or
entirely different from the original photolysis reaction. Sometimes a photolysis degradation may produce a catalyst that will start the thermal degradation.

The intensity and wavelength of light, size, shape, color, and type of
tablet container will greatly affect the rate of photolysis degradation.
Ultraviolet radiation, which has the greatest energy supply, is more effective in initiating photolysis degradation.

Free radicals are important in photolysis degradation as they undergo
subsequent reactions. The reaction is said to be photochemical if the molecules absorbing the radiation react, whereas it is said to be photosensitive
if the absorbing molecules do not participate directly in the reaction but
pass on their energy to other molecules that are reacting.

The method commonly used to protect tablets from light is the use of
colored glass or opaque plastic containers. The USP specifies the light
transmission of different glass and plastic containers. It has been demonstrated that when fading of tablet surface penetrates to a depth of 0.03 cm,
the tablet surface appears white and the faded layer does not change upon
further light exposure [31−36]. Drugs that are prone to photolysis degradation are folic acid [37], ascorbic acid [38], benzodiazepines derivatives
[39], sulfonamide [15], and steroids [40].

D. Racemization

Racemization is a reaction whereby an optically active drug substance
changes to an optically inactive mixture of the corresponding dextro and
levo forms. This degradation reaction is important because some actives
are more therapeutically effective in certain optical forms or the optical
isomer has a different biological effect. For example, 1-hyoscyamine is
three times as active as the dl form, atropine. In general, racemization
follows a first-order degradation reaction and is dependent upon temperature, solvent, catalyst, and light. The racemization of a compound appears to depend on the functional group bound to the asymmetrical carbon
atom, with aromatic groups tending to accelerate the racemization. Tablet
formulation that contains 1-hyoscyamine should be as dry as possible and
avoid the use of alkaline excipients [41].

XI. CONTAINER-CLOSURE SYSTEM

Tablet container-closure systems must provide functional protection against
such factors as moisture, oxygen, light, volatility, and drug/package

interaction. The choice of container and closure system for a tablet product can affect the stability of the active's chemical or physical characteristics. Regulations require that stability data for the solid dosage form be provided in the container in which it is to be marketed. The Code of Federal Regulations, Title 21, Section 250.300 restricts the dispensing of nitroglycerin tablets to the original, unopened container because of volatility problems encuntered in repackaging this product [42]. The USP/NF has provided definitions for various types of containers based on their capability to provide protection: light-resistant, well-closed, and tight-closed containers.

The USP/NF describes quantitative tests to measure the permeation and/or light resistance of a container-closure system and establishes limits for each test to define tight, well-closed, and light-resistant containers (Table 6). As mentioned before, the compendia have also provided definitions for the storage conditions stipulated in tablet product monographs: cold, cool, room temperature, excessive heat, and protect from freezing. There is a wide choice available for tablet packaging from among different kinds of glass, plastic, unit dose, blister, and closure systems. An understanding of the properties of the container-closure system and the types of protection necessary for the tablet product will be needed to establish the package selection. Glass and plastic are the commonly used components for tablet packaging.

Glass shows a high degree of chemical inertness, resistance to decomposition by atmosphereic conditions, and is completely impermeable to all gases, solutions, and solvents. It is transparent to light when clear or

Table 6 USP/NF Limits for Glass Types I, II, and III and Plastic Classes I to VI Used for Oral Dosage Forms

Nominal size (ml)[a]	Maximum percentage light transmission at any wavelength between 290 and 450 nm (closure-sealed containers)
1	25
2	20
5	15
10	13
20	12
50	10

[a] Any container of size intermediate to those listed above exhibits a transmission not greater than that of the next larger size container listed above. For containers larger than 50 ml, or type NP glass, the limits for 50 ml apply.

flint, but amber- or green-shaded glass offers good resistance to ultraviolet light, and amber glass shows the greater absorbance to infrared
rays. Tablet products that are physically or chemically unstable as an effect of radiant energy should be packaged in amber glass containers.
Flint glass is transparent to light rays above 300 nm, whereas amber glass
shuts out light rays up to 470 nm (Fig. 10). Since photolysis degradation
decreases with increasing wavelength, it is expected that amber glass
would protect tablets against light.

The use of plastic or polymeric material packages for tablets has become very popular, especially with unit-dose hospital packages for which
aluminum foil is sometimes used. Polyethylene, high- and low-density,
polystyrene, polyvinylchloride, and polypropylene are among the commonly
used polymeric materials to fit different shape and sizes of tablet packages.

The USP/NF has provided test procedures and limits for high-density
polyethylene packaging. Polymeric materials are available in different densities or certain additives which affect its chemical and physical properties.
Stability data should specify the type, properties, and commercial supplier
of plastic container that was used during tablet stability studies. The
major disadvantage of plastic containers is two-way permeation through the
walls. The degree of permeation varies from one polymeric material to
another. Chemical and physical stability of the tablet dosage form can be
influenced by penetration of atmospheric water vapor or loss of moisture
from the formulation. Gases such as oxygen and carbon dioxide in the air
can permeate the plastic container walls, catalyzing drug degradation in
tablets vulnerable to oxidation.

Polymeric materials commonly used in strip and blister tablet unit-dose
packages include cellophane, polyethylene, cellulose acetate, polyvinylchloride, polypropylene, vinyl, and fluorinated hydrocarbon. In strip and

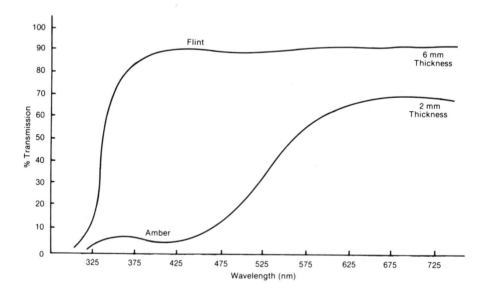

Figure 10   Transmission curves for flint and amber glass.

blister tablet unit-dose packages aluminum foil is sometimes used to obtain the desired tensile strength. Aluminum has a number of excellent properties that can add to tablet product stability: it reflects 90−95% of infrared radiation and 80−85% of white light and is impermeable to moisture vapor.

Closure is an important feature of the container and will contribute to the stability of the product in terms of contamination, or to the ingress of moisture or oxygen. The primary objective of a closure system is to effect a seal. This is usually achieved by using adhesives, achieved by fusion or separate devices such as screw caps. Screw-cap closure seals consist of a threaded shell containing a liner and facing. Threaded shells may be fabricated from metals such as tin plate or aluminum or from plastics such as phenol, urea, or melamine formaldehydes. Liners are generally made from pulpboard, polymeric material, and aluminum, or any of these combinations with suitable adhesive. In all cases, the facing material which comes in direct contact with the tablets must be compatible.

Tablet unit-dosage forms are usually sealed by fusion. Fusion is the welding by heat and pressure of the thermoplastic materials of which the container itself is made. Strict quality assurance procedures to ensure that the proper closure system is always used for a specific tablet product is a must to attain the maximum shelf life of the product.

Publications on the properties and applications of different types of container-closure systems, including the relation of the tablet to the package, are numerous [15,43−51].

XII. EXPIRATION DATING

A. Stability Studies

Expiration dating on tablets can be based on accelerated stability and/or long-term storage stability at the recommended label storage condition. Tablet stability studies can be classified as follows:

1. Research tablets: Initial formulation(s) of new drug substance(s)
2. Proposed tablets: May include investigational new drugs or new combination of drugs
3. New marketed tablets: Newly marketed tablets for which the first three production lots are required for stability study
4. Established tablets: Marketed tablets for which at least one lot per year is required for stability study
5. Revised tablets: Tablets with formulation changes, such as color replacement, new packaging closing system component changes, or a revised manufacturing process
6. Special tablet studies: Studies used to answer a specific problem for a tablet product, such as the investigation of the effect of humidity on special tablet blister packaging, or any item which does not fall into any of the above five classifications.

Recommended testing stability protocols or appropriate variations for tablets are as follows.

A. Research Tablets

5°C	25°C	40°C	50°C	60°C
0, 3, 6, 12, and yearly thereafter	0, 3, 6, 12, 18 months, and yearly thereafter	0 initial 12 weeks 6 months 12 months	0 initial 4 weeks 8 weeks 12 weeks	0 initial 4 weeks 8 weeks 12 weeks

37°C/70% RH	37°C/80% RH	Light (600 fc)
0 initial 4 weeks 12 weeks	0 initial 4 weeks 8 weeks 12 weeks	0 initial 8 weeks 12 weeks

B. Proposed Tablets

5°C	25°C	40°C	50°C	60°C
0, 3, 6, 12, and yearly thereafter	0, 3, 6, 12, 18 months, and yearly thereafter	0 initial 12 weeks 6 months	0 initial 8 weeks 12 weeks	0 initial 8 weeks 12 weeks

37°C/70% RH	37°C/80% RH	Light (600 fc)
0 initial 4 weeks 8 weeks 12 weeks	0 initial 8 weeks 12 weeks	0 initial 8 weeks 12 weeks

C. New Marketed Tablets

Store at controlled room temperature condition (targeted at 25°C) for 1 year after expiration date. Sample initially and at yearly intervals.

D. Established Tablets

Store at controlled room temperature condition (targeted at 25°C) for 1 year after expiration date. Sample initially and at yearly intervals.

E. Revised Tablets

5°C	25°C	40°C	50°C	60°C
0, 3, 6, 12 months, and yearly thereafter	0, 3, 6, 12 months, and yearly thereafter	0 4 weeks 8 weeks 12 weeks 6 months	0 4 weeks 8 weeks 12 weeks	0 4 weeks 8 weeks

37°C/80% RH	Light (600 fc)
0	0
8 weeks	8 weeks
12 weeks	12 weeks

Examples of appropriate variations of the previously mentioned protocols are given in Tables 7-9.

As a general guideline, the following two principles should be taken into consideration in formulating such tablet stability protocols:

1. Less stable tablet materials and formulas would require more frequent testing.
2. The amount of testing required for an active or tablet product depends on the amount of data already available.

A stability-indicating assay should be used for testing at the appropriate scheduled intervals. Tablets in final packing closure systems intended for marketing will be submitted to such tests. An assay will be considered stability indicating if it specifically determines the intact active material or determines the degradation product(s) in the presence of the intact active material or determines both the intact active material and its degradation product(s). The ideal approach is the third one. The reason is mainly that a normal stability-indicating assay will generally have a precision of ±2% coefficient of variation. This means that a difference of 4% from the initial 100% value will not be detected by analytical variation as it will be considered statistically insignificant. On the other hand, if an assay procedure for the degradation was developed with the same coefficient of variation, then less than 1% variation in the same 4% degradation can be detected and estimated.

If the stability-indicating assay was initially developed on the intact active raw material, then it is necessary to show that such an assay procedure is applicable in the presence of formulation-inactive materials or their degradation product(s), if any.

F. Label Storage Conditions

The appropriate label storage condition for a tablet product can be based on a long-term shelf-stability study at the recommended label storage condition or short-term studies at accelerated stress conditions. Assuming that the degradation reaction(s) is constant in the range from the highest temperature studied to the anticipated shelf-storage temperature, t_{90}, estimation could be used for calculating the label storage condition.

Data from at least three temperatures are evaluated and the t_{90} values are estimated. If each t_{90} value versus reciprocal temperature point (1/T) falls above 10 kcal (Fig. 11), or a minimum t_{90} was achieved after at least 12 weeks at 50°C and 26 weeks at 40°C, then the label storage condition of store at room temperature is recommended. If one or more t_{90} value versus 1/T falls between 10 kcal and 17 kcal, or a minimum of t_{90} was achieved after at least 12 weeks, but less than 24 weeks at 40°C and more than 4 weeks at 50°C, then the label storage condition of store at room temperature and protect from temperature above 40°C is recommended. If t_{90}

Table 7   Stability Protocols, Tablets

Retrieve option	Decode key					Date: Packaging	Protocol no.	
Temperature	004	025	037	045	056	025	037	
R. Humidity	00	00	00	00	00	00	90	
Other						Light (600 fc)		
000 month	T	T	*	*	*	*	*	*
001 month	*	*	T	T	T	T	T	*
002 month	*	*	T	T	T	T	*	*
003 month	*	T	T	T	T	T	*	*
006 month	*	T	T	*	*	*	*	*
012 month	*	T	*	*	*	*	T	*
024 month	*	T	*	*	*	*	T	*
036 month	*	T	*	*	*	*	*	*
048 month	*	T	*	*	*	*	*	*
060 month	*	T	*	*	*	*	*	*
*** ***	*	*	*	*	*	*	*	*
*** *.*	*	*	*	*	*	*	*	*
*** ***	*	*	*	*	*	*	*	*
*** ***	*	*	*	*	*	*	*	*
*** ***	*	*	*	*	*	*	*	*

Table 8   Stability Protcols, Tablets

Retrieve option	Decode key					Date:		
Temperature R. humidity Other	004 00	025 00	037 00	045 00	056 00	Packaging	Protocol no.	
000 month	T	T	*	*	*	*	*	*
003 month	*	T	T	T	T	*	*	*
006 month	*	T	T	*	*	*	*	*
012 month	*	T	T	*	*	*	*	*
024 month	*	T	*	*	*	*	*	*
036 month	*	T	*	*	*	*	*	*
047 month	*	T	*	*	*	*	*	*
060 month	*	T	*	*	*	*	*	*
*** ***	*	*	*	*	*	*	*	*
*** ***	*	*	*	*	*	*	*	*
*** ***	*	*	*	*	*	*	*	*
*** ***	*	*	*	*	*	*	*	*
*** ***	*	*	*	*	*	*	*	*
*** ***	*	*	*	*	*	*	*	*

Table 9   Stability Protocol, Tablets

Retrieve option	Decode key			Date: Packaging	Protocol no.
	004 00	025 00	037 00		
Temperature					
R. humidity					
Other					
00 month	T	T	*	*	*
012 month	*	T	T	*	*
024 month	*	T	*	*	*
036 month	*	T	*	*	*
048 month	*	T	*	*	*
060 month	*	T	*	*	*
*** ***	*	*	*	*	*
*** ***	*	*	*	*	*
*** ***	*	*	*	*	*
*** ***	*	*	*	*	*
*** ***	*	*	*	*	*
*** ***	*	*	*	*	*
*** ***	*	*	*	*	*

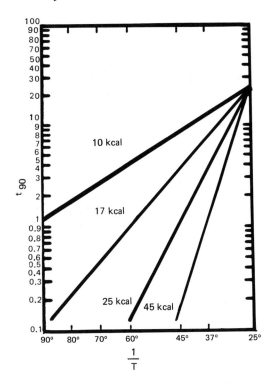

Figure 11 Accelerated stability plot.

value versus 1/T are above 75 kcal, but one or more is below 17 kcal or a minimum of t_{90} was achieved after at least 52 weeks at 30°C, then the label storage condition of store at controlled room temperature is used. If t_{90} value versus 1/T is lower than 25 kcal and above 45 kcal, or a minimum of t_{90} was achieved after at least 4 weeks at 40°C and 1 week at 50°C, then the label storage condition of store below 30°C is used. Other label storage conditions, like protect from freezing or protect from light, should be used as necessary.

G. Stability During Shipment

Appropriate labeling conditions derived from suitable stability studies must be described to assure proper protection of tablet products during shipment. Periods of time that a tablet product may be exposed to extreme high or low temperature should be determined and appropriate label recommendations are used accordingly, e.g., may be adversely affected by exposure to 50°C more than 3 weeks.

XIII. COMPUTER APPLICATION

Computer programs are an efficient means of assisting in the design of stability studies, especially complex models, and the interpretation of data.
A typical computer program can provide an efficient control of sample
storage at given conditions, control inventory, schedule test intervals,
sample at schedule intervals, test requirements and analytical procedure
for each sample, determine manpower required for sample testing, review
data, evaluate statistical data, highlight out-of-limits results, maximize research and development capabilities, interpret data, plot results, estimate
shelf life, prepare reports for regulatory submission or commitments and
product stability trend analysis. Implementation of computer use in stability programs will allow efficient statistical evaluation of the kinetic data,
handling of complex administrative functions, organization of voluminous
amounts of data, and reduce the potential for human errors. Several stability computer programs are commercially available from pharmaceutical as
well as specialized computer companies. Example for such computer forms
and stability reports are presented in Figures 12 and 13. Stability data
listed in these two figures are filled according to the instructions per the
coding letter mentioned beneath each requirement as follows:

a = Computer transaction code
b = Product list number
c = Product lot number
d = Assay type: chemical or biological, etc.
e = Assay name
f = Date of assay as per the stability protocol
g = Time of the stability point
h = Number of assay code as per the written stability-indicating assay
     monograph
i = Number of monograph code as per the written stability-indicating
     assay monograph
j = % RH
k = Temperature in °C
l = Other stability conditions, e.g., light
m = Date assay was performed
n = Chemist or technician name/or initial who performed the assay
o = Number of tests performed
p = All results of assay performed
q = Average assay results
r = Previous assay results reported
s = Units the assay is to be run by, e.g., average tablet weight
     (ATW)
t = Number of samples analyzed
u = Total time for stability study as per the stability protocol
v = Product release limit
w = In-house or action limit
y = Name of supervisor who checked and approved the analysis
z = Date of supervisor approval

F/C	List no.	Lot no.	Assay type	Assay name	Scheduled assay date	Time of stability point Y M D	Assay code	Monograph code	% R.H.	Temp. (°C)	Other
10	1234	SAH	C	Vit. A	80 10 21	00 12 00	01	02	40	37	00
a	b	c	d	e	f	g	h	i	j	k	1

Assay date Y M D	Chemist	Test	Result calculation	Assay result	Previous assay result	Assay units	Sample no.	Stability schedule
80 10 21	HAS	1	81 80 79	80	90	mg/ATW	03	3Y
m	n	o	p	q	r	s	t	u

Product limit	In-house limit	Approval	Approval date
90–110	95–105	SAH	80 10 27
v	w	y	z

Figure 12 Computer stability assay report.

Report date	List no.	Lot no.	Exp. date	Months of schedule	Stability time	Assay code	Monograph code	Chemist	Product
80 10 27	1234	SAH	83 09 20	01	3Y	01	02	HAS	Vit. tab.

Assay name		Assay date	Assay units	Assay results	Assay % of initial
	01	80 10 20	mg/ATW	24.90	99.6
Vit. A	02	80 10 20		25.00	100.0
	03	80 10 20		24.30	97.2
	01	80 10 21	mg/ATW	128.00	102.0
Vit. E	02	80 10 21		130.00	104.0
	03	80 10 21		128.00	102.0

Figure 13   Computer stability detail report.

REFERENCES

1. Garrett, E. R., Schumann, E., and Grostic, M., *J. Am. Pharm. Assoc., Sci. Ed., 48*:684 (1959).
2. Carstensen, J. and Musa, M., *J. Pharm. Sci., 61*:1112 (1972).
3. Jacobs, A. L., Dilatush, A. E., Weinstein, S., and Windheuser, J. J., *J. Pharm. Sci., 55*:893 (1966).
4. Troup, A. and Mitchner, H., *J. Pharm. Sci., 53*:375 (1964).
5. Blang, S. M. and Huang, V., *J. Pharm. Sci., 61*:1770 (1972).
6. Wai, K. N., Dekay, H. G., and Banker, G. S., *J. Pharm. Sci., 51*: 1076 (1962).
7. Bandelin, F. J. and Malesh, W., *J. Am. Pharm. Assoc., Pract. Pharm. Ed., 19*:152 (1958).
8. Zazareth, M. R. and Huyck, C. L., *J. Pharm. Sci., 50*:608 (1961).
9. Zazareth, M. R. and Huyck, C. L., *J. Pharm. Sci., 50*:620 (1961).
10. Robeiro, D., Stevenson, D., Samyn, J., Milosovich, G., and Mattocks, A. M., *J. Am. Pharm. Assoc., Sci. Ed., 44*:226 (1955).
11. Naggar, V. F., Khalil, A. S., and Ellis, L. F., *Pharmazie, 26*:636 (1971).
12. Szabo, S. and Kovacs, B., *Gyogyszereszet, 14*:464 (1970).
13. Costello, R. A. and Mattacks, A. M., *J. Pharm. Sci., 51*:106 (1962).
14. Goodhart, F. W., Everhard, M. E., and Dickcins, D. A., *J. Pharm. Sci., 53*:338 (1964).
15. Lachman, L., *J. Pharm. Sci., 54*:1519 (1965).
16. Finhalt, P., Kristiansen, H., Kyowezynski, L., and Higuchi, T., *J. Pharm. Sci., 55*:1435 (1966).
17. Guttman, D. E. and Meister, P. D., *J. Am. Pharm. Assoc., Sci. Ed., 47*:773 (1958).
18. Rubin, S. H., DeRitter, E., and Johnson, J. B., *J. Pharm. Sci., 65*:963 (1976).
19. Carstensen, J. T., Osadca, M., and Rubin, S. H., *J. Pharm. Sci., 58*:549 (1969).
20. Carstensen, J. T., *J. Pharm. Sci., 53*:839 (1964).
21. Carstensen, J Johnson, J., Spera, D., and Frank, M., *J. Pharm. Sci., 57*:23 (1968).
22. Ravin, L. J., Kennon, L., and Swintosky, J. V., *J. Am. Pharm. Assoc., Sci. Ed., 47*:760 (1958).
23. Fletcher, G. and Davis, D. G. G., *J. Pharm. Pharmacol., 20*:108 (1968).
24. Haynes, J., Carstensen, J., Calahan, J., and Card, R., *Stevens Symp. Stat. Meth. Chem. Ind., 3*:1 (1959).
25. Svirblis, P., Socholitsky, I., and Kandritzer, A., *J. Pharm. Sci., 45*:450 (1956).
26. Kelly, C. A., *J. Pharm. Sci., 59*:1053 (1970).
27. Tardif, R., *J. Pharm. Sci., 54*:281 (1965).
28. Hon, J. P. and Poole, J. W., *J. Pharm. Sci., 60*:503 (1971).
29. Yamana, T. and Tsuji, A., *J. Pharm. Sci., 65*:1563 (1976).
30. Gardner, L. A. and Goyan, J. E., *J. Pharm. Sci., 62*:1026 (1973).
31. Lachman, L., Swartz, C. J., and Cooper, J., *J. Am. Pharm. Assoc., Sci. Ed., 49*:213 (1960).
32. Lachman, L., Weinstein, S., Swartz, C., Urbanzi, T., and Cooper, S., *J. Pharm. Sci., 50*:141 (1961).

33. Lachman, L., Urbanzi, T., Weinstein, S., Cooper, J., and
     Swartz, C., *J. Pharm. Sci.*, *51*:321 (1962).
34. Kuramoto, R., Lachman, L., and Cooper, J., *J. Am. Pharm. Assoc.*,
     Sci. Ed., *47*:175 (1958).
35. Swartz, C., Lachman, L., Urbanzi, T., and Cooper, J., *J. Pharm.
     Sci.*, *50*:145 (1961).
36. Swartz, C., Lachman, L., Urbanzi, T., Weinstein, S., and
     Cooper, J., *J. Pharm. Sci.*, *51*:326 (1962).
37. Guven, C. K. and Kauber, S., *Eczocilik Bull.*, *11*:161 (1969).
38. Seth, S. K. and Mital, H. C., *Ind. J. Pharm.*, *27*:119 (1965).
39. Felmeisher, A. and Dischler, C. A., *J. Pharm. Sci.*, *53*:756 (1964).
40. Chulski, E. W., Johnson, R. H., and Wagner, J. G., *J. Am. Pharm.
     Assoc.*, *Sci. Ed.*, *49*:253 (1960).
41. Rosenblum, E. I. and Taylor, W. S., *J. Pharm. Pharmacol.*, *7*:328
     (1955).
42. Shangraw, R. F. and Contractor, A. M., *J. Am. Pharm. Assoc.*,
     NS 512, 633 (1972).
43. Bull, A. W., *J. Pharm. Pharmacol.*, *7*:806 (1955).
44. Dean, D. A., *Drug Dev. Commun.*, *2*:109 (1976).
45. Huebner, G., *Pharm. Ind.*, *37*:930 (1975).
46. Spingler, E., *Pharm. Ind.*, *33*:831 (1971).
47. Cloche, J. R., *Labo-Pharma. Prob. Technol.*, *22*:291 (1974).
48. Arbona, B. and Douchairie, B., *Prob. Technol.*, *22*:135 (1974).
49. DeWilde, J. H., *Pharm. Weekbl.*, *107*:724 (1972).
50. Spingler, E., *Pharm. Weekbl.*, *107*:813 (1972).
51. Cooper, J., Plastic Containers for Pharmaceuticals: Testing and
     Control WHO Offset Publ. No. 4 (1974).
52. *United States Pharmacopeia/National Formulary*, 21st Ed./16th Ed.,
     Mack Publishing Co., 1985.
53. *Guideline for Submitting Documentation for the Stability of Human
     Drugs and Biologics*, Washington, D.C., FDA, 1987.
56. Martin, A. N., *Physical Pharmacy*, 3rd Ed., Philadelphia, Lea &
     Febiger, 1983.

9
Quality Assurance

Samir A. Hanna

Bristol-Myers Squibb Company, Syracuse, New York

I. INTRODUCTION

The total control of quality requires the organized effort of an entire
company to assure the specified quality in each lot of drug product manufactured. The quality of oral solid-dosage forms as well as any drug
dosage form must be built in during plant construction, product research
and development, purchasing of materials, production, testing, inspection,
labeling, storage, and distribution. It cannot be assumed that end-product testing alone will ensure product quality.

Nearly all drug substances dispensed in the oral solid-dosage form are
stable under ordinary conditions. The essential qualities of a good compressed tablet are characterized by a number of specifications. These include the appearance, size, shape, thickness, weight, homogeneity, stability, hardness, dissolution time, and disintegration time. The appearance, size, shape, and thickness of the tablet are generally used to distinguish and identify the active ingredients which they contain. The remaining specifications assure the manufacturer that the tablets do not
vary from allowable limits within the same lot or from one production lot to
another. All such qualities are designed to ensure a safe, therapeutically
effective oral solid-dosage form.

II. QUALITY ASSURANCE SYSTEM

Since manufacturing produces the tablets, they should have prime responsibility for quality results. Removal of the responsibility from manufacturing for producing a quality product results in lackluster product quality
performance. Quality assurance, however, must establish control points

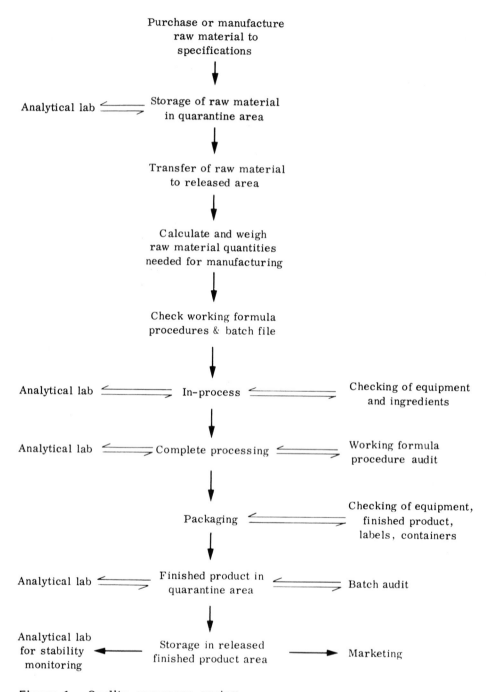

Figure 1   Quality assurance system.

to monitor the quality of the product as it is processed and on the final product. With experience, these control points are located at the critical points in the process flow. These include raw materials, in-process, complete processing, packaging line, finished product, and stability monitoring.

The quality assurance system is diagrammed in Figure 1. This system can vary in details, but not in principle, from company-to-company, and will depend on the nature and size of the manufacturing facility and on the types of oral solid-dosage forms produced.

III. GOOD MANUFACTURING PRACTICES REQUIREMENTS

Most governments promulgate regulations governing the manufacture, processing, packaging, and distribution of finished pharmaceuticals. International standards have been published by the World Health Organization, but each country prefers to promulgate regulations that fit its own needs. Examples of such regulations in the United States are found in Part 211, Title 21 of the Code of Federal Regulations, Current Good Manufacturing Practices in Manufacturing, Processing, Packaging, or Holding of Drugs (CGMPs). These regulations were originally published in the *Federal Register* of June 20, 1963, by the Food and Drug Administration (FDA); and over the past 12 years these regulations have been revised several times. On February 13, 1976, the FDA published in the *Federal Register* proposals for revising drug CGMPs to update them in light of current technology and to adopt more specific requirements to better assure the quality of finished products. The final regulation was published in the *Federal Register* on March 28, 1979. The current CGMPs are enforced by the FDA, and it is on the basis of these regulations that the FDA has insisted on the proper manufacturing of drugs. The regulations extend into the area of finished pharmaceuticals, buildings, equipment, personnel, components, master production and control records, batch production, production and control procedures, product containers and their components, laboratory controls, distribution records, stability, expiration dating, and complaint files.

Regulations for good manufacturing practices during tablet manufacturing are aimed at assuring that only those tablets which have met the established specifications and are packed and labeled under proper controls are distributed.

IV. COMPENDIAL REQUIREMENTS

Since the first officially recognized tablet appeared in the *United States Pharmacopeia* (USP IX) (1916), the number has steadily increased. Presently, the USP XXII and the *National Formulary* (NF) XVII officially recognizes 560 different tablets. Specifications published in the official compendia are designed to assure a pharmaceutically elegant and therapeutically effective dosage form. The acceptable limits of deviation are dependent upon the special problems associated with the production of the particular tablet.

Individual monographs for tablets include tablet dosage-form uniformity by either weight variation or content uniformity, and limits on disintegration time or dissolution besides the stated drug quantity. It is a compendial requirement that any sampling within a specific batch of tablets would reveal the tablets to be in compliance with respect to the individual monograph specifications.

A. Uniformity of Tablets Dosage Units

The uniformity of tablets dosage units can be demonstrated by either weight variation or content uniformity test. Weight variation test is required when tablets to be tested are uncoated and contains 50 mg or more of a single active ingredient comprising 50% or more, by weight of the tablet dosage-form unit. Content uniformity test is required for coated tablets, and all other cases except for special tablets as stated above.

Weight Variation

Tablet dosage-form uniformity by weight variation is determined by selecting not less than 30 tablets from each production batch and weighing accurately 10 tablets individually and calculating the average weight. From the results of the assay obtained as directed in the individual compendial monograph, the content of active ingredient in each of the individual 10 tablets is calculated.

The USP/NF weight variation requirements are met if the amount of the active ingredient in each of the 10 tablets under test lies within the range of 85−115% of the label claim and the relative standard deviation is less than or equal to 6%. If one tablet is outside the above-mentioned range and no other tablet is outside the range of 75−125% of label claim and/or if the relative standard deviation is greater than 6%, the extra 20 tablets should be tested. USP/NF tablet dosage-form uniformity test requirements are met if not more than one tablet of the 30 individual tablets tested is outside the range of 85−115% of label claim and no tablet is outside the range of 75−125% of label claim and the relative standard deviation of the 30 tablets tested does not exceed 7.8%.

Content Uniformity

Tablet dosage-form content uniformity is determined by selecting not less than 30 tablets from each production batch and assaying 10 tablets individually as directed in the assay of the individual compendial monograph. If the amount of the active ingredient in the individual tablet is less than required in the assay, make necessary dilution of the solutions and/or volume of aliquots so that the concentration of the active ingredients in the final solution is the same as that in the assay procedure. In case of a titrimetric assay, make necessary dilution to use adequate volume of titrant and appropriate corresponding changes in the calculation formula and titration factor.

Where special procedure is specified in the test for content uniformity in the individual monograph, make any necessary correction of the results obtained as follows:

1. Prepare a composite specimen of a sufficient number of dosage units to provide the amount of specimen called for in the assay in

the individual monograph plus the amount required for the special procedure given in the test for content uniformity in the monograph by finely powdering tablets in single-unit containers to obtain a homogeneous mixture. If a homogeneous mixture cannot be obtained in this manner, use suitable solvents or other procedures to prepare a solution containing all of the active ingredient, and use appropriate aliquot portions of this solution for the specified procedures.

2. Assay separate, accurately measured portions of the composite specimen of tablets in single-unit containers, both (a) as directed in the assay, and (b) using the special procedure given in the test for content uniformity in the monograph.

3. Calculate the weight of active ingredient equivalent to one average dosage unit by (a) using the results obtained by the assay procedure, and by (b) using the results obtained by the special procedure.

4. Calculate the correction, F, by the formula $F = P - A$, in which P is the weight of active ingredient equivalent to one average dosage unit obtained by the special procedure, and A is the weight of active ingredient equivalent to one average dosage unit obtained by the assay procedure.

5. Calculate the ratio F/P. If it is greater than 0.030, subtract the weight represented by F from each of the results obtained by the special procedure. If it is less than -0.030, add the weight represented by F to each of the results obtained by the special procedure. If it is between -0.030 and 0.030, inclusive, no correction is to be applied.

The USP/NF content uniformity requirements are met if the amount of the active ingredient in each of the 10 tablets under test lies within the range of 85–115% of the label claim and the relative standard deviation is less than or equal to 6%. If one tablet is outside the above-mentioned range and no other tablet is outside the range of 75–125% of label claim and/or if the relative standard deviation is greater than 6%, the extra 20 tablets should be tested. USP/NF tablet dosage-form uniformity test requrements are met if not more than one tablet of the 30 individual tablets tested is outside the range of 85–115% of label claim and no tablet is outside the range of 75–125% of label claim and the relative standard deviation of the 30 tablets tested does not exceed 7.8%.

Label claim average limits specified in the potency definition in the individual tablet product compendial monograph should be appropriately adjusted if greater than 100%.

B. Disintegration Time

A tablet is generally formulated with a disintegration agent which will cause the tablet to rupture and fall apart in water or gastric fluid. Factors affecting the disintegration of tablets are the physical and chemical properties of the granulation, the hardness, the porosity, and the disintegrating agent used. Disintegration does not imply complete solution of the tablet or even its active constituent. Complete disintegration is defined as that state in which any tablet residue remaining on the screen of a disintegration apparatus is a soft mass having no palpably firm core.

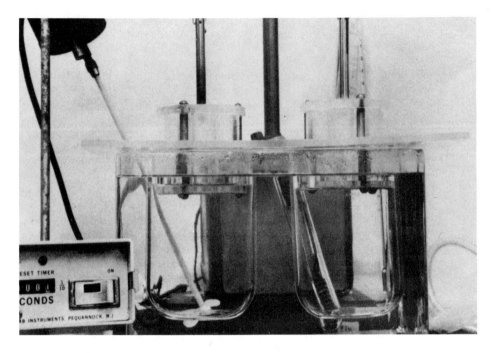

Figure 2   USP disintegration apparatus.

The principal function of the test is to assure product uniformity. The
USP XXI and NF XVI disintegration apparatus (Fig. 2) consists of a
basket-rack holding six open-end glass tubes, each 7.75 ± 0.25 cm long
and having an inside diameter and wall thickness of approximately 21.5
and 2.0 mm, respectively. Attached by screws to the underside of the
lower plate holding the tubes is 10-mesh stainless steel wire cloth. The
basket rack is immersed in a 1 L beaker containing an appropriate fluid
at 37 ± 2°C. The basket rack is raised and lowered through a distance
of 5–6 cm at the rate of 28–32 cps. The volume of fluid used is such
that during the operation the basket rack is never less than 2.5 cm below
the surface of the fluid or above the bottom of the beaker. Each tube is
provided with a slotted and perforated cylindrical, transparent plastic
disk which is placed on top of the tablet.

Uncoated Tablets

One uncoated tablet is placed into each glass tube and a disk is added to
each tube. The basket rack is immersed and moved in water as the immersion fluid, unless another fluid is specified in the individual monograph.
At the end of the time limit specified in the monograph, the basket rack is
lifted; and all tablets should have disintegrated completely. If one or two
tablets fail to disintegrate completely, the test is repeated with 12 additional tablets. Not less than 16 of the total 18 tablets tested must disintegrate completely.

Plain-Coated Tablets

Plain-coated tablets are tested by first placing a tablet in each glass tube and immersing the basket rack in water at room temperature for 5 min; then a disk is added to each tube, and the apparatus is operated for 30 min using simulated gastric fluid at 37 ± 2°C as the immersion fluid, and this is observed. If the tablets have not disintegrated completely, they are immersed in a simulated intestinal fluid at 37 ± 2°C, and the test is continued for the time specified in the monograph plus 30 min. If one or two of the tablets fail to disintegrate completely, the test is repeated with 12 additional tablets. Not less than 16 of the total 18 tablets tested must disintegrate completely.

Enteric-Coated Tablets

One tablet is placed in each glass tube, and the basket rack is immersed in water at room temperature for 5 min, if the tablet has a soluble external coating. Then the apparatus is operated without adding the disks for 1 h using simulated gastric fluid at 37 ± 2°C as the immersion fluid, and this is observed. No tablets should show evidence of disintegration, cracking, or softening. Then a disk is added to each tube, and the apparatus is operated using simulated intestinal fluid at 37 ± 2°C as the immersion fluid for 2 h plus the time specified in the monograph, or where only an enteric-coated tablet, for only the time limit specified in the monograph. The basket is lifted from the fluid and is observed. All tablets should have disintegrated completely. If one or two tablets fail to disintegrate completely, the test is repeated with 12 additional tablets. Not less than 16 of the total 18 tablets tested must disintegrate completely.

C. Dissolution Test

The test is intended to measure the time required for a given drug in an oral solid-dosage form to go into solution under a specified set of conditions. It affords an objective means toward the evaluation of the physiological availability of the drug. Since drug absorption and physiological availability are largely dependent upon having the drug in the dissolved state, suitable dissolution rates are an important property of a good tablet product. However, dissolution rate is not necessarily a measure of safety or therapeutic efficacy, which must be initially established through appropriate in vivo studies and clinical evaluation. However, in some cases it was possible to correlate dissolution rates with physiological availability of the drug.

The USP XXII and NF XVII dissolution apparatus 1 (Fig. 3) consists of a 1-L glass or other inert, transparent vessel with a slightly concave bottom, fitted with a variable speed motor and a cylindrical stainless steel basket. The whole assembly is immersed in a water bath at 37.0 ± 0.5°C. The motor shaft is placed in the center of the vessel to which the top part of the basket is attached. The detachable part of the basket is made of welded seam, 40-mesh stainless steel cloth formed into a cylinder 3.66 cm high and 2.5 cm in diameter. The motor is regulated between 25 and 200 rpm and is maintained at the rate specified in the individual monograph within ±5%. The vessel is immersed in the constant temperature bath and 900 ml of the dissolution medium specified in the individual monograph is

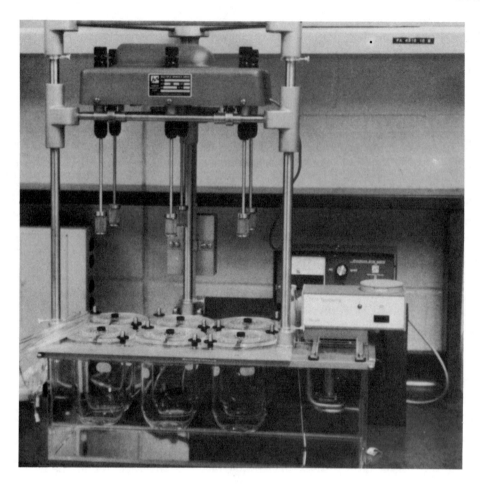

Figure 3   USP dissolution apparatus, 1.

placed in it. When the dissolution medium comes to a temperature of 37.0 ± 0.5°C one tablet is placed in the basket and is immersed to a distance of 2.0 ± 0.2 cm between the basket and the concave bottom of the vessel. The basket is rotated and the samples are withdrawn for analysis as directed in the individual tablet product compendial monograph at the rate and time specified in the monograph.

Apparatus 2, the stainless steel basket is replaced by a stirring blade 3 − 5 mm thick, eccentrically mounted on a shaft 10.0 ± 0.5 mm in diameter. The blade is immersed to a distance of 2.5 ± 0.2 cm between the blades lower edge and the spherical bottom of the vessel. The blade is rotated, and the samples are withdrawn for analysis at the rate and time specified in the monograph.

Apparatus 1 and 2 must comply with the USP suitability test using one tablet each of the USP dissolution calibrator-disintegrating and -non-disintegrating type. Dissolution test requirements are met if the quantities of active ingredient dissolved from each tablet tested conform to the acceptance criteria in Table 1-A. Testing should continue through the

Table 1-A USP/NF Dissolution Test Acceptance Criteria

Stage	Number tested	Acceptance criteria
S_1	6	Each unit is not less than Q + 5%
S_2	6	Average of 12 units (S_1 + S_2) is equal to or greater than Q, and no unit is less than Q − 15%
S_3	12	Average of 24 units (S_1 + S_2 + S_3) is equal to or greater than Q, and not more than 2 units are less than Q − 15%

Q = Amount of dissolved active ingredient specified in the tablet product individual monograph expressed as a percentage of labeled content.
Source: Technicon Instrument Corp., Tarrytown, New York; Hanson Research Corp., Northridge, California; Beckman Instruments, Inc., Fullerton, California.

three stages unless the results conform to either S_1 or S_2. Automation of either procedure that can perform dissolution testing of six tablets at a time is commercially available from Technicon Instrument Corp., Hanson Research Corp., and Beckman Instruments, Inc.

Extended-release and enteric-coated tablets active ingredient USP compendial release requirements are tested using same dissolution apparatus 1 or 2 and procedure as specified in the individual tablet product monograph.

Enteric-coated tablets are tested using method A or B that incorporates the use of acid phase of 0.1 N hydrochloric acid and buffer phase of pH 6.8 phosphate buffer.

Extended-release and enteric-coated tablets USP compendial requirements are met if the quantities of active ingredient dissolved from each tablet tested conform to the acceptance criteria in Tables 1-B, 1-C, and 1-D.

Table 1-B USP/NF Extended-Release Acceptance Criteria

Level	Number tested	Criteria
L_1	6	No individual value lies outside each of the stated ranges and no individual value is less than the stated amount at the final test time.
L_2	6	The average value of the 12 units (L_1 + L_2) lies within each of the stated ranges and is not less than the stated amount at the final test time; none is more than 10% of labeled content outside each of the stated ranges; and none is more than

Table 1-B   (Continued)

Level	Number tested	Criteria
L_2 (cont.)		10% of labeled content below the stated amount at the final test time.
L_3	12	The average value of the 24 units ($L_1 + L_2 + L_3$) lies within each of the stated ranges, and is not less than the stated amount at the final test time; not more than two of the 24 units are more than 10% of labeled content outside each of the stated ranges; not more than two of the 24 units are more than 10% of labeled content below the stated amount at the final test time; and none of the units is more than 20% of labeled content outside each of the stated ranges or more than 20% of labeled content below the stated amount at the final test time.

Table 1-C   USP/NF Enteric-Coated Acid Phase Testing Acceptance Criteria

Level	Number tested	Criteria
A_1	6	No individual value exceeds 10% dissolved.
A_2	6	Average of the 12 units ($A_1 + A_2$) is not more than 10% dissolved, and no individual unit is greater than 25% dissolved.
A_3	12	Average of the 24 units ($A_1 + A_2 + A_3$) is not more than 10% dissolved, and no individual unit is greater than 25% dissolved.

Table 1-D   USP/NF Enteric-Coated Buffer Phase Testing Acceptance Criteria

Level	Number tested	Criteria
B_1	6	Each unit is not less than Q + 5%.
B_2	6	Average of 12 units ($B_1 + B_2$) is equal to or greater than Q, and no unit is less than Q − 15%.

Table 1-D (Continued)

Level	Number tested	Criteria
B_3	12	Average of 24 units (B_1 + B_2 + B_3) is equal to or greater than Q, not more than 2 units are less than Q − 15% and no unit is less than Q − 25%.

V. RAW MATERIALS

The storage conditions of raw materials for tablets manufacturing, particularly hydroscopic substances, are important. Because of the great number of potential sources of contamination, strict sanitation of the plant warehouse is an absolute necessity. Quality assurance should make periodic sanitation inspections and follow-up to assure that deficiencies are corrected.

An extensive and varied microbial flora is usually associated with raw materials from natural sources; for example, gum arabic and tragacanth. Synthetic raw materials, on the other hand, are normally free or low in microbial contamination.

A. Sampling of Raw Materials

Samples of raw materials are to be collected in clean containers using a disinfected sampling "thief" or scoop, observing aseptic technique for microbiological analysis or clean container and clean technique for analytical laboratory. The number of containers to sample in a given lot can be determined by using MIL-STD-105D, as shown in Table 2.

Samples are to be labeled as to lot number, receiving number, supplier, container size and type, name of raw material, and date of receipt. Samples are than submitted to quality assurance analytical and microbiological laboratories.

B. Chemical and Microbiological Attributes

In the development of raw material specifications, the analytic research and development chemist should strive for the following:

Ascertain which chemical, physical, and biological characteristics are critical for assuring reproducibility from lot-to-lot of raw materials to be used for evaluating each lot of raw material produced or purchased.

Establish the test methods and acceptable tolerance of the attributes to be evaluated.

Establish the supplier's ability to supply raw materials of consistent quality.

Good raw material specifications must be written in precise terminology, be complete, and provide details of test methods, type of test instruments to use, manner of sampling, and proper identification. Figure 4 lists

Table 2   Number of Containers of Raw Materials to Be
Sampled per Lot

Inactive raw materials	
Containers	No. samples
1	All
2 – 8	2
9 – 15	3
16 – 90	5
91 – 150	8
151 – 280	13
281 – 500	20
501 – 1200	32
1201 – 3200	50

Active raw materials	
Containers	No. samples
1 – 5	All
6 – 10	6
11 – 18	7
19 – 28	8
29 – 100	9
> 101	10

Packaging components		
Cases, rolls, or boxes (no. per lot)	Cases, rolls, or boxes (no. samples)[a]	Units sample no.
1 – 8	2	
9 – 15	3	
16 – 90	5	
91 – 150	8	
151 – 280	13	
281 – 500	20	
501 – 1200	32	
1201 – 3200	50	
3201 – 10,000	80	
10,001 – 35,000	125	315
35,001 – 150,000	200	500
150,001 – 500,000	315	1250
> 500,001	500	1250

[a]Across pallet.

A. (Raw Material Name)
   1. Structural formula, molecular weight
   2. Chemical name(s)
   3. Item number
   4. Date of issue
   5. Date of superseded, if any, or new
   6. Signature of writer
   7. Signature of approval

B. Samples
   1. Safety requirement
   2. Sample plan and procedure
   3. Sample size and sample container to be used
   4. Reservation sample required

C. Retest Program
   1. Retesting schedule
   2. Reanalysis to be performed to assure, identity, strength, quality, and purity

D. Specifications (wherever applicable)
   1. Description
   2. Solubility
   3. Identity
      a. specific chemical tests as related alkaloids; organic nitrogenous basis; acid moiety or inorganic salt tests; sulfate, chloride, phosphate, sodium, and potassium; spot organic and inorganic chemical tests
      b. infrared absorption
      c. ultraviolet absorption
      d. melting range
      e. congealing point
      f. boiling point or range
      g. thin-layer, paper, liquid, or gas chromatography
   4. Purity and quality
      a. general completeness of solutions, pH, specific rotation, nonvolatile residue, ash, acid-insoluble ash, residue on ignition, loss on drying, water content, heavy metals, arsenic, lead, mercury, selenium, sulfate, chloride, carbonates, acid value, iodine value, saponification value
      b. special quality tests, particle size, crystallinity characteristics, and polymorphic forms
      c. special purity tests, ferric in ferrous salts, peroxides and aldehydes in ether and related degradation products
   5. Assay, calculated either on anhydrous or hydrous basis
   6. Microbial limits, especially for raw materials from natural sources

E. Test Procedures
   1. Compendial, USP, or NF references.
   2. Noncompendial, detailed analytical procedure, weights; dilutions; extractions; normality; reagents; instrumentation used and procedure, if any; calculations

F. Approved Suppliers
   1. List of prime suppliers and other approved alternative suppliers, if any

Figure 4   Raw material quality assurance monograph.

Item number	Date of issue		Superseded	Written by	Approved by

Sampling plan   Preservation sample   Retest program
                                      4 oz   Schedule   Tests
                                                                1 year   Identity
                                                                            specific-
                                                                            rotation

                                                                            Assay

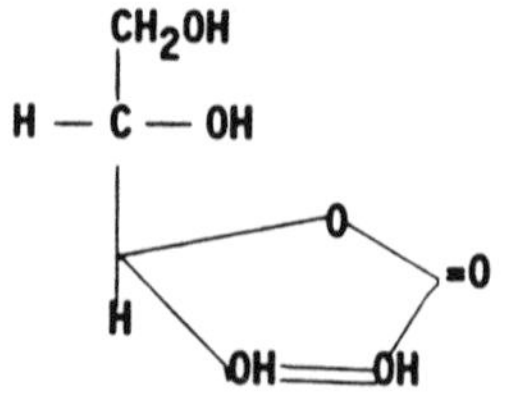

$C_6H_8O_6$ Mol. wt. 176.13   L - Ascorbic Acid

Specifications

Description
White or slightly yellow crystals or powder; on exposure to light gradually darkens; in the dry state, it is reasonably stable in air, but in solution rapidly oxidizes; melts at about $190^\circ C$

Solubility
Freely soluble in water; sparingly soluble in alcohol, insoluble in chloroform, ether, and benzene

Identification
Infrared
The infrared absorption spectrum of a potassium bromide dispersion of it exhibits maxima only at the same wavelength as that of a similar preparation of USP Ascorbic Acid RS.

Alkaline
cupric
tartrate
Color reduces slowly at room temperature but more readily upon heating

Specific-
rotation
Between $+20.5^\circ$ and $+21.5$

Residue on
ignition
NMT 0.1%

Heavy metals
NMT 0.002%

Assay
99.0-100.5% on anhydrous basis

Completeness
of solution
10 g per 20 ml of water for injection is not less clear than an equal volume of water for injection examined similarly

Test Procedures: for all tests, see USP

Approved supplier
1. Roche Laboratories, Division of Hoffmann-LaRoche, Inc., Nutley, NJ
2. Pfizer, Inc., New York, NY

Figure 5   Ascorbic acid, USP.

general tests, limits, and other physical or chemical data for raw materials related to identity, purity, strength, and manner of quality assurance. Figure 5 provides a quality assurance monograph for acetominophen, USP, as an example of a specific raw material.

The current FDA GMPs covering raw material handling procedures are found in the Code of Federal Regulations, Title 21, Section 211.42. It simply states that "components" be received, sampled, tested, and stored in a reasonable way, that rejected material be disposed of, that samples of tested components be retained, and that appropriate records of these steps be maintained. In practice, the manufacturer will physically inspect and assign lot numbers for all raw materials received and will quarantine them until they are approved for use. Each raw material is sampled according to standard sampling procedures and is sent to the quality control laboratory for testing according to the written procedures (Fig. 5). If acceptable, it is moved to the release storage area and properly labeled to indicate the item number, name of material, lot number, date of release, reassay date, and signature of a quality assurance inspector. The raw material is retested as necessary according to an established schedule to assure that it still conforms to specifications at time of use. Quality assurance should reserve samples from active and inactive raw materials required to determine whether the material meets the established specification. These reserve samples should be retained for at least 5 years. Approved components shall be rotated in such a manner that the oldest stock is used first.

Any raw material not meeting specifications must be isolated from the acceptable materials, labeled as rejected, and returned to the supplier or disposed of promptly. To verify the supplier's conformance to specifications, further supporting assurance by means of on-site periodic inspections is pertinent to the total quality of raw materials. This will assure that cross-contamination does not take place owing to improperly cleaned equipment or poor housekeeping practices, since contaminants may go undetected because specifications generally are not designed to control the presence of unrelated materials. In general, raw materials may be classified into two basic groups: those that are active or therapeutic ingredients, and those that are inactive, inert materials.

VI. ACTIVE OR THERAPEUTIC MATERIALS

A. Antibiotics

Antibiotics are one of the few drugs for which the official analytic method appears in the Code of Federal Regulations. The USP XXI and NF XVI refer to the Code of Federal Regulations for specifications and analytic methods given in the individual monographs for each antibiotic. The Code of Federal Regulations, Title 21, Chapter 1, Parts 436 to 436.517 and Parts 442 and 455, contains the analytic method specifications for all antibiotics approved for human use in the United States. The number of tests required varies from one antibiotic to another. The data in Table 3 provide the tests required by the Code of Federal Regulations for some

Table 3   Tests of Some Antibiotic and Antibiotic-Containing Tablets

	LOD	Moisture	pH	Crystallinity	Iodometric assay[a]	Hydroxylamine col. assay[a]	Residue on ignition	Heavy metals	Melting range or temperature	Disintegration	Nonaqueous titration	Special test	Microbial limits	ID	Specific rotation
Ampicillin	NMT 2%		3.5–6.0	X	X	X					X		Potency[c] safety	X	
Tablets[b]					X					NMT 15 min			Potency[c]		
Cephalexin monohydrate	4–8%		3.0–5.0	X	X								Potency[c] safety	X	
Tablets[b]	NMT 9%				X					NMT 30 min			Potency[c]		
Neomycin sulfate	NMT 8%		5.0–7.5										Potency[c] safety	X	
Tablets[b]		NMT 10%								NMT 1 hr			Potency		
Tetracycline		NMT 13%	3.0–7.0	X								Absorption at 380 nm	Potency[c]	X	
Tablets[b]		NMT 3% NMT 6%								NMT 1 hr			Potency[c]	X	
Zinc bacitracin		NMT 5%	6.0–7.5							NMT 1 hr			Potency[c] NMT 10% Zn safety	X	

Product	Loss on drying	Content	Melting range	Heavy metals	pH / Content	Disintegration	UV absorption / Specific surface area	Assay	Specific rotation
Tablets[b]	NMT 5%					NMT 1 hr		Potency[c]	
Griseofulvin	NMT 1%	NMT 0.2%	217–224°C	NMT 25 ppm			UV absorption, Specific surface area	Potency[c] safety	X +348° to +364°
Tablets[b]	NMT 5%					NMT 1 hr		Potency[a] (spect.)	
Erythromycin	NMT 10%	NMT 2%		NMT 50 ppm	8.0–10.5 X			Potency[c] safety	X −50° to −58°
Tablets[b]	NMT 7.5%					NMT 1 hr		Potency[c]	
Sodium novobiocin Tablets	NMT 6%	10.5–12%			6.5–8.5	NMT 1 hr		Potency[c]	X
						NMT 1 hr		Potency[c]	

[a]Chemical methods of assay as alternative to microbiological assay are allowed for special antibiotics: iodometric and hydroxylamine colorimetric for most penicillin, cephalothin, and cephaloridine; GLC for lincomycin and clindamycin; ultraviolet spectrophotometry for chloramphenicol succinate and palmitate, clactinomycin, and griseofulvin; colorimetric for cycloserine and troleandomycin.

[b]Antibiotic raw materials used for tablet manufacturing must conform to the standards listed in the CFR for each specific antibiotic.

[c]Potency is determined microbiologically using the turbidimetric assay and the diffusion plate assay.

Source: Code of Federal Regulations, 21 Food and Drugs, U.S. Govt. Printing Office, 1981.

antibiotics and antibiotics prepared as tablets. Testing of antibiotics is generally performed by chemical, microbiological, or biological methods, or by all three methods. Caution must be exercised during antibiotic raw material sampling for testing to assure that it is not altered during the sampling procedure. The sample must be taken in a relatively dry atmosphere, relatively free from dust, and free from both chemical and microbial airborne contamination, and exposure must be reduced to a minimum during sampling. Special attention should be given to the assay for potency of antibiotic raw materials. Since the potency value in terms of micrograms per milligram obtained for this material is used in calculating the number of grams or kilograms required for the working formula procedures, it is recommended that at least two separate weighings of such antibiotic raw material powder be assayed on each of three different days (six different assays using six differing weighings). If all the individual results are not within the normal distribution of the group or show too much variance, additional assays should be done until a mean potency is obtained with confidence limits of ±2.5% (or better) at p = 0.05.

B. Activities Other than Antibiotics

The current editions of the USP XXII and NF XVII contain monographs on most therapeutically active materials used in tablet manufacturing. Since there is such a wide variance in the nature of the active ingredients used in tablet manufacturing, it is impossible to summarize briefly the testing of those raw materials. One of the most important decisions to be made in raw material control is the degree of purity that will be maintained for each material. It is not uncommon to find an appreciable variation in the degree of purity between samples of the same raw material purchased from different commercial sources. The selection then must be one which results in the highest purity practical for each raw material, consistent with safety and efficacy of the final oral dosage form. A typical raw material currently existing in a compendia has a purity requirement of generally not less than 97%. Its specifications normally consist of a description, solubility, identification, melting range, loss on drying, residue on ignition, special metal testing, specific impurities that are pertinent to the method of synthesis of each individual raw material and assay. The methods of assay are usually chemical in nature. However, it should be indicated that these compendial tests are intended as the minimum required from the legal point of view.

For certain tablet products, it may be necessary to obtain an active ingredient with special specifications far tighter than those of the comparable compendial standard. Raw materials cannot be adequately evaluated and controlled without special instrumentation such as spectrophotometry; infrared spectrophotometry; potentiometric titrimetry; column, gas, paper, thin-layer, and high-pressure liquid chromatography; polarography; x-ray diffraction; x-ray fluorescence; spectrophotofluorimetry; calorimetry; and radioactive tracer techniques. No less demanding are the tests required for microbiological assay, pharmacological assay, and safety testing. For certain tablet products, even when highly purified and well-characterized raw materials are involved, specifications should include additional critical features such as particle size, crystal shape, and other peculiarities such as crystalline versus amorphous forms. Any of these characteristics could have an effect on the safety or effectiveness of the final oral dosage form. It is a GMP requirement that all raw materials, active or inactive, be assigned a reassay date, meaningful or indicative, that would assure purity and potency. Tests are performed at reassay times to confirm continued suitability of each raw material.

VII. INACTIVE OR INERT MATERIALS

A. Diluent

Diluents used in tablet formulations include lactose, sucrose, koalin, sodium chloride, dicalcium phosphate, calcium sulfate, and calcium carbonate. Mannitol and crystalline sorbitol are often used as diluents for chewable tablets.

Diluents usually make up the major portion of the tablet. Therefore, its physical characteristics, such as color, odor, and foreign matter, are as important as its chemical purity. This is especially important if the final dosage form is an uncoated, white tablet. Among other important specifications of diluents are particle size, powder uniformity, heavy metal content, water content, and microbial limit.

B. Binders

The following materials are used as binders: water, alcohol, starch paste (10 – 18%), gelatin solutions (10 – 20%), tragacanth (1 – 3%), sodium alginate, methyl cellulose, ethylcellulose, carboxymethylcellulose, polyethylene glycol 4000 or 6000, and povidone.

The binding force of the binding agent used is important to assure that granules form with the proper holding power to prevent possible picking and sticking of the tablet. A suitable test, such aas viscosity, will ascertain such property. Other physical and chemical tests of binders are foreign matter, residue on ignition, pH, and microbial limit.

C. Lubricants

The most frequently employed materials are magnesium stearate, calcium stearate, talc, stearic acid, starch, mineral oil, sodium chloride, sodium benzoate, 8,1-leucine, and carbowax 4000 or 6000.

Lubricants are most effective when used in a very fine powder, 100 mesh or finer. An accurate, precise particle size determination, preferably using advanced instrumentation procedures, is recommended. If soluble lubricants are used, a completeness of solution test to assure its water solubility is to be performed. Heavy metals, water content, melting range, and microbial limit, specifically for talc is also important, as it is a mining product. Talc, if used, should be tested and must comply with the FDA's lead, arsenic, and asbestos limits published in the *Federal Register*, Vol. 38, No. 118.

D. Disintegrating Agents

Disintegrating agents that are currently in use include dried corn or potato starch; cellulose derivatives such as methylcellulose, sodium carboxymethyl-cellulose, alginic acid, microcrystalline cellulose, and certain gums.

Disintegrating agents are tested for foreign matter, specially those of plant origin such as starches, water content, viscosity, cellulose derivatives, heavy metals, and microbial limit for starches and alginic acid. Starch, USP, has a limit of not more than 14% for water content, low-moisture starch, which has a water content as low as 5%, is commercially available.

E. Coloring Agents

Approved certified water-soluble Food, Drug and Cosmetics (FD&C) dyes, or mixtures thereof, or their corresponding lakes, may be used to color tablets. Color in tablets mainly serves as a means of identification. The FDA determines and approves colorants for use in food and drugs with recommendation of limits, if any. Table 4 lists selected colors and FDA restrictions on their use. The FDA also certifies and releases colors batch by batch for human use. A typical analysis of a color will contain identity tests, total volatile matter, heavy metals, water-insoluble matter, synthesis impurities, arsenic, lead, and total color. An FD&C color lake analysis will contain additional tests for chloride, sulfate, and inorganic matter.

F. Flavoring Agents

If a flavored tablet is desired, flavors or volatile oils may be sprayed as an alcoholic solution onto the dry granules or dry flavors may be used by blending with other tablet constituents. If dry flavors are used, a tight limit for water content will assure the quality of the dry flavors. For the same reason, dry flavors should be stored in tightly closed containers away from excessive heat and retested for water content every 6 months.

Flavors are usually tested for refractive index, specific gravity, solubility, and alcohol content, if any. A GLC chromatogram that can be used as a "fingerprint" for each specific flavor will help in assuring the supplier's continuous compliance to specifications. A knowledge of any synthetic FD&C dyes in the flavor formula is important for the formulator to keep up with FDA colorants regulations.

G. Sweetening Agents

The most popular sweetening agents used are mannitol, lactose, crystalline sorbitol, and artificial sweetening agents like saccharin, sodium saccharin, calcium saccharin, aspartame. Chewable tablets often use mannitol or crystalline sorbitol as a diluent and sweetening agent simultaneously.

Testing for unwanted impurities resulting from synthesis side reaction in the manufacturing procedure is essential in the analysis of sweetening agents; for example, furfuraldehyde in lactose, reducing and total sugars in sorbitol, reducing sugars in mannitol. Sweetening agents are usually tested for water content, heavy metals, residue on ignition, arsenic, and other special tests such as specific rotation, melting range, selenium, and readily carbonizable substances.

Table 4 Colorants

Colorant	Restriction on use
FD&C Blue #1	Permanent listing for use in foods, drugs, and cosmetics
Blue #2	Permanent listing for use in foods, drugs, and cosmetics
Green #2	Provisional listing for use in foods, drugs, and cosmetics
Red #40	Provisional listing for use in foods, drugs, and cosmetics
Yellow #5	Permanent listing for use in foods, drugs, and cosmetics
Yellow #6	Provisional listing for use in foods, drugs, and cosmetics
D&C Blue #6	Provisional listing for use in drugs and cosmetics with requirement for label declaration
Green #5	Provisional listing for use in drugs and cosmetics
Green #6	Provisional listing for use in drugs and cosmetics
Orange #5	Provisional listing for use in drugs and cosmetics
Orange #10	Provisional listing for use in drugs and cosmetics
Orange #17	Permanent listing for use in drugs and cosmetics
Red #6	Provisional listing for use in drugs and cosmetics
Red #7	Provisional listing for use in drugs and cosmetics
Red #21	Provisional listing for use in drugs and cosmetics
Red #22	Provisional listing for use in drugs and cosmetics
Red #27	Provisional listing for use in drugs and cosmetics
Red #28	Provisional listing for use in drugs and cosmetics
Red #30	Provisional listing for use in drugs and cosmetics
Red #8	Provisional listing for use in drugs and cosmetics with restriction of NMT 0.75 mg to be ingested on a daily basis
Red #12	Provisional listing for use in drugs and cosmetics with restriction of NMT 0.75 mg to be ingested on a daily basis
Red #19	Permanent listing for use in drugs and cosmetics with restriction of NMT 0.75 mg to be ingested on a daily basis
Red #33	Provisional listing for use in drugs and cosmetics with restriction of NMT 0.75 mg to be ingested on a daily basis
Red #36	Provisional listing for use in drugs and cosmetics with restriction of NMT 0.75 mg to be ingested on a daily basis
Yellow #10	Provisional listing for use in drugs and cosmetics

Lakes of the above

Annetto	Permanent listing for use in foods, drugs, and cosmetics
Carotene	Permanent listing for use in foods, drugs, and cosmetics
Caramel	Permanent listing for use in foods, drugs, and cosmetics and provisional listing for use in cosmetics
Caramine	Permanent listing for use in foods, drugs, and cosmetics
Titanime dioxide	Permanent listing for use in drugs and cosmetics

Source: Food and Drug Administration, *Federal Register*.

H. Coating Materials

Raw materials mainly used in sugar-coating formulations are arsenic-free shellac, sugar, acacia, gelatin, starch, calcium carbonate, talc, white bees-wax, and cranberry wax. Film-coating materials which have been used are mainly povidone, methyl- and ethylcellulose, carboxymethylcellulose, cellulose acetate phthalate, natural gums, and various nonaqueous solvents such as polyethyleneglycols, methanol, and methylene chloride. Raw materials that are usually used for enteric coating are mixtures of fats and fatty acids, shellac, and cellulose acetate phthalates.

Coating materials are usually tested for foreign matter, water content, melting range, pH, viscosity (if needed), arsenic, heavy metals, acid value, saponification value and iodine value (for fats and fatty acids), and microbial limits.

VIII. CONTAINER

The compendium defines the container as that device that holds the drug and that is or may be in direct contact with the drug. The immediate container is that which is in direct contact with the drug at all times. The closure is a part of the container.

Container components should not interact physically or chemically with tablet product to alter the strength, quality, or purity beyond the specified requirements. The compendium provides specifications and test procedures for light resistance: well-closed, tight-closed, and four different types of glass containers.

Specifications and test methods are designed for containers on the basis of tests performed on the product in the container. The following features are to be considered in developing container specifications:

Properties of container tightness
Moisture and vapor tightness regardless of container construction
Toxicity, chemical, and physical characteristics of materials needed in container construction
Physical or chemical changes of container upon prolonged contact with tablet
Compatibility between container and tablet

Good manufacturing practices require that stability data be submitted for any new drug substance for the finished dosage form of the drug in the container in which it is to be marketed.

The use of plastics in rigid containers, film and blister packs, especially in single-dose containers, for tablet packaging has increased in the last 15 years. Obviously this is because of cost reduction in transportation and dispensing convenience. Plastics generally used in tablet packaging are polyethylenes, polypropylenes, cellulose plastics, polystyrene, and polyvinylchloride. Table 5 lists some characteristics and uses of these plastics. Regardless of end use or fabrication method of polymer, additives must be compounded or dry blended into the base resin. These additives can be classified as stabilizers, plasticizers, lubricants, colorants, fillers, impact modifiers, and processing aids. Not all polymers contain all of these additives. Polyethylene is one of the most thermally stable thermoplastics available. This means that polyethylene bottles offer the best

Table 5   Characteristics and Uses of Plastics

Polymer	Uses				Permeability				Effect of laboratory reagents			
	Rigid cont.	Films	Blister packs	Clarity	O_2	N_2	CO_2	H_2O	Weak acid	Strong acid	Weak alkalis	Strong alkalis
Polyethylenes	X	X	–	O	H	L	H	L	R	OAA	R	R
Polypropylenes	X	X	–	T	H	L	H	L	R	OAA	–	R
Cellulose acetate	–	X	X	C	L	L	H	H	A	D	A	D
Polystyrene	X	X	–	C	L	L	H	H	–	OAA	–	–
Polyvinylchloride	X	X	X	C	L	–	H	H	–	–	–	–

Note: O = opaque, T = translucent, C = clear, L = low, H = high, R = resistant, A = attacked, D = decomposes, OAA = oxidizing acids attack.

Source: Cooper, J., Plastic Containers for Pharmaceuticals, Testing and Control, WHO, Geneva, 1974.

Table 6   High-Density and Low-Density
Polyethylene

Description:

Identification:

    A: Density by displacement
    B: Multiple internal reflective spectrum (MIR)
    C: Thermal analysis

Light transmission:

Water vapor transmission:

Extractable:

    A: Alcohol extraction
    B: Chloroform extraction

Nonvolatile residue:

Heavy metals:

---

possible protection from breakage at an economical cost. This, along with other desirable processing and packaging properties, is the reason why high-density polyethylene (HDPE) is used for most tablet packaging in plastic bottles. The Pharmaceutical Manufacturers Association, the Society of the Plastics Industry, and the USP prepared a monograph for polyethylene containers to be used for dry drug packaging. Table 6 lists a prepared quality control monograph for high-density and low-density polyethylene polymer. Tablets are protected from adverse moisture conditions, for example, vitamins and aspirin tablets, by the use of a tack seal adhesive. Generally a synthetic resin, emulsion-based material, such as formulated polyvinyl emulsion adhesive, is used. Table 7 outlines a quality control monograph for such adhesives.

Table 7   Formulated Polyvinyl Adhesive

Description:

Identification:

    Multiple internal reflective spectrum (MIR)

Odor:

Total solids:

Viscosity at 25°C:

    By using Brookfield Synchro-Lecteric Viscometer or equivalent

pH (1/10 in water)

Table 8 Moisture Properties of Blister Materials

Material	Water-vapor transmission[a] (gm)
Polyvinyl chloride, 1 mil	4.00
Polyvinylidine chloride, 1 mil	0.200
Polychlorotrifluorethylene, 1 mil	0.055

[a]Loss per 24 h/in^2/mil at 95°F and 90% RH.

The requirement for tamper-resistant OTC packaging was enacted by FDA regulations 21 C.F.R. Parts 211, 314, and 700 in 1982. As defined by this legislation

a tamper-resistant package is one having an indicator or barrier to entry which, if breached or missing, can reasonably be expected to provide visible evidence to consumers that tampering has occurred. Tamper-resistant packaging may involve immediate-container/closure systems or secondary-container/carton systems or any combination thereof intended to provide a visual indication of package integrity when handled in a reasonable manner during manufacture, distribution, and retail display.

The FDA also requires either that the tamper-resistant feature be designed from materials that are generally not readily available, or that barriers made from readily available materials carry a distinctive design or logo that cannot be readily reproduced by an individual attempting to restore the package. The following package configurations have been used by tablet manufacturers to comply with FDA tamper-resistant regulation: blister package, strip package, bubble pack, foil or plastic pouches, bottle seals, shrink seals or bands and film wrappers. Blister package is the most widely used single-dose container for tablets. It provides users with convenience, pleasing appearance, and tamper resistance. The blister package is composed of a semirigid thermoplastic resin blister filled with tablet and lided with a heat-sealable backing material. The backing material is usually heat-seal-coated aluminum foil. The coating material on the foil must be compatible with the blister material to ensure satisfactory sealing for tamper resistance. Polyvinylchloride alone or laminated with polyvinylidene or polychlorotrifluroethylene is commonly used for blister material. Laminated polyvinyl chloride is a superior moisture barrier to polyvinylchloride resin alone, as shown in Table 8. It should be noted that good manufacturing practices classify packaging components, such as cartons, bottles, caps, film seal, adhesives, and labeling, as raw materials. Therefore, all previous quality assurance procedures for raw materials are to be followed for packaging components.

IX. IN-PROCESS QUALITY ASSURANCE

Conformance to compendial standards as the sole basis for judging an oral dosage form to be perfectly satisfactory will be grossly misleading. Obviously, a compendial monograph could never cover all possibilities which might adversely affect the quality of a product. The difficulty lies in part in the fact that oral dosage forms are frequently produced in batches of hundreds of thousands or even millions of tablets, so that the numbers of tablets assayed at the end of the process is not likely to represent more than a tiny fraction of the actual production.

There is a real and significant difference between a finished tablet product compendia standard and manufacturing quality assurance procedure. The CGMP guidelines emphasize environmental factors to minimize cross-contamination of products, labeling, and packaging errors, and the integrity of production and quality control records; but they do little to minimize within-batch and batch-to-batch variation in the output of production. Therefore, it is an important function of the in-process quality assurance program to ensure that tablets have uniform purity and quality within a batch and batch-to-batch.

X. QUALITY ASSURANCE BEFORE START CHECKING

A. Environmental Control and Sanitation

To assure that tablet dosage forms meet high standards of quality and purity, an effective sanitation program is required at all facilities where such products are manufactured. A successful extermination program must be enforced within and outside the plant to control insects and rodents. People are the mainstay of any plant housekeeping and sanitation program. Consequently, personal cleanliness, proper hair covering, and clothing with appropriate pockets should be demanded. Floors, walls, and ceilings should be resistant to external forces, capable of being easily cleaned, and in good repair. Adequate ventilation, proper temperature, and proper humidity are other important factors. Ventilation in granulating, coating, and compression departments is usually designed such as to be able to absorb and remove dust. In such departmental operations, dust collectors, air filters, and scrubbers to clean the air are checked on a routine schedule. Air quality monitoring and foot candle measurements at the work station could be an indication of the adequacy of these elements.

The water supply may be potable, distilled, or deionized and under adequate pressure to keep the water flowing clean. Deionization units should be checked and changed frequently to deliver water of consistently high chemical and microbial quality as per written compendial or in-house specifications.

Quality assurance must review and check, based on written procedures that specify the details of the testing procedures and schedules, the following:

> Sanitation (Fig. 6)
> Cleaning records
> Ventilation system: filter conditions and changes, pressure gage, humidity monitoring, temperature monitoring, microbial monitoring (Fig. 7), light intensity, foot candle measurement

Page	No.	
Date	Supersedes NEW	Sanitation Control — Pest Control
Written by	Checked by	

Certox: insecticide

Type of action
  Kills on contact

Formula	Approximate %
Petroleum distillates	71.8
Technical piperonyl butoxide*	12.0
Pyrethrine	1.2
Inert ingredients	15.0

Dilution
  Dilute 1 gallon of concentrate with 4 gallons of water.

Time interval
  To be used once weekly after working hours on Friday evenings.

Area designation
  Floor and drains

Equipment
  Spray unit for Certox
  The Certox concentrate
  Safety equipment

Removal of waste materials
  Removal of waste materials remaining in the spray units after exterminating shall be the responsibility of the exterminator.

Effectiveness inspection
  It will be the responsibility of the quality assurance department to perform routine area checks to ascertain the effectiveness of the frequency of spraying.
  It will, however, be the responsibility of the area supervisor to take necessary action immediately upon seeing any infestation.

Special restrictions and cautions
  1. Foods should be removed or covered during treatment.
  2. Do not store or use near heat or open flame.
  3. Apply only as designated on area designation assignments.

Toxicity in humans
  Can cause severe allergic dermatitis and systemic allergic reactions.

Toxic symptoms
  Large amounts may cause nausea, vomoting, tinnitus, headache, and other CNS disturbances.

Government status
  EPA Registration Number: 1748-110
  Since Certox presents no significant toxicity problem, no tolerance data are available.

*Equivalent to 9.6% (butylcarbityl)(6-propyl-piperonyl)ether and 2.4% related compounds.

Figure 6 Quality assurance operating procedure.

Product _____   Lot no. _____

Room _____   Date exposed _____

Media _____   Time of   Incubation   Date
                   exposure _____ temperature _____ °C   read _____

1 — Location of plate exposure	Plate no.	Colony count

2 — Location of air sampler (m^3 air/hr)	Plate no.	Colony count

Comments

Microbiologist _____   Supervisor _____

Date Reported _____

Figure 7   Environmental control tablet manufacturing.

Water system: released sticker on point of use of water after checking
and release from quality control laboratories, proper flushing period,
and/or volume before water use

B. Manufacturing Working Formula Procedures

Documentation of the component materials and processing steps, together with
with production operation specifications and equipment to be used, make up
the manufacturing working formula procedures (MWFPs).

A working formula procedure should be prepared for each batch size
that is produced. To attempt expansion or reduction of a batch size by
manual calculations at the time of production cannot be considered good
practice.

Quality assurance must review and check the working formula procedures
for each production batch before, during, and after production operation
for:

Signed and dated when issued by a responsible production person
Proper identification by name and dosage form, item number, lot num-
ber, effective date of document, and reference to a superseded
version, if any, amount, lot, and code numbers of each raw mate-
rial utilized
Each step initiated by two of the operators involved
Calculations of both active and inactive materials, especially if there
were any corrections for 100% potencies for actives used
Reassay dates of components used
Starting and finishing times of each operation
Equipment to be used and specification of its setup
Proper labeling of released components and equipment indicating product
name, strength, lot number, and item number

C. Raw Materials

Quality assurance must check if any released raw material is to be taken to
the production department in its original container; such containers should
be cleaned. However, most raw materials are weighed in an environmental
control weighing area where they are transferred to a secondary container
that only circulates inside the production department. This secondary container should also be properly labeled with a sticker that bears all the information that was on the original container label. Only released raw materials with proper reassay dates are allowed in the production department.
Raw materials intended for use in specific products should be stacked and
isolated together with proper identification, name, dosage form, item number, lot number, weight, and signatures.

D. Manufacturing Equipment

Quality assurance must ensure that manufacturing equipment be designed,
placed, and maintained in such a way as to facilitate thorough cleaning, be
suitable for its intended use, and minimize any contamination of drugs and
their containers during manufacture. Manufacturing equipment and utensils
should be thoroughly cleaned and maintained in accordance with specific

written directions. Whenever possible, equipment should be disassembled and thoroughly cleaned to preclude the carryover of drug residues from previous operations. Adequate records of such procedures and tests, if any, should be maintained by quality assurance. It is good manufacturing practice to use laboratory checks whenever possible to detect trace quantities of drugs if products containing such drugs had been produced on a specific equipment.

Prior to the start of any production step, the quality assurance personnel should ascertain that the proper equipment and tooling for each manufacturing stage are being used. Equipment must be identified by labels bearing the name, dosage form, item number, and lot number. Equipment used for special batch production should be completely separated in the production department, and all dust-producing operations should be provided with adequate exhaust systems to prevent cross-contamination and recirculation of contaminated air.

Weighing and measuring equipment used in production and quality assurance, such as disintegration apparatus (unit and thermometer), friability testers, and balances, should be calibrated and checked at suitable intervals by appropriate methods; records of such tests should be maintained by quality assurance. Examples of such calibration methods are given in Figure 8.

Page	No.	
Date	Supersedes	Calibration of Disintegrator Apparatus
Written by	Checked by	

a. Disintegration time (to be checked each shift)
  1. The water in the beaker in the water bath is at $37 \pm 2°C$.
  2. The volume of the water in the beaker is such that at the highest point of the upward stroke, the wire mesh remains at least 2.5 cm below the surface of the water and descends to not less than 2.5 cm from the bottom of the beaker on the downward stroke.
b. Thermometers (to be checked every six months)
  1. Employ suitable USP melting point standards for the range of the thermometer to be tested.
  2. Use USP method class I to determine the actual melting range of the standards.
  3. Tag the thermometer with date calibrated, next calibration date, temperature correction, and signature of the person conducting the test.

Figure 8   Quality assurance calibration procedures.

E. Sampling Procedure

Sampling procedures of finished tablet products can be based either on attribute inspection that grades the product as defective or nondefective or inspection by variables for percentage defective. The focal point of any sampling plan is the acceptable quality level (AQL). The second important step is to decide on the inspection level of the sampling plan, which will determine the relationship between the lot size and the sample size (N/n). The principal purpose of the sampling plan is to assure that tablets produced are of quality at least as good as the designated AQL. This means that as long as the fraction defective (r) is less than the AQL designated for a specific production procedure, then a large percentage of the lots of tablets produced will be accepted. Sampling procedures for inspection by variables for percentage defective may be used if a quality characteristic can be continuously measured and is known to be normally distributed, such as mean of the sample or the mean and standard deviation of the sample. The assumption of a specific distributional form is a special feature of variable sampling. A separate plan must be employed for each quality characteristic that is being inspected or a common sampling plan is used, but the allowable number of defects varies for each quality characteristic; that is, no critical defects are allowed (c), but some minor defects are allowed. Also, the fraction defective yielded by a given process mean and standard deviation should be calculated to assure a normal distribution of sample statistics.

For practical purposes, MIL-STD-414 for inspection by variables for percentage defective and MIL-STD-105D for inspection by attributes for defective or nondefective products are often used to design a sample plan.

In tablet manufacturing, sampling procedures for inspection by attributes are generally used, for the following reasons.

Variables sampling, as compared with attributes sampling, requires more mathematical understanding and clerical calculation.

Switching procedures from different inspection levels in variables sampling are more cumbersome.

For large lot sizes, which is the case in tablets manufacturing, producer's risk is larger in variables sampling than in attributes sampling plan.

The smaller sample size required by variables sampling sometimes costs more, depending on the type of quantitative test performed, than a large sample size required by a comparable attributes plan because of the precise measurements required by the variable plan.

Variables data can be converted to attributes data, but the reverse is not possible.

There are three types of attributes sampling plans: single sampling, double sampling, and multiple sampling.

Single Sampling Plan

A single-sampling plan specifies the sample size that should be taken from each lot of tablets and the number of defective units that cannot be exceeded in this sample. For example, a sample of 100 (n) is taken from a lot; if 2 (c) or fewer defective units are found, the lot is accepted. The discriminatory power of a sampling plan is explained by its operating

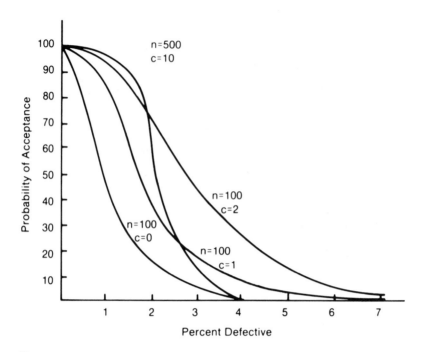

Figure 9   Operating characteristic curves for sampling plan for samples of different sizes and different acceptance numbers.

characteristic (OC) curve. This curve serves to show how the probability of accepting a lot will vary with the quality of the sample of tablets inspected. The operating characteristic curves for a single sampling plan that gives the probability of accepting a lot from a randomly operating process turning out products of average quality at various defective levels for samples of different sizes and different acceptance numbers are given in Figure 9.

From this figure, the OC curve of the above-mentioned example of single-sampling plan, n = 100 and c = 2, shows that if tablets quality (per centage defective) is 5, the probability of lot acceptance is 12; if it is 1, the probability of acceptance is 92. Again, Figure 9 shows that QC curves vary with the number of n as c in this example is kept proportional to n. This example shows that the precision of a sampling plan increased with the size of a sample (n). The three OC curves for sampling plan n = 100, c = 2, n = 100, c = 1; and n = 100, c = 0 illustrate that a plan varies with the acceptance number alone (c). The smaller the c, the tighter is the plan; as c is increased, the plan becomes more lax and the OC curve is raised. The schematic instructions for a single-sampling plan are shown in Figure 10.

Double-Sampling Plan

The first sample is smaller than a comparable single-sample plan. The second sample size is generally twice the size of the first. Consequently, if the lot is accepted or rejected on the first sample, there may be a

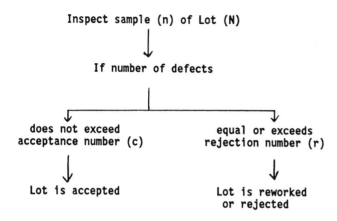

Figure 10 Schematic instructions for MIL-STD-105D single-sample plan.

considerable savings in total inspection cost. If the results of the first sample fall within the acceptance and rejection values, a second sample is taken. The results of the two samples are combined and compared with the final acceptance or rejection values. For example, a first sample of 50 ($n_1 = 50$) is taken from a lot, if 2 ($c_1 = 2$) or fewer defective units are found, the lot is accepted; if 7 or more defective units are found, the lot is rejected. If the number of defective units is 3 but not more than 6 ($c_2 = 6$), a second sample of 100 ($n_2 = 100$) is taken; if in the combined sample ($n_1 + n_2 = 150$) the number of defective units is 6 or less, the lot is accepted; if 7 or more defective units are found, the lot is rejected. Operating characteristic curves of double-sampling plans showing the probability of acceptance or rejection on the first sample and combined first and second samples for the above-mentioned example are shown in Figure 11. Curve II in this figure gives the principal operating characteristic curve for the plan, since it gives the probability of final acceptance. The difference between curve II and curve I gives the probability of acceptance on the second sample; the difference between curve II and curve III gives the probability of rejection on the second sample. To illustrate, for the previously mentioned example, for a lot of tablets with a fraction defective of 5, the probability of acceptance on the second sample is 59 and the probability of final acceptance is 63.5. The schematic instructions for double-sampling plan are shown in Figure 12.

Multiple-Sampling Plan

This plan allows for more than two samples when necessary for a final decision. For standardized sampling, the plan is tied to a maximum of seven equal samples. For nonstandardized sampling, the sample size may vary between inspection checks depending on the proximity of the sample results to the acceptance or rejection values. For example, in a multiple standardized sampling plan, if from a given lot the cumulative sample sizes, acceptances, and rejection numbers of 20, 40, 60, 80, 100, 120, and 140; 0, 1, 3, 5, 8, 9, and 10; 4, 5, 6, 8, 10, 11, and 12 are assigned, respectively, the lot is rejected if the number of defective units at any

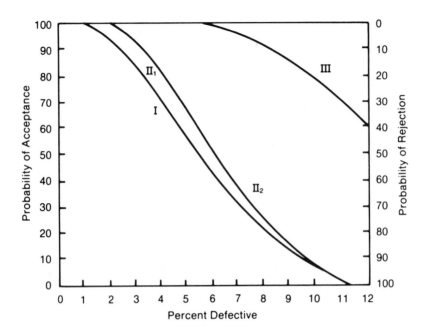

Figure 11 Operating characteristic curves of double-sampling plan: (I) probability of acceptance on first sample (left scale); (II) probability of acceptance on combined samples (left scale); (II$_2$) probability of rejection on combined samples (right scale); (III) probability of rejection on first sample (right scale).

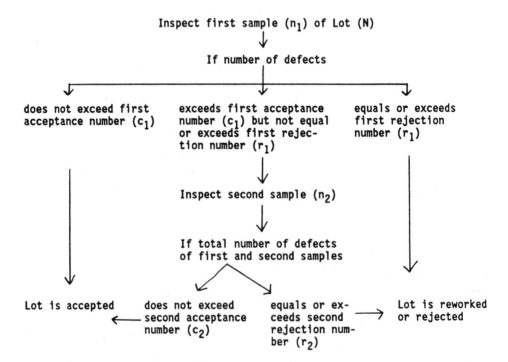

Figure 12 Schematic instructions for MIL-STD-105D double-sampling plan.

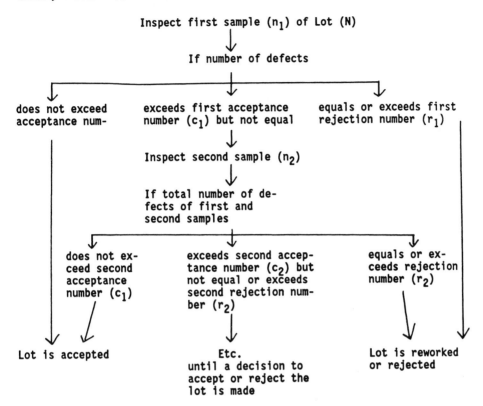

Figure 13   Schematic instructions for MIL-STD-105D multiple sampling plan.

sampling stage equals or exceeds the rejection number. If not, the multiple sampling procedure continues until at least the seventh sample is taken when a decision to accept or reject the lot is to be made. The schematic instructions for multiple sampling plan are shown in Figure 13.

Military standard sampling procedures for inspection by attributes (MIL-STD-105D) was issued by the U.S. Government in 1963. The focal point of MIL-STD-105D is the acceptable quality level. In applying MIL-STD-105D it is necessary also to decide on the inspection level. This determines the relationship between the lot size and the sample size. For a specified AQL and inspection level and a given lot size, MIL-STD-105D gives a reduced, a normal, or a tightened sampling plan. The switch from the normal plan to the tightened plan is made if two of five consecutive lots have been rejected on original inspection. Switching back from tightened to normal plans is made if five consecutive lots have been accepted on original inspection. Switching from normal to reduced sampling plan is made if 10 consecutive lots have been accepted on original normal inspection and the total number of defectives is less than a value set forth in a special table. Figure 14 shows the operation characteristic curves for both normal and tightened plans for a single sampling plan with an AQL of 1% and sampling size of 50 (n = 50). If the lot has a fraction defective of 1, the probability of acceptance on the normal inspection is 92.5; if the tightened inspection is used, this probability will decrease to 82.

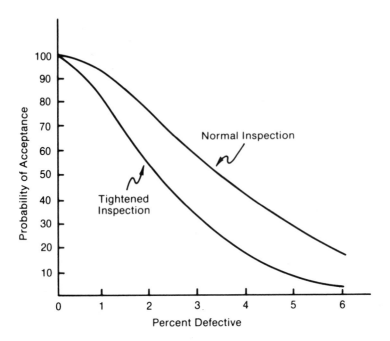

Figure 14   Operating characteristic curves for a MIL-STD-105D single-sampling plan.

The construction of a sampling plan normally requires four quality standards be specified: acceptable quality level, unacceptable quality level (UQL), producer's risk (α), which is the probability of rejecting good quality, and consumer's risk (β), which is the probability of accepting poor quality. Figure 15 defines these parameters for projections for a sampling plan. The usual approach is the determination of desirable AQL, UAL, α, and β subsequent computation of sample size and acceptable values by applying the tables of MIL-STD-105D. For low-dosage or highly toxic tablets, as in the case of digoxin or warfarin tablets, it is desirable that the AQL and UAL be kept close together and α and β be very small; consequently, a large sample will be required for a suitable sampling plan. Conversely, the plan will call for a very few samples if the AQL and UQL are quite far apart and α and β are large, as in the case of aspirin tablets. For example, a lot of 50,000 tablets is required to contain no more than 1% defective tablets and the single normal inspection level of MIL-STD-105D is used. Entering Table 1 of MIL-STD-105D (Table 9), find letter N under column II for the general inspection levels for lot size of 35,000 – 150,000. Entering Table 11-A (Table 10), find the sample size of 500 and at an AQL 1, 10 for acceptance and 11 for rejection.

In practice, this means that a 500-tablet sample is taken from the lot at random and tested; the lot is accepted if 10 or fewer are defective and rejected if 11 or more are defective. If tightened inspection is used for the same example, it would call for a sample size code of P for the general inspection level III. From Table II-B (Table 11), a sample size of 800 would now have to be used, instead of 500, and at an AQL 1, 12 for acceptance

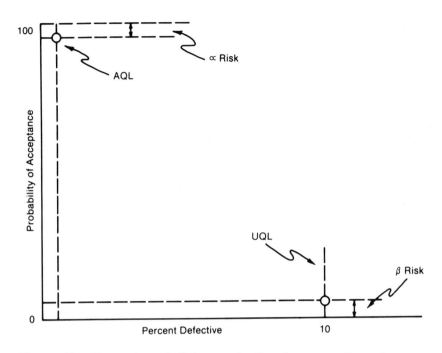

Figure 15   Parameters defining projection for a sampling plan.

Table 9   Sample Size Code Letters

Lot or batch size	Special inspection levels				General inspection levels		
	S-1	S-2	S-3	S-4	I	II	III
2 – 8	A	A	A	A	A	A	B
9 – 15	A	A	A	A	A	B	C
16 – 25	A	A	B	B	B	C	D
26 – 50	A	B	B	C	C	D	E
51 – 90	B	B	C	C	C	E	F
91 – 150	B	B	C	D	D	F	G
151 – 280	B	C	D	E	E	G	H
281 – 500	B	C	D	E	F	H	J
501 – 1200	C	C	E	F	G	J	K
1201 – 3200	C	D	E	G	H	K	L
3201 – 10,000	C	D	F	G	J	L	M
10,001 – 35,000	C	D	F	H	K	M	N
35,001 – 150,000	D	E	G	J	L̲	N̲	P̲
150,001 – 500,000	D	E	G	J	M	P	Q
500,001 and over	D	E	H	K	N	Q	R

Source: From Military Standard, Sampling Procedures and Tables for Inspection by Attributes, U.S. Dept. of Defense, MIL-STD-105D, 1963.

Table 10 Master Table for Normal Inspection

Acceptable quality levels (normal inspection, single sampling)

Sample size code letter	Sample size	0.010		0.015		0.025		0.040		0.065		0.10		0.15		0.25		0.40		0.65		1.0		1.5		2.5		4.0		6.5		10		15		25		40		65		100		150		250		400		650		1000	
		A	R	A	R	A	R	A	R	A	R	A	R	A	R	A	R	A	R	A	R	A	R	A	R	A	R	A	R	A	R	A	R	A	R	A	R	A	R	A	R	A	R	A	R	A	R	A	R	A	R	A	R
A	2	↓		↓		↓		↓		↓		↓		↓		↓		↓		↓		↓		↓		↓		↓		↓		↓		0	1	1	2	2	3	3	4	5	6	7	8	10	11	14	15	21	22	30	31
B	3	↓		↓		↓		↓		↓		↓		↓		↓		↓		↓		↓		↓		↓		↓		↓		0	1	1	2	2	3	3	4	5	6	7	8	10	11	14	15	21	22	30	31	44	45
C	5	↓		↓		↓		↓		↓		↓		↓		↓		↓		↓		↓		↓		↓		↓		0	1	1	2	2	3	3	4	5	6	7	8	10	11	14	15	21	22	30	31	44	45	↑	
D	8	↓		↓		↓		↓		↓		↓		↓		↓		↓		↓		↓		↓		↓		0	1	1	2	2	3	3	4	5	6	7	8	10	11	14	15	21	22	30	31	44	45	↑		↑	
E	13	↓		↓		↓		↓		↓		↓		↓		↓		↓		↓		↓		↓		0	1	1	2	2	3	3	4	5	6	7	8	10	11	14	15	21	22	30	31	44	45	↑		↑		↑	
F	20	↓		↓		↓		↓		↓		↓		↓		↓		↓		↓		↓		0	1	1	2	2	3	3	4	5	6	7	8	10	11	14	15	21	22	30	31	44	45	↑		↑		↑		↑	
G	32	↓		↓		↓		↓		↓		↓		↓		↓		↓		↓		0	1	1	2	2	3	3	4	5	6	7	8	10	11	14	15	21	22	30	31	44	45	↑		↑		↑		↑		↑	
H	50	↓		↓		↓		↓		↓		↓		↓		↓		↓		0	1	1	2	2	3	3	4	5	6	7	8	10	11	14	15	21	22	30	31	44	45	↑		↑		↑		↑		↑		↑	
J	80	↓		↓		↓		↓		↓		↓		↓		↓		0	1	1	2	2	3	3	4	5	6	7	8	10	11	14	15	21	22	30	31	44	45	↑		↑		↑		↑		↑		↑		↑	
K	125	↓		↓		↓		↓		↓		↓		↓		0	1	1	2	2	3	3	4	5	6	7	8	10	11	14	15	21	22	30	31	44	45	↑		↑		↑		↑		↑		↑		↑		↑	
L	200	↓		↓		↓		↓		↓		↓		0	1	1	2	2	3	3	4	5	6	7	8	10	11	14	15	21	22	30	31	44	45	↑		↑		↑		↑		↑		↑		↑		↑		↑	
M	315	↓		↓		↓		↓		↓		0	1	1	2	2	3	3	4	5	6	7	8	10	11	14	15	21	22	30	31	44	45	↑		↑		↑		↑		↑		↑		↑		↑		↑		↑	
N	500	↓		↓		↓		↓		0	1	1	2	2	3	3	4	5	6	7	8	10	11	14	15	21	22	30	31	44	45	↑		↑		↑		↑		↑		↑		↑		↑		↑		↑		↑	
P	800	↓		↓		↓		0	1	1	2	2	3	3	4	5	6	7	8	10	11	14	15	21	22	30	31	44	45	↑		↑		↑		↑		↑		↑		↑		↑		↑		↑		↑		↑	
Q	1250	↓		↓		0	1	1	2	2	3	3	4	5	6	7	8	10	11	14	15	21	22	30	31	44	45	↑		↑		↑		↑		↑		↑		↑		↑		↑		↑		↑		↑		↑	
R	2000	↓		0	1	1	2	2	3	3	4	5	6	7	8	10	11	14	15	21	22	30	31	44	45	↑		↑		↑		↑		↑		↑		↑		↑		↑		↑		↑		↑		↑		↑	

A = Acceptance number, R = rejection number, ↓ = use first sampling plan below arrow (if sample also equals or exceeds lot or batch size, do 100% inspection), ↑ = use first sampling plan above arrow.

Source: MIL-STD-105D.

Table 11 Master Table for Tightened Inspection

Acceptable quality levels (tightened inspection, single sampling)

Sample size code letter	Sample size	0.010		0.015		0.025		0.040		0.065		0.10		0.15		0.25		0.40		0.65		1.0		1.5		2.5		4.0		6.5		10		15		25		40		65		100		150		250		400		650		1000	
		A	R	A	R	A	R	A	R	A	R	A	R	A	R	A	R	A	R	A	R	A	R	A	R	A	R	A	R	A	R	A	R	A	R	A	R	A	R	A	R	A	R	A	R	A	R	A	R	A	R	A	R
A	2	↓		↓		↓		↓		↓		↓		↓		↓		↓		↓		↓		↓		↓		↓		↓		↓		↓		0	1	1	2	2	3	3	4	5	6	8	9	12	13	18	19	27	28
B	3	↓		↓		↓		↓		↓		↓		↓		↓		↓		↓		↓		↓		↓		↓		↓		↓		0	1	1	2	2	3	3	4	5	6	8	9	12	13	18	19	27	28	41	42
C	5	↓		↓		↓		↓		↓		↓		↓		↓		↓		↓		↓		↓		↓		↓		↓		0	1	1	2	2	3	3	4	5	6	8	9	12	13	18	19	27	28	41	42	↑	
D	8	↓		↓		↓		↓		↓		↓		↓		↓		↓		↓		↓		↓		↓		↓		0	1	1	2	2	3	3	4	5	6	8	9	12	13	18	19	27	28	41	42	↑		↑	
E	13	↓		↓		↓		↓		↓		↓		↓		↓		↓		↓		↓		↓		↓		0	1	1	2	2	3	3	4	5	6	8	9	12	13	18	19	27	28	41	42	↑		↑		↑	
F	20	↓		↓		↓		↓		↓		↓		↓		↓		↓		↓		↓		↓		0	1	1	2	2	3	3	4	5	6	8	9	12	13	18	19	27	28	41	42	↑		↑		↑		↑	
G	32	↓		↓		↓		↓		↓		↓		↓		↓		↓		↓		↓		0	1	1	2	2	3	3	4	5	6	8	9	12	13	18	19	27	28	41	42	↑		↑		↑		↑		↑	
H	50	↓		↓		↓		↓		↓		↓		↓		↓		↓		↓		0	1	1	2	2	3	3	4	5	6	8	9	12	13	18	19	27	28	41	42	↑		↑		↑		↑		↑		↑	
J	80	↓		↓		↓		↓		↓		↓		↓		↓		↓		0	1	1	2	2	3	3	4	5	6	8	9	12	13	18	19	27	28	41	42	↑		↑		↑		↑		↑		↑		↑	
K	125	↓		↓		↓		↓		↓		↓		↓		↓		0	1	1	2	2	3	3	4	5	6	8	9	12	13	18	19	27	28	41	42	↑		↑		↑		↑		↑		↑		↑		↑	
L	200	↓		↓		↓		↓		↓		↓		↓		0	1	1	2	2	3	3	4	5	6	8	9	12	13	18	19	27	28	41	42	↑		↑		↑		↑		↑		↑		↑		↑		↑	
M	315	↓		↓		↓		↓		↓		↓		0	1	1	2	2	3	3	4	5	6	8	9	12	13	18	19	27	28	41	42	↑		↑		↑		↑		↑		↑		↑		↑		↑		↑	
N	500	↓		↓		↓		↓		↓		0	1	1	2	2	3	3	4	5	6	8	9	12	13	18	19	27	28	41	42	↑		↑		↑		↑		↑		↑		↑		↑		↑		↑		↑	
P	800	↓		↓		↓		↓		0	1	1	2	2	3	3	4	5	6	8	9	12	13	18	19	27	28	41	42	↑		↑		↑		↑		↑		↑		↑		↑		↑		↑		↑		↑	
Q	1250	↓		↓		↓		0	1	1	2	2	3	3	4	5	6	8	9	12	13	18	19	27	28	41	42	↑		↑		↑		↑		↑		↑		↑		↑		↑		↑		↑		↑		↑	
R	2000	↓		↓		0	1	1	2	2	3	3	4	5	6	8	9	12	13	18	19	27	28	41	42	↑		↑		↑		↑		↑		↑		↑		↑		↑		↑		↑		↑		↑		↑	
S	3150	↓		0	1	1	2	2	3	3	4	5	6	8	9	12	13	18	19	27	28	41	42	↑		↑		↑		↑		↑		↑		↑		↑		↑		↑		↑		↑		↑		↑		↑	

A = acceptance number, R = rejection number, ↓ = use first sampling plan below arrow (if sample size equals or exceeds lot or batch size, do 100% inspection), ↑ = use first sampling plan above arrow.
Source: MIL-STD-105D.

Table 12   Master Table for Reduced Inspection

Acceptable quality levels (reduced inspection,* single sampling)

In the table below each acceptable quality level heading covers two sub‑columns, **A** = acceptance number and **R** = rejection number; each cell is written "Ac Re". ↓ = use first sampling plan below arrow; ↑ = use first sampling plan above arrow.

Sample size code letter	Sample size	0.010	0.015	0.025	0.040	0.065	0.10	0.15	0.25	0.40	0.65	1.0	1.5	2.5	4.0	6.5	10	15	25	40	65	100	150	250	400	650	1000
A	2															0 1	↑	↑	1 2	2 3	3 4	5 6	7 8	10 11	14 15	21 22	30 31
B	2														0 1	0 2	↑	↑	1 3	2 4	3 5	5 6	7 8	10 11	14 15	21 22	30 31
C	2													0 1	0 2	1 3	↑	↑	1 4	2 5	3 6	5 8	7 10	10 13	14 17	21 24	↑
D	3												0 1	0 2	1 3	1 4	2 5	3 6	5 8	7 10	10 13	↑	↑	↑	↑	↑	↑
E	5											0 1	0 2	1 3	1 4	2 5	3 6	5 8	7 10	10 13	↑	↑	↑	↑	↑	↑	↑
F	8										0 1	0 2	1 3	1 4	2 5	3 6	5 8	7 10	10 13	↑	↑	↑	↑	↑	↑	↑	↑
G	13									0 1	0 2	1 3	1 4	2 5	3 6	5 8	7 10	10 13	↑	↑	↑	↑	↑	↑	↑	↑	↑
H	20								0 1	0 2	1 3	1 4	2 5	3 6	5 8	7 10	10 13	↑	↑	↑	↑	↑	↑	↑	↑	↑	↑
J	32							0 1	0 2	1 3	1 4	2 5	3 6	5 8	7 10	10 13	↑	↑	↑	↑	↑	↑	↑	↑	↑	↑	↑
K	50						0 1	0 2	1 3	1 4	2 5	3 6	5 8	7 10	10 13	↑	↑	↑	↑	↑	↑	↑	↑	↑	↑	↑	↑
L	80					0 1	0 2	1 3	1 4	2 5	3 6	5 8	7 10	10 13	↑	↑	↑	↑	↑	↑	↑	↑	↑	↑	↑	↑	↑
M	125				0 1	0 2	1 3	1 4	2 5	3 6	5 8	7 10	10 13	↑	↑	↑	↑	↑	↑	↑	↑	↑	↑	↑	↑	↑	↑
N	200			0 1	0 2	1 3	1 4	2 5	3 6	5 8	7 10	10 13	↑	↑	↑	↑	↑	↑	↑	↑	↑	↑	↑	↑	↑	↑	↑
P	315		0 1	0 2	1 3	1 4	2 5	3 6	5 8	7 10	10 13	↑	↑	↑	↑	↑	↑	↑	↑	↑	↑	↑	↑	↑	↑	↑	↑
Q	500	0 1	0 2	1 3	1 4	2 5	3 6	5 8	7 10	10 13	↑	↑	↑	↑	↑	↑	↑	↑	↑	↑	↑	↑	↑	↑	↑	↑	↑
R	800	0 2	1 3	1 4	2 5	3 6	5 8	7 10	10 13	↑	↑	↑	↑	↑	↑	↑	↑	↑	↑	↑	↑	↑	↑	↑	↑	↑	↑

*If the acceptance number has been exceeded, but the rejection number has not been reached, accept the lot, but reinstate normal inspection.

A = Acceptance number, R = rejection number, ↓ = use first sampling plan below arrow, ↑ = use first sampling plan above arrow.

and 13 for rejection. On the other hand, if reduced inspection is to be used for the same example, it would call for a sample size code of L for the general inspection level I. From Table II-C (Table 12), a sample size of only 80 will be required and at an AQL 1, 2 for acceptance and 5 for rejection.

To examine the kind of sampling job one accomplishes with these three sampling plans, one has to examine the OC curves for code letters N, P, and L at an AQL level of 1.0% defective in the same MIL-STD-105D. These curves indicate that, at sampling size code letter N, one would accept lots containing 3% defectives 12% of the time. At a sample size code letter P, however, one would accept lots with 3% defectives only 2% of the time. In reduced inspection, with a sample size code letter L, one would accept lots with 3% defectives 46% of the time.

MIL-STD-105D gives four additional special inspection levels — S-1, S-2, S-3, and S-4 — which may be used when relatively small sample sizes are necessary, such as might be the case with costly destructive testing.

In summary, the steps necessary for the use of MIL-STD-105D are as follows:

Choose the AQL.
Choose the inspection level.
Determine lot size.
Find sample size code letter from the table.
Choose the type of sample plan, and find its table.
Use the tightened or reduced inspection table for the same type of plan whenever it is required.

A continuous sampling plan with in-process testing clearly can yield more valuable information on the homogeneity of the production procedure to increase the opportunity to detect and correct any production difficulties. Such testing is facilitated by the fact that the entire lot is accessible and the sample may be obtained entirely at random. Actually, the same procedures described before for sampling plans may be applied to continuous sampling as well.

XI. AFTER START CHECKING

A. Bulk Granulation and/or Raw Materials Processing

Only released, properly labeled raw materials are allowed in the granulation area. Depending upon the nature of the product, quality assurance should check and verify that the temperature and humidity in the area are within specified limits required for the product. If the temperature and/or humidity is beyond the specified limits, production is to be informed and corrective actions must be taken.

The specified granulation procedure is to be checked, at each step in the process, according to written in-process quality assurance procedures.

Quality assurance should verify and document the proper equipment, the proper addition of ingredient, proper mixing time, proper drying time, and screening with proper mesh size sieves.

At certain points, samples are to be taken for the quality control laboratory for potency assay of the granulation and any other testing that is necessary to ensure batch uniformity.

Drums of in-process granulation or raw materials are labeled with product name, item number, lot number, gross, and tare and net weights of the contents.

B. Compression Processing

It is quality assurance's responsibility to ascertain that all drums of granulation or raw materials are properly labeled and staged in the compression machine staging area, that they are clean, and that the compression machine is properly identified as to the product, strength, item number, and lot number.

The production process begins with the setup of the compression machine to prepare tablets within the specified limits for the particular product. Quality assurance at each step in the setup procedures verifies the addition of granulation and/or raw materials to the tablet press hopper and performs visual appearance, weight measurement and hardness, friability, and disintegration tests as required to adjust the compression machine. Tablets produced during the compression machine setup period are rejected, accounted for, and destroyed.

A variable group of tests including tablet physical appearance, color, odor, thickness, diameter, friability, hardness, weight variation, and disintegration time are widely used for in-process tablet controls. Such in-process tests are designed to ensure control of problems that can arise during tablet granulation or when raw materials are compressed into tablets. These problems are distribution of active materials in the tablet, poor flow properties, cross-contamination, lamination or capping of tablets, faulty lubrication, higher or lower moisture content, high proportion of "powder."

In-process sampling plans will require a fast measuring method suited for testing single units. Weight, hardness, friability, and thickness can be measured rapidly. The Cahn Instrument Co. (California) and the Mettler Instrument Corp (New Jersey) have automatic balances that can operate in the weight range from below $1-10$ gm at about 50 tablets per minute, thus making single-tablet weighings easy and fast. By using such in-process automatic weighings, tablets from a full revolution of a multiple-punch compression machine with more than one hopper can be weighed in a few minutes to check for uniform punch performance and variance between left and right sides of the tablet machine.

Good manufacturing practices requires that in-process quality assurance be adequately documented throughout all stages of manufacturing. Throughout the compression run, in-process samples are removed, tested, and data recorded on special forms (Figs. 16 and 17; Table 13) as specified in the product's in-process monograph. The number of samples taken for testing and the type of testing is obviously dependent upon the size of the batch and the type of product. If deviation from the specified limits occurs, the necessary corrective action is taken, recorded, and a resample is taken and tested to determine whether the quality attribute of the product is now within limits. In some instances, as in the case of compendial weight variation or disintegration time specifications, the deviation is such that all tablets produced prior to the corrective action are isolated, accounted for, and rejected. In some tablet compression machines, tablets are ejected from more than one side. If this is the case, samples must be taken, tested, and recorded separately from all sides of the compression machine.

I. General information

Product: __Acetaminophen tablets__ Time/date start: __3/15/77__
Strength: __500 mg__ Time/date finish: __3/18/77__
Lot number: __A__ Upper punch set no.: __100__
Tablet press location: __10__ Lower punch set no.: __101__
Tablet press identity no.: __10A__ Die set no.: __10 - 100__
Compression control monograph code no./date: __001/ 1/1/77__

II. Tablet weight information

Target weight: __500__ mg
Machine adjustment values: Low __496.2__ mg High __503.8__ mg
Monograph limits: __475__ mg to __525__ mg

III. Tablet thickness limits

__5.0__ mm ± __3__ mm

IV. Tablet hardness information

Tablet hardness: __7-10__ SCA units
Machine adjustment values: Low __8__ SCA units
High __9__ SCA units

V. Tablet disintegration time limit

NMT __10__ min

Submitted by: __T. Jones__

Date: __3/18/77__

Figure 16 Quality assurance department tablet compression in-process tests.

In addition to the above, portions of the initial, final, and in-process samples are used for collecting average run samples for the quality control laboratory for final batch analysis and release.

For antibiotic tablets, the Code of Federal Register specifies the number of samples and frequency of collection, for each individual antibiotic, that must be collected and sent to the quality control laboratory for testing and subsequent release of the batch.

There is no limit as to the ingenuity a quality assurance department can use in devising in-process controls. The following sampling and testing schedule is often used for in-process quality assurance tablet production monitoring:

An initial and final sample is tested for physical appearance, tablet weight, thickness, diameter, hardness, friability, and disintegration.

An hourly sample for physical appearance testing.

Product name <u>Acetaminophen</u> Product code <u>   001   </u> Production bulk number <u>   A   </u>

Inspection	Date	Quality assurance inspector	Remarks
Initial	3/15/77	M. Groel	
Composite	3/18/77	R. Orlando	

| Bulk sample | Count | Number of Dosage Forms Rejected ||||||||||
		Broken	Capped	Chipped	Color	Cracked	Dirty	Size	Edge	Imprint	Mottled
Initial	1000	0	0	0	0	0	3	0	0	0	0
%		0	0	0	0	0	0.03	0	0	0	0
	1000	2	0	0	0	0	0	0	0	0	0
%		0.02	0	0	0	0	0	0	0	0	0
	1000	0	0	0	0	0	0	0	0	0	0
%		0	0	0	0	0	0	0	0	0	0
Composite	1000	3	0	0	0	0	7	0	0	0	0
%		0.03	0	0	0	0	0.07	0	0	0	0

Comparison to   Approved for packaging
house standard <u>   M. Groel   </u>
(initial sample)   <u>   R. Orlando   </u>

<u>Tablet</u>

[x] Diameter   [x] Lower

[x] Upper   [x] Color

Figure 17   Quality assurance inspection report, bulk tablets.

Table 13   Product Acetaminophen   Strength 500 mg   Lot # A   Technician T. Jones

	L/1	R/2	L/3	R/4	L/9	R/10	L/11	R/12	L/17	R/18	L/23	R/24
Time and date of sample	3/15/77		3/15/77		3/15/77		3/15/77		3/15/77		3/15/77	
Tab. wt. 1 (mg)	505.0	502.0	500.0	500.0	494.0	500.0	500.0	492.0	506.0	500.0	506.0	500.0
Tab. wt. 2 (mg)	504.0	503.0	500.0	497.0	498.0	500.0	492.0	491.0	507.0	505.0	499.0	500.0
Tab. wt. 3 (mg)	498.0	500.0	500.0	494.0	505.0	501.0	496.0	495.0	505.0	500.0	502.0	500.0
Tab. wt. 4 (mg)	503.0	497.0	500.0	492.0	500.0	497.0	496.0	492.0	503.0	504.0	505.0	500.0
Tab. wt. 5 (mg)	505.0	491.0	500.0	496.0	500.0	506.0	492.0	490.0	500.0	503.0	500.0	500.0
Avg. tab. wt. (mg)		498.6	500.0	495.8	499.4	500.8	495.2	492.0	504.2	502.0	502.4	500.0
Hardness 1 (SCA)	8.5	8.4	8.9	9.0	9.2	8.9	8.8	8.4	8.5	9.0	9.0	8.6
Hardness 2 (SCA)	8.2	8.3	8.8	8.9	9.0	9.5	8.5	8.5	8.5	9.2	8.8	9.1
Hardness 3 (SCA)	8.2	8.9	9.0	9.1	9.0	9.5	8.5	8.9	8.8	9.4	8.9	8.8
Avg. hardness (SCA)	8.3	8.5	8.9	9.0	9.1	9.3	8.6	8.6	8.6	9.2	8.9	8.9
Thickness (mm)	5.09	5.11	5.13	5.12	5.12	5.12	5.16	5.16	5.12	5.11	5.14	5.12
Friability wt. (start)	9.942				9.989						9.568	
Friability wt. (end)	9.912				9.958						9.527	
% Loss	0.3				0.31						0.42	
Disintegration time	40.0 sec				45.0 sec						40.0 sec	

REMARKS

Every second hour sample is tested for tablet friability, hardness, thickness, diameter, weight, and disintegration.

The homogeneity of the physical appearance of tablets is judged by visual examination and/or instrumentation. Speckled or mottled tablets indicate improper and incomplete blending resulting in uneven distribution of ingredients. Colors of compressed and coated tablets are usually compared to a reference standard. The surface of coated tablets is checked for smoothness before imprinting. In some cases, deterioration of some tablet ingredients may be gross and can be detected visually or by odor, such as acetic acid in hydrolyzed aspirin tablets.

A ±5% is usually allowed for tablet thickness, depending on the size of the tablet. Tablet thickness may vary from lot-to-lot due to the difference in density of the granulation, the pressure applied to the tablets, or the speed of the compression machine. Tablet thickness and diameter is important to ensure in filling equipment that uses tablet thickness as its counting mechanism. Tablet thickness is determined with a caliber as its thickness gauge in millimeters, for example, Ames (Ames G., Division of Miles Laboratory, Inc., Elkhart, Indiana) thickness gauge.

Tablets must be fabricated to withstand chipping, abrasion, and breakage during the expected tablet life under conditions of storage, transportation, and handling. The hardness of a tablet is expressed as that force required to break the tablet. Hardness can be measured by the Schleuniger (Schleuniger, Vicor Corp., Marion, Iowa) (Strong Cobb), Pfizer (Pfizer, Inc., New York, New York), and the Stokes (Division of Pennwalt Corp., Warminster, Pennsylvania) Hardness Testers (Fig. 18). The hardness values of the Strong Cobb is not equivalent to the Pfizer or the Stokes instruments. A maximum breaking load of four Strong Cobb units or

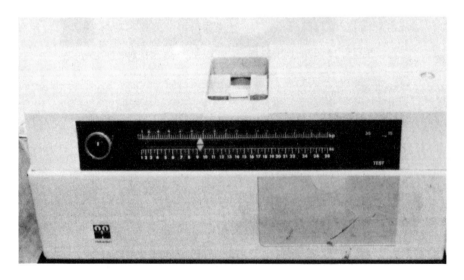

(A)

Figure 18   (A) Hardness tester, Schleuniger. (Courtesy of Vicor Corporation.) (B) Hardness tester, Pfizer, U.S. Patent 2975630. (Courtesy of Pfizer Corporation.)

equivalent is essential in order to ensure sufficient hardness. Exceptionally soft tablets may not withstand handling, whereas excessively hard tablets may chip or fracture or not disintegrate in the required period of time.

The Roche (Roche Laboratories, Division of Hoffman-LaRoche, Inc., Nutley, New Jersey) Friabilator represents a device to determine tablet friability. The instruments are designed to measure the wearing qualities of tablets. A number of tablets are weighed and placed in the tumbling apparatus. After a given number of rotations, the tablets are weighed; and the loss in weight is a measure of the ability of the tablets to withstand this type of wear (Fig. 19). Actually, it is a common practice to trial-ship tablets using different methods of transportation to check the tablet's ability to withstand transportation handling.

The use of control charts is increasingly becoming an essential part of any quality assurance operation. Figures 20 and 21 represent a graphical control chart plotting of the data presented previously in Table 13. Control charts may be classified as attributes or variable types. Variable charts are based on the normal distribution of actual numerical measurements of quality attributes, whereas attribute charts refer to some other attributes of quality that are present or absent in which each sample inspected is tested to determine if it conforms to the requirements. Variable charts, or the X, R (mean and range) charts, are undoubtedly the most generally used charts in quality assurance of tablets. The most common and usual application of variable charts in tablet manufacture is in hardness and weight control. Routinely, in-process results are plotted on a control

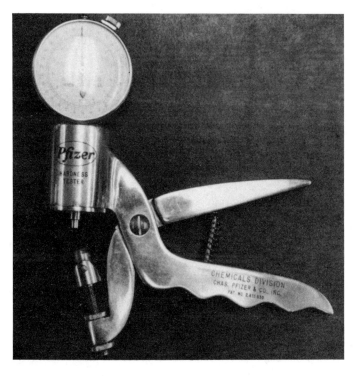

(B)

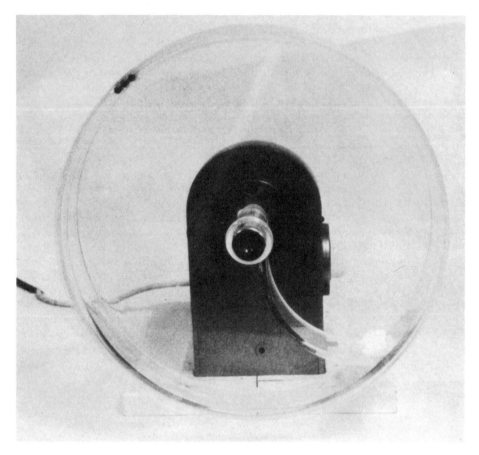

Figure 19   Roche Friabilator.

chart so that a complete picture of any possible fluctuation during the entire compression operation can be readily detected.

The control limits or process capability can be determined by sampling, measuring, and recording weights in subgroups that cover the compression operation. The range within each subgroup; that is, the absolute number difference between the lowest and highest individual tablet reading, and the average number difference between the lowest and highest individual tablet reading, and the average range are calculated for the total number of groups. The average tablet-reading plots can detect movements toward limits that will allow making necessary corrections before limit values are exceeded. While the subgroup's sample range plots will allow the monitoring of the sample range trend, an increase in sample range values or general high variability indicates possible control problems.

When the tablet-manufacturing process has been completed, the theoretical yields to be expected from the formulation at different stages of manufacture and the accountability calculations are checked for comparison with the practical and the permissible yield limits. Such information is recorded

TABLET WEIGHT CONTROL CHART

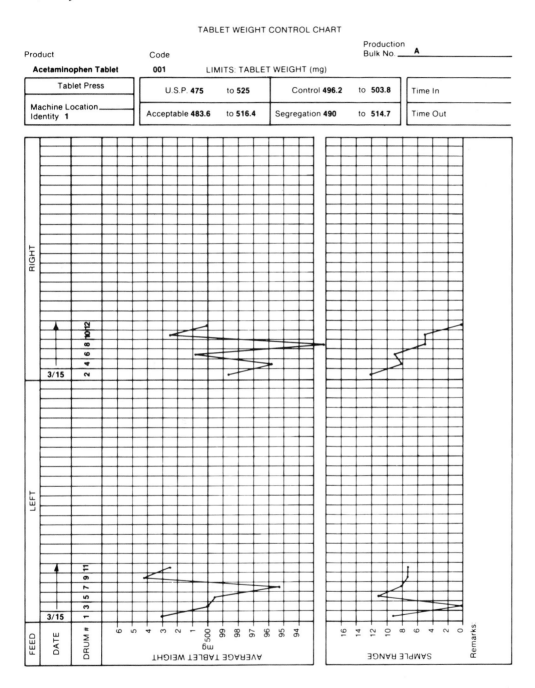

Figure 20   Tablet weight control chart.

TABLET HARDNESS CONTROL CHART

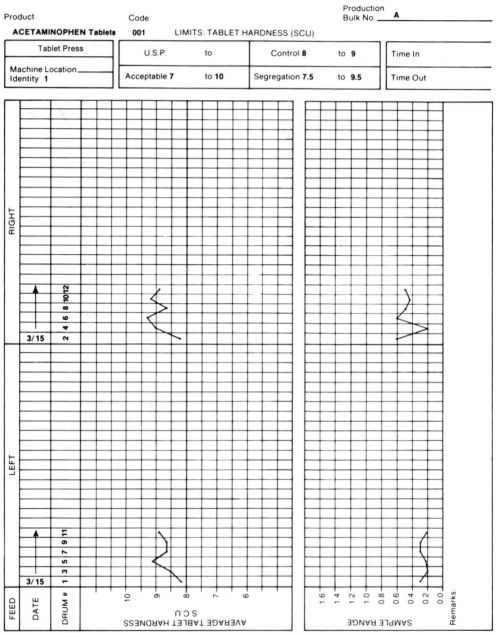

Figure 21   Tablet hardness control chart.

Product ___Acetaminophen tablets___ Page _____ Product description _____ Lot __A__ Code __001__

A Production grams or tablets ___2900000___

+ Samples grams or tablets ___50000___

+ Rejects grams or tablets ___4184___

= Total material out grams or tablets ___2954184___

÷

B Total material introduced grams or tablets ___2974663___

Yield

$\frac{A}{B} \times 100 = $ ___97.75___ %

Accountability

$\times 100 = $ ___99.3___ %

Production stage	Seq.	Foreman	Date
Supervisor	Date	QC audit	Date

<u>Check</u>

☐ Spiked ☐ Combined lot

☐ Trial ☒ Packaged directly into final container

Production	Comments
	Distribution

Figure 22   Product accountability.

on appropriate forms (Fig. 22), and any discrepancy must be reconciled if beyond process allowable variation.

XII. QUALIFICATION/VALIDATION

The FDA in CGMPs and guidelines has stated that sampling and testing of finished products alone cannot provide the necessary assurance of drug product quality. Finished product testing does not provide sufficient statistical data to verify product quality within and between batches of tablet product. Consequently, the FDA requires the validation of manufacturing process and qualification of equipment, facilities, and personnel used during manufacture of a product.

Qualification is to generate the data necessary to assure that equipment operates as it was designed to within predetermined range in a reproducible manner. Validation of a process is to demonstrate that a certain manufacturing process used defined parameters, materials, equipment, and personnel would result in product of repeatable acceptable quality. System validation can be accomplished by identifying the critical steps of a process and implementing necessary tests to control them to provide a high degree of assurance that this system will consistently produce a tablet product that meets its predetermined specifications. The FDA defines a validated manufacturing process as:

> A validated manufacturing process is one that has proved to do what it purports or is represented to do. The proof of validation is obtained through collection and evaluation of data, preferably, beginning from the process development phase and continuing through into the production phase. Validation necessarily includes process qualification (the qualification of materials, equipment, systems, building, personnel), but it also includes the control of the entire process for repeated batches or runs.

The FDA usually mandates three consecutive successful runs as the minimum acceptable data to validate a process.

XIII. FINISHED PRODUCT

A. Specification

Final testing of tablets is made in the quality control laboratories. These tests are designed to determine compliance with specifications. Thus, the testing of the finished product for compliance with predetermined standards prior to release of the tablets for packaging and subsequent distribution is a critical factor for quality assurance. The purpose of establishing these specifications and standards is to ensure that each tablet contains the amount of drug claimed on the label, that all of the drug in each tablet is available for complete absorption, that the drug is stable in the formulation in its specific final container for its expected shelf life, and that the tablets themselves contain no toxic foreign substances. Normally, the design of test parameters, procedure, and specifications are done during product development. It is a good manufacturing practice to base

Table 14 Quality Control Physical, Chemical, and Microbial Attributes for the Evaluation of Tablets

1. Appearance, odor, color, taste	10. Identification tests for the active ingredient and possible contaminants
2. Hardness	
3. Disintegration	11. Content uniformity
4. Friability	12. Dissolution
5. Thickness uniformity	13. Microbial limits, e.g., total microbial count
6. Weight uniformity	
7. Assay of the active ingredient	14. Stability of the active ingredient in the formula and marketed container
8. Moisture content	
9. Light stability	

such parameters on experiences developed from several pilot and production batches. Furthermore, the results of these studies should be subjected to statistical analysis in order to correctly appraise the precision and accuracy of each procedure for each characteristic. In the long run, with additional production experience it is possible that specifications be modified for perfection and upgrade of product specifications. The complexity of quality control testing of tablets can be clearly understood from the quality control attributes outlined in Table 14. Essential qualities of a good tablet as required by USP XXII/NF XVII are presented in Table 15.

B. Bulk Tablets Testing

Each lot of tablets should be tested to ensure identity, quality, potency, and purity. Quality assurance will authorize the release for further processing based on actual laboratory testing: physical, chemical, and/or biological.

Different assay limits are test methods for some tablet products listed in the USP XXI and NF XVI are presented in Table 16. Tests required by the official compendia on the ingredients and the dosage form applies to all manufacturers of a specific compendia tablet product. The manufacturer frequently employs alternative methods that are more accurate, specific, or economical than those in the compendia. For example, in Table 17, the sodium nitrate titrimetric assay method for amino salicylic acid tablets, USP XXI, is compared to a specific nonaqueous assay method. The results in Table 18 clearly illustrates the importance of the specificity of the assay procedure before the market introduction of a tablet product. Amino salicylic acid tablets, product A, B, and C, pass the NF limits using the sodium nitrate titrimetric assay method, while product A fails to meet the same NF limits when the specific nonaqueous titration assay method is used.

The manufacturer is not required to employ the official analytical procedures as long as the quality of his product complies with the compendium requirements. However, in the case of a legal action, the compendium procedures are the basis for determining compliance. Table 17 lists

Table 15 USP/NF Requirements for Tablets

Test	Procedure
1. Identification	Specific color test, infrared spectrum, UV spectrum
2. Impurities or degradation products	See Table 17
3. Weight variation	Sec. III.A
4. Content uniformity	For tablet that contains highly toxic or 50 mg or less of active ingredient
5. Disintegration	Sec. III.C
6. Dissolution	Sec. III.D
7. Moisture	See Table 3
8. Microbial limit	Negative salmonella as in digitalis, pancreatin, and Rauwolfia serpentina tablets
9. Assay	See Table 14
10. Packaging and storage	Well-closed container, e.g., codeine phosphate tablets
	Tight-closed container, e.g., diazepam tablets
	Light-resistant container, e.g., colchicine tablets
	Avoid exposure to excessive heat, e.g., tetranitrite tablets
	Preferably in glass containers, e.g., nitroglycerine tablets
	Protect from heat and moisture, e.g., oxytriphyline tablets

Source: U.S. Pharmacopeia/National Formulary.

Table 16 Difference in Assay Limits and Test Methods for Tablets in USP/NF

Product	USP/NF limit (%)	Method of assay
1. Aminosalicylic acid tablets	95 – 105	Potentiometric titration with 0.1 M $NaNO_2$
2. Codeine sulfate tablets	93 – 107	Aqueous titration with 0.02 N H_2SO_4
3. Belladonna extension tablets	90 – 110	Aqueous titration with 0.02 N H_2SO_4
4. Digitalis tablets	85 – 102	Biological
5. Menadiol sodium phosphate tablets	95 – 110	Potentiometric titration with 0.01 N ceric sulfate
6. Methyl prednisolone tablets	92.5 – 107.5	Colorimetric with tetrazolium blue
7. Oxyphenbutazone tablets	94 – 106	UV absorbance in NaOH
8. Oxandrolone tablets	92 – 108	GLC
9. Pancreatin tablets	NLT 90	Enzymetric assay
10. Penicillin V potassium tablets	90 – 120	Microbiological
11. Tetracycline HCl tablets	NLT 85	Microbiological
12. Penicillin G potassium tablets	90 – 120	Microbiological
13. Rauwolfia serpentina tablets	0.15 – 0.2 as reserpine	Colorimetric with sulfamic acid
14. Theophylline sodium glycinate	47 – 54	Aqueous titration with 0.1 N ammonium thiocyanate

Source: U.S. Pharmacopeia/National Formulary.

Table 17 Aminosalicylic Acid Tablet Analysis

Product	USP method of analysis[a]	Nonaqueous titration	Limit
A	95.6 ± 0.5	89.1 ± 0.1	95 – 105
B	100.3 ± 0.8	97.8 ± 0.4	95 – 105
C	101.4 ± 0.4	98.9 ± 0.8	95 – 105

[a]Mean of three determinations.
Source: Watson, J. R., Yokonama, F., and Pernarowski, M., *J. Assoc. Offic. Anal. Chemists* 44, 1961.

Table 18   Assay Limits of Impurities or Degradation Products in Some
USP/NF Tablets

Product	Impurities or degradation products	Limits
Prednisolone tablets	Total steroids	NMT 4%
Ergonovine maleate tablets	Related alkaloids	NMT 5%
Ergotamine tartrate and caffeine tablets	Water-soluble ergot alkaloids	Negative
Methyl ergonovine maleate tablets	Related alkaloids	NMT 5%
Aminosalicylic acid tablets	m-Aminophenol	NMT 1%
Sodium aminosalicylic acid tablets	m-Aminophenol	NMT 0.75%

Source: U.S. Pharmacopeia/National Formulary.

impurities or degradation product limits and test methods for some USP
XXII and NF XVII tablet products.

C. Quality Assurance During Packaging Operation

If the quality control laboratory analysis confirms that the product complies
with specifications and quality assurance audit of manufacturing operations
are satisfactory, the bulk tablet product is released to the packaging department and production control is notified. Production control issues a
packaging form which carries the name of the tablet product, item number,
lot number, number of labels, inserts, packaging materials to be used, operations to be performed, and the quantity to be packaged. A copy of
this form is sent to the supervisor of label control, which in turn will count
out the required number of labels. Since labels may be spoiled during the
packaging operation, a definite number in excess of that actually required
is usually issued. However, all labels must be accounted for before its
destruction. If the lot number and expiration date of the tablets product
are not going to be printed directly on the line, the labels are run through
a printing machine which imprints the lot number and expiration date. The
labels are recounted and placed in a separate container with proper identification for future transfer to the packaging department. The packaging
department then requests, according to the packaging form, the product to
be packaged and all packing components, such as labels, inserts, bottles,
caps, seals, cartons, and shipping cases. Quality assurance inspects and
verifies all packaging components, equipment to be used for the packaging
operation to ensure that it has the proper identification and the line has
been thoroughly cleaned and that all materials from the previous packaging
operation have been completely removed.

Packaging operations should be performed with adequate physical segregation from product-to-product. Tablets of similar shape should not be

scheduled on the neighboring packaging lines at the same time. Quality assurance should periodically inspect the packaging line and check filled and labeled containers for compliance with written specification, for example, absence of foreign drugs and labels, adequacy of the containers and closure system, and accuracy of labeling. Some packaging operations, especially those using high-speed equipment, are fitted with automated testing equipment to check each container for fill and label placement. Alternatively, an operator may visually inspect all packages fed into the final cartons. Proper reconciliation and disposition of the unused and wasted labels should occur at the end of the packaging operation. Quality assurance should select finished preservation samples at random from each lot. The preservation samples should consist of at least twice the quantity necessary to perform all tests required to determine whether the product meets its established specifications. These preservation samples should be retained for at least 2 years after the expiration date and stored in their original package under conditions consistent with product labeling.

Quality assurance should also select a finished sample and send it to the analytical control laboratory for final testing, which is usually an identification test.

D. Auditing

Good Manufacturing Practice requires that the manufacturing process be adequately documented throughout all stages of the operation. The history of each task from the starting materials, equipment used, personnel involved in production and control until completed packaging is complete, should be recorded. Preservation samples are to be stored for at least 2 years beyond the labeled expiration date of each product. The areas of recordkeeping are:

Individual components, raw materials, and packaging
Master formula
Batch production
Container and labeling
Packaging and labeling operation
Laboratory control testing, in-process and finished
Proper signing and dating by at least two individuals independently for each operation in the proper spaces
Reconciliation of materials supplied with amount of tablets produced, taking into account allowable loss limits

Before releasing the product for distribution, quality assurance should evaluate the batch records of all in-process tests and controls and all tests of the final product to determine whether they conform to specification.

Index